SYNOPSIS OF PRESCRIPTIONS OF THE GOLDEN CHAMBER WITH 300 CASES

— A Classic of Traditional Chinese Medicine with Ancient and Contemporary Case Studies

Written by Zhang Zhongjing
Compiled and Translated by Luo Xiwen, Ph.D.

NEW WORLD PRESS

First Edition 1995

ISBN 7-80005-291-5

Published by
NEW WORLD PRESS
24 Baiwanzhuang Road, Beijing 100037, China

Distributed by
CHINA INTERNATIONAL BOOK TRADING CORPORATION
35 Chegongzhuang Xilu, Beijing 100044, China
P.O. Box 399, Beijing, China

Printed in the People's Republic of China

CONTENTS

PREFACE

Synopsis of Prescriptions of the Golden Chamber with 300 Cases is a further presentation of my research on the application of classical prescriptions. Doctors and scholars of traditional Chinese medicine are familiar with the two famous works, *Treatise on Febrile Diseases Caused by Cold* (*Shanghan Lun*) and *Synopsis of Prescriptions of the Golden Chamber* (*Jinkui Yaolue*), which were written by Master Zhang Zhongjing, a famous ancient Chinese medical practitioner and researcher, and both have been used as a medical textbook for more than 1,700 years. In the preface of *Treatise on Febrile Diseases Caused by Cold with 500 Cases* I explained the background of the present book:

"My first translation of TCM classic is *Treatise on Febrile Diseases Caused by Cold* (*Shanghan Lun*), which was published by *New World Press*, Beijing in 1986. Shortly after the book was in circulation, I received a lot of letters of appreciation. Among my readers there have been some scholars who are interested in Chinese medicine but do not have a good command of the theory, and felt that it would be much better if the book could be accompanied by some case studies, so they can better understand the real meaning of such an ancient treatise. I thus decided to write another book of CASE STUDIES. The present book, *Treatise on Febrile Diseases Caused by Cold with 500 Cases,* is written for those scholars who wish to see how *Shanghan Lun* is still in use in China."

Synopsis of Prescriptions of the Golden Chamber with 300 Cases is a logical development of the original idea conceived when I began to write *Treatise on Febrile Diseases Caused by Cold with 500 Cases*. Originally, I planned to collect another 500 cases demonstrating *Jinkui Yaolue*, but in the end 300 cases were selected, because about one-third of the prescriptions in *Jinkui Yaolue* also appears in *Shanghan Lun*. I refer readers to the comparison volume *Treatise on Febrile Diseases Caused by Cold with 500 Cases* for further information.

I wish to draw the attention of my readers to the following points:

a. Many Chinese scholars of medicine suggest that students read *Shanghan Lun* and *Jinkui Yaolue* in succession. This has been advanced many times in the past millennium, and I believe it is valid to this day.

b. In all prescriptions that appear in *Shanghan Lun* and *Jinkui Yaolue*, a note refers to relevant clauses and cases in *Shanghan Lun*. An asterisk indicates that part of it also appears in *Shanghan Lun*.

c. Sources of cases recorded are given in brackets.

For example: (01-100) means the case is quoted from Book No. 01, page 100. In the Bibliography, books are listed in numerical order. In cases, when the original source is listed, it appears as follows:

In Case 1 under Clause 18-8, we read:

Case 1 (64-732): Case Recorded in Dr. Ran Xuefeng's Case Studies

This means the case was originally recorded in Dr. Ran Xuefeng's Case Studies, then quoted by bibliographic item number 64, which can be found in the Bibliography, i.e., Book 64: *Collection of Annotations to the Synopsis of the Golden Chamber*.

d. The bracket system (01-100) is applicable to all NOTES in the book.

In the preface of *Treatise on Febrile Diseases Caused by Cold with 500 Cases*, the following passage also appears:

"I feel that the 500 cases recorded here can be helpful to readers in their understanding of TCM theory. Moreover, these cases can also be taken as references in their treatment of various cases in their professional activities. By this I mean that doctors should not use prescriptions or cases as an example to treat their patients in the same way. Since cases are always varied, you will never find a ready-to-use prescription in this book as you may in a Western medical book. Rather they are hints in diagnosing syndromes and principles or directions whenever the doctor encounters a similar case in his professional activities. Direct copying of any prescriptions is considered wrong and may cause problems."

I wish to express my thanks and gratitude to Yuzhen, my wife, for her assistance and encouragement.

I also wish to thank the publisher, New World Press, for their efforts which have made this publication possible.

Luo Xiwen, Ph.D.
Chinese Academy of Social Sciences

February 1989
Beijing, China

CHAPTER I

ON PULSE, SYMPTOM COMPLEX AND TRANSMISSION OF DISEASES OF THE VISCERA, BOWELS, CHANNELS AND COLLATERALS*

CLAUSE 1-1

Question: Would you kindly explain the meaning of "A superior doctor (1) will cure a disease before its onset?"

Master: "To cure a disease before its onset" means that when the Liver is affected, a prescription is chosen to tonify the Spleen, as the doctor knows the Liver disease will be transmitted into the Spleen (2). During the last periods of each season, the Spleen Vital Energy is strong enough to resist transmission of the pathogenetic factors (3), so the Spleen does not need to be tonified. A mediocre doctor would not know about the transmission. So he would not tonify the Spleen when the Liver is affected.

*This chapter deals with the pulse, symptom complex of diseases affecting the Viscera, Bowels, Channels and Collaterals, as well as the onset, development and transmission of diseases. Serving as an outline for the whole book, it states the essential of Master Zhang Zhongjing's thinking regarding the mechanism, pathology, diagnosis and treatment of diseases.

NOTES

1. Superior doctor: A doctor with a cure rate of ninety percent is termed a superior doctor, a doctor with a cure rate of seventy percent is called a mediocre doctor. (01-7)

2. According to the interacting (conquering or checking) relationships between the Five Evolutive Phases or Five Elements (*Wuxing*) in the following sequence:

Water —	Fire —	Metal —	Wood —	Earth
(Kidney)	(Heart)	(Lung)	(Liver)	(Spleen)

Each Element will check (or conquer) the subsequent one. So when the Liver is affected, pathogenetic factors will be transmitted to the Spleen.

3. During the last periods of every season: During the last eighteen days

(*ii*) of the last months of the four seasons (the third, sixth, ninth and twelfth months of the lunar year), the Spleen Vital Energy is strong and does not need to be tonified. (01-7)

For a case of Liver disease, drugs with a sour taste should be used to tonify the deficient Liver. Scorched, bitter and sweet ingredients should be used as an adjuvant to harmonize the syndrome (1).

NOTES

1. According to the theory of the Five Elements, Wood (Liver) is the mother (producing factor) of the Fire (Heart). And bitterness is the taste of the Heart. So serve drugs of bitter taste is to tonify the Heart. Once the Heart (the son, the produced) is reinforced, the mother (the Liver) is also tonified. That is why when Liver is deficient, drugs of bitter taste should also be used for its assisting effect. (64-12)

Ingredients with a sour taste (1) function on the Liver, scorched and bitter drugs (2) function on the Heart, and sweet ingredients (3) function on the Spleen. When the Spleen is tonified with sweet drugs, the Kidney will be checked. Then the restricted Kidney will be weak in Vital Energy, rendering it unable to circulate Water. While the Water stagnates, the Heart Vital Energy will be strong enough to curb the Lung. A deficient Lung will not check the Liver. So the Liver Vital Energy will be strong enough to heal the Liver syndrome. By tonifying the Spleen, the Liver disease will be healed. This marvelous treatment is suitable for Liver diseases of a deficient nature. It is not applicable to Liver diseases of an excessive nature (4).*

Medical classic states: "Purging the Deficiency and tonifying the Excess will make a deficient case more deficient and an excessive case more excessive. It is therefore a set principle." The statement, "When the Liver is affected, the Spleen should be tonified" quoted above, is a case in conformity with this principle. For diseases of all the other Viscera, this principle is always applicable.

*According to You Yi, this passage is not in the original text. It is possible a later annotation. (02-1)

NOTES

1. Such as Radix Paeoniae Alba, Fructus Schisandrae, Fructus Corni and Semen Ziziphi Spinosae. (64-12)

2. Such as Radix Rehmanniae (fried) and Flos Chrysanthemi (fried). (64-12)

3. Such as Radix Glycyrrhizae Praeparata, Fructus Tritici and Fructus Ziziphi Jujubae. (64-12)

4. Liver disease of an excessive nature will bear the following symptoms at its onset: costal pain, vertigo, chest distress with tight pulse. Then anorexia, abdominal distention, general fatigue, watery stool with tight pulse and white-greasy tongue coating will be observed. This is a typical case of Liver conquering Spleen syndrome, which should be treated by purging the Liver and tonifying the Spleen. *Xiaoyao San** is the cure. Among the ingredients, Poria, Rhizoma Atractylodis Macrocephalae, Radix Glycyrrhizae Praeparata are those that could tonify the Spleen.

**Xiaoyao San*: Radix Angelicae Sinensis, Radix Bupleuri, Radix Paeoniae Alba, Rhizoma Atractylodis Macrocephalae, Radix Glycyrrhizae Praeparata, Rhizoma Zingiberis Recens and Herba Menthae. (64-12)

Commentary: The principle discussed in this clause is still applicable in present-day practice. At the first stage of the Liver disease, symptoms and signs of dizziness, costal pain, stuffiness in the chest and tight pulse will appear. Symptoms of Spleen disease will then follow: Lack of appetite, general fatigue, watery stool, white and thick tongue coating. Satisfactory effects will refult only when the prescription includes ingredients that function on the Spleen.

The Spleen is the source of acquired essence (food essence), and the source of nutrients for growth and development. The functioning of the Spleen is of vital importance in determining the course of the disease. (02-2)

CASES

Case 1 (65-15): Excessive Liver Checking the Deficient Spleen

Zhai, female, 38, first treatment on March 1, 1981.

The patient had distention and pain over costal region and abdomen, with anorexia and belching for two months. Three years ago, she suffered from icterohepatitis. Recently the following symptoms began after an attack of mental depression: distended and painful chest and abdomen, anorexia and distention after meals, belching with anorexia, irritation and anger, bitterness in the mouth, loose stool or constipation and scanty urine.

Diagnosis: This syndrome is caused by stagnated Liver with decline of Vital Energy and deficient Spleen under the checking of the Liver, with invasion of pathogenetic Humidity.

Treatment: To regulate stagnated Vital Energy in the Liver, replenish the Spleen and dissolve the Humidity.

Prescription:

Radix Bupleuri	6 grams
Radix Angelicae Sinensis	9 grams
Radix Paeoniae Alba	12 grams
Rhizoma Atractylodis Macrocephalae	9 grams
Poria	9 grams
Pericarpium Citri Reticulatae	9 grams
Radix Aucklandiae	3 grams
Fructus Amomi	6 grams
Fructus Hordei	9 grams
Rhizoma Corydalis	9 grams
Fructus Citri Sarcodactylis	9 grams
Radix Glycyrrhizae Praeparata	3 grams

Second treatment on March 8. After six doses, all symptoms were subsiding, but insomnia was reported. Six grams of Semen Ziziphi Spinosae were added and after twelve doses, the syndrome was relieved.

CLAUSE 1-2

Man lives in a world with Five Evolutive Phases (Five Elements, *Wuxing*) (1) and grows up in a suitable climate (2). The climate can promote and give birth to all creatures under heaven, but may also injure and hurt these creatures, similar to the way water keeps a boat afloat, but can also overturn it. Good health results when the Congenital Vital Energy (3) of the Five Viscera circulates normally.

NOTES

1. Five Evolutive Phases, or Five Elements (*Wuxing*)— Wood, Fire, Earth, Metal and Water— are the five essential substances that constitute the material world, and are also indispensable to the daily life of human beings. They are interrelated through mutual production and mutual conquest (checking), and undergo endless changes and movement.

2. Climate: The original text is "Wind Vital Energy" (*Fengqi*). When the six climatic factors (Wind, Cold, Summer-heat, Humidity, Dryness and Fire) are normal, they are termed the six (normal) climatic factors. While they exist in an abnormal state, they become pathogenetic (climatic) factors.

3. Congenital Vital Energy: The original text is *Yuanzhen*. It may indicate: a) Body Resistance (01-9), and b) Original (inborn) Vital Energy, stored in the Kidney and energizes all visceral functions (02-2).

When man is strongly influenced by exogenous pathogenetic climatic factors, he will perish. All human catastrophes fall within the following three categories of causa morbi:

1) When pathogenetic factors invade the Channels and Collaterals and are transmitted into the Viscera and Bowels, this is an endogenous causa morbi;

2) Exogenous pathogenetic factors invade the four extremities and the nine body orifices (1) and then circulate through the blood vessels, thus obstructing the normal flow of Vital Energy. This is an exogenous causa morbi from the Exterior;

3) Intemperance in sexual life, various traumata, animal and insect bites.

These cover the causes of all diseases (2).

NOTES

1. Nine body orifices or openings: a) two eyes, two ears, two nostrils, mouth and urethral orifice and anus; or b) two eyes, two ears, two nostrils, mouth, tongue and throat.

2. According to Chen Yan, the author of *Treatise on Three Categories of Pathogenetic Factors and Symptoms (San Yin Ji Yi Bing Zheng Fang Lun)*, there are three types of causa morbi: exogenous causa morbi caused by the six climatic pathogenetic factors; endogenous causa morbi caused by impairment of the spiritual depression to the Five Viscera; and non-exogenous, non-endogenous causa morbi caused by intemperance in sexual life, traumata, animal and insect bites. (02-3)

One should carefully protect one's Body Resistance and avoid the attack of climatic pathogenetic factors. Otherwise, Channels and Collaterals will be violated and health endangered. In case pathogenetic factors have invaded the Channels and Collaterals, medical treatment should be given in time to stop the transmission of pathogenetic factors into the Viscera and Bowels. If there is heaviness and uneasiness in the extremities, *Daoyin* (1), *Tuna* (2), acupuncture and *Gaomo* (3) therapies should be practiced to clear the nine orifices. Besides, one should avoid violation of his Majesty's law, avoid animal bites and all accidents and injuries. One should also regulate sexual life, wear clothing suitable to season and maintain moderate diet with bitter, sour, pungent and sweet flavors. In this way, one can maintain good health and prevent the intrusion of pathogenetic factors through *Couli* (4). *Cou* is a juncture where the Triple Burners (5) and Body Resistance converge and a Channel wherein the Vital Energy and the Blood flow. *Li* is the texture on skin, Viscera and Bowels.

NOTES

1. *Daoyin*: Breathing and physical exercise therapy used in ancient times, similar to present-day *Qigong* therapy. (01-9)
2. *Tuna*: Breathing therapy practiced in ancient times. (01-9)
3. *Gaomo*: Rubbing areas affected with rheumatic or skin diseases with ointment. (01-9)
4. *Couli*: a) Texture of the skin, muscles and internal organs; b) Juncture of the skin and muscles. (11-375)
5. Triple Burners (*Sanjiao*): Three Portions of Body Cavity. See notes under Clause 1-6.

CLAUSE 1-3

Question: Different facial complexions indicate different diseases. Could the Master explain this in detail?

Master: Take the nose as an example.

When the tip of the nose is blue-purple (cyanosis) (1) this indicates abdominal pain. If the patient is sensitive to cold, it will be a fatal case (2).

When the tip of the nose is black-dark (3), this indicates stagnation of the pathogenetic Water.

Yellow nose (4) indicates Cold stagnation in chest.

White nose (5) indicates hemorrhage.

Slightly red nose (6) appearing at an inappropriate season (7) indicates a fatal case.

Jing (8) disease indicated by the patient's staring is difficult to cure.

Different complexions manifest diseases as follows:

Blue-purple (cyanosis) complexion indicates pain; black-dark complexion manifests internal injury caused by overstrain; red complexion signifies pathogenetic Wind; and yellowish complexion is a sign of constipation.

Bright-colored complexion suggests stagnant Fluid-retention.

NOTES

1. Blue-purple color (cyanosis, *qing*) of the skin or complexion, caused by stagnation or obstruction of the Vital Energy and the Blood, indicating symptoms of cold, pains, blood stasis or convulsions. (11-414)

2. In another edition, the text reads: "When the patient senses cold in the abdomen and suffers pain, case is fatal." (01-9)

3. Black-dark (*hei*) of the skin or complexion seen usually in severe and chronic cases due to stagnation of the Vital Energy and the Blood, indicating Cold, pains, and reduced Vital function of the Kidney. (11-389)

4. Yellow color (sallow, *huang*) of the skin or complexion, caused by dysfunction of the Spleen or Blood Deficiency, indicating presence of Humidity. (11-392)

5. White color (pallor, *bai*) of the skin or complexion caused by debility, indicating Cold and Deficiency of the Blood. (11-367)

6. Red color (*chi*) of the skin or complexion caused by excessive filling of capillaries, indicating presence of Heat. (11-374)

7. Appearing at an inappropriate season: Red is the color of Fire, which is of Yang nature. It should appear in spring and summer. When red appears in autumn or winter, then it is appearing at an inappropriate season. According to the checking sequence of the Five Evolutive Phases, the case will end in death. (01-10)

8. *Jing* (or *chi*) disease: Febrile disease with such symptoms as opisthotonus, convulsions, trismus, etc. For details see Chapter II.

Commentary: Canon of Medicine states: "Eyesight, complexion of five colors* are the manifestations of Vital Energy." The Vital Energy, the Blood and Essence of the Five Viscera and the Six Bowels have their manifestations exposed on the surface of the body. Therefore, the sturdiness or weakness of the Viscera and the Bowels, and the sufficiency and insufficiency of the Vital Energy and the Blood can also be diagnosed by watching the color of the patient's complexion. Thus, observing the patient's complexion is an important means of diagnosis. In this clause, the Master observed the color of the nose with reference to the facial complexion, presenting the readers with guide-lines for observing skin colors. He also pointed out the importance of differentiating various parts of the nose in the observation of colors. This is because colors in different parts of the body (e.g. face**) represent different diseases or disease of different organs.

*Five colors: Blue-purple (*qing*), black-dark (*hei*), yellow (*huang*), white (*bai*) and red (*chi*).

**Color in different parts of the face may indicate diseases of different body organs (according to location) and different syndromes (according to the color in each location). See the following diagram:

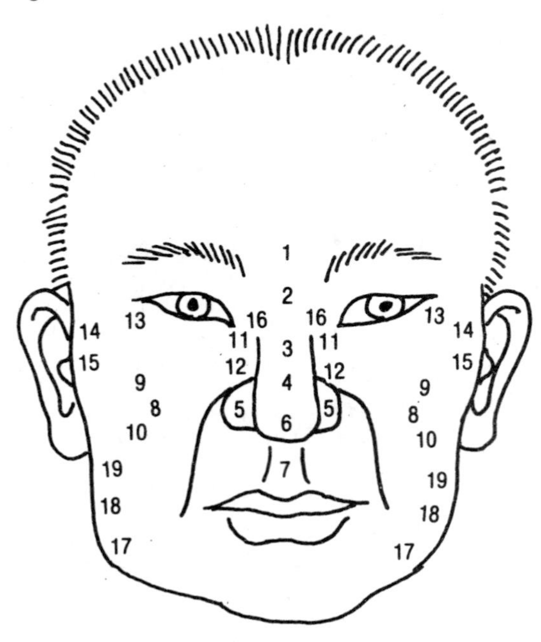

1. Throat	8. Large Intestine	15. Hand
2. Lung	9. Kidney	16. Breast
3. Heart	10. Navel	17. Foot
4. Liver	11. Gall Bladder	18. Knee
5. Stomach	12. Small Intestine	19. Back
6. Spleen	13. Shoulder	
7. Urinary Bladder	14. Arm	

(23-16)

CLAUSE 1-4

Master: The patient usually remains still but cries out occasionally. This is an indication of joint disease. If the patient speaks in a low murmuring voice, he is suffering from an ailment of the chest and diaphragm. Or if he speaks in a faint, long and clear voice, he is suffering from a headache.

Commentary: This clause deals with auscultation, one of the four methods of diagnosis.* Joint diseases include arthralgia and rheumatalgia. When the patient suffers from such diseases, he cannot move normally, so he usually remains still. In case patient must move, joint disease will cause great pain and make patient cry out suddenly. Disease in chest and diaphragm indicates Blocked-up Chest,** fullness and distention of the gastric region, or heartburn.*** When a patient is suffering from a headache, he dares not speak out loud as this might aggravate his headache. He speaks in a faint, long and clear voice, as he is not suffering from any disease of the respiratory tract or chest. (02-6)

*The four methods of diagnosis: observation; auscultation and olfaction; interrogation (history taking); pulse feeling and palpation.

**Blocked-up Chest (*Jiexiong*): Excessive harmful factors accumulated in the chest with tenderness and sensation of fullness in the costal regions. Details see *Treatise on Febrile Diseases Caused by Cold* (hereinafter *Shanghan Lun*), Clauses 128-138.

***Heartburn (*Ao' nong*): Burning sensation in the Stomach with restlessness, seen in acute febrile diseases or gastroenteritis.

CLAUSE 1-5

Master: The patient shrugs his shoulders when breathing. This signifies existence of excessive pathogenetic factors in the chest (1). Breath ascending to the throat while the patient breathes is a symptom of cough. When the patient must open his mouth to breathe and still feels short of breath, it is an indication of pulmonary asthenia (2) accompanied by copious salivation and sputum.

NOTES

1. Pathogenetic factor in chest obstructs normal respiration, forcing the pa-

tient to shrug shoulders to aid breathing.

2. Pulmonary asthenia, or withered Lung (*Feiwei*): Consumptive pulmonary disease due to deficient Yin. See Chapter VII.

Commentary: This clause discusses diagnosis by observation of patient's respiration and physical appearance.

CLAUSE 1-6

Master: If the patient's inspiration is a bit rapid, it can be diagnosed as excessive pathogenetic factors in the Middle Portion of Body Cavity (1). A purgative will provide the cure. When the patient is in a state of deficient nature (of weak build), the case will be difficult to cure. When the pathogenetic factors in the Upper Portion of Body Cavity (2) make the patient inspire with short and rapid breaths, or when the pathogenetic factors in the Lower Portion of Body Cavity (3) make the patient inspire with long and deep breaths, both cases will be difficult to treat. While the patient has to shake his body to aid in respiration, then he is suffering from an incurable disease.

NOTES

1. The Middle Portion of Body Cavity: located between the diaphragm and umbilicus of the body cavity, housing the Spleen and the Stomach.

2. The Upper Portion of Body Cavity: located above the diaphragm, housing the Heart and the Lung.

3. The Lower Portion of Body Cavity: located below umbilicus of the body cavity, housing the Liver, the Kidney, the Urinary Bladder and the Intestines.

CLAUSE 1-7

Master: Pulse at *cunkou* (1) will follow the changes in Vital Energy of a certain Viscus in different seasons (2). Vital Energy of the Viscera will appear as different colors when they are strong in certain seasons (3). For example, blue-purple (cyanosis) signifies strong Vital Energy in the Liver. Under normal conditions, the four seasons will give birth to their respective colors (4). When blue-purple (cyanosis) of the Liver Vital Energy does not appear as it should, but white (pallor) color appears, it is an indication of disease. In all cases when unseasonal colors or pulses appear, they can be diagnosed as symptoms and signs of diseases. (5)

NOTES

1. *Cunkou*: Point on the wrist over the radial artery where pulse is felt. Inch (*cun*), Bar (*guan*) and Cubit (*chi*) are three spots on the wrist over the radial artery where the pulse is felt. The Bar is located above the head of the radius at the wrist where the physician places the tip of his middle-finger; the Inch lies next to it on the distal side, where the tip of the physician's index-finger rests; the Cubit is on the proximal side where the tip of the physician's ring-finger is placed. The Inch, the Bar and the Cubit on the left wrist indicate the pulse condition of the Heart, the Liver and the Kidney respectively, while those on the right indicate the pulse condition of the Lung, the Spleen and the "Vital Gate" (*mingmen*). (11-375)

2. Vital Energy of different Viscera will vary in the four seasons; for example, the Liver Vital Energy is strong in spring. At the same time, the pulse changes with the four seasons, four example, the pulse rises and is full in spring and summer, while it sinks and becomes consolidated in autumn and winter.

3. See the following diagram:

Viscera Vital Energy	*Strong in (season)*	*Color*
Liver	Spring	Blue-purple (cyanosis)
Heart	Summer	Red
Spleen	Long-summer*	Yellow
Lung	Autumn	White (pallor)
Kidney	Winter	Black-dark

4. The four seasons have their respective colors: blue-purple in spring, red in summer, white in autumn and black-dark in winter. (01-12)

5. This clause deals with diagnosis by observation of color (complexion) and pulses. As the seasons change, human physiological functions change correspondingly with visible manifestation of colors and pulses. When an unseasonal pulse or color appears, it generally foretells certain pathological changes in a disease.

*Spleen Vital Energy is also said to be strong during the last eighteen days of the third, sixth, ninth and twelfth months of the lunar year. See Clause 1-1. (40-5)

CLAUSE 1-8

Question: Could you explain the following: premature arrival, late arrival, late departure and excessive temperature.

Master: On the midnight of the first day of the first *Jiazi* (1) (sixty-day cycle) after the Winter Solstice, Lesser Yang begins to germinate (2) and the weather gradually becomes warm. If the weather begins to warm up before the onset of Lesser Yang, this is termed "premature arrival" (*wei zhi er zhi*). On the other hand, if the weather does not warm up after the germination of Lesser Yang, it is a case of "late arrival" (*zhi er bu zhi*). When the weather remains severe after the start of Lesser Yang, it is a case of "late departure" (*zhi er bu qu*). And when the weather turns as hot as summer just after the beginning of the first *Jiazi*, it is termed "excessive temperature" (*zhi er tai guo*).

NOTES

1. This occurs sixty days after the Winter Solstice (approximately December 21), which would place it in the Rain Water (approximately February 19). (02-4)

The twenty-four Solar Terms (*jieqi*) in the year:

Approximate dates	*Solar Terms (jieqi)*
February 5	Beginning of Spring
February 19	Rain Water
March 5	Waking of Insects
March 20	Spring Equinox
April 5	Pure Brightness
April 20	Grain Rain
May 5	Beginning of Summer
May 21	Grain Full
June 6	Grain in Ear
June 21	Summer Solstice
July 7	Slight Heat
July 23	Great Heat
August 7	Beginning of Autumn
August 23	Limit of Heat
September 8	White Dew
September 23	Autumn Equinox
October 8	Cold Dew
October 23	Frost's Descent
November 7	Beginning of Winter
November 22	Slight Snow
December 7	Great Snow

December 21	Winter Solstice
January 6	Slight Cold
January 21	Great Cold

2. In ancient times, the year was divided into six periods, i.e., Lesser Yang (starting from the Rain Water, approximately February 19), Greater Yang, Initial Yang, Initial Yin, Lesser Yin and Greater Yin, each consisting of sixty days. (01-13)

Commentary: This clause deals with normal and abnormal weather conditions. Though this might bear no direct relationship with clinical practice, it is an important factor in the treatment and diagnosis of all diseases, especially epidemic diseases.

CLAUSE 1-9

Master: When the pulse is floating at the front (1), it indicates a syndrome at the Exterior (2). When the pulse is floating at the back, the syndrome is located in the Interior with symptoms of lumbago and stiffness in the back that make it difficult for the patient to move and cause a serious shortness of breath.

NOTES

1. Inch, Bar and Cubit (*cun, guan* and *chi*) are points on the wrist over the radial artery when the pulse is felt. Since the Bar is in the middle, the Inch is considered the front of the pulse. Thus "the pulse is floating at the front" means "the pulse at the Inch point or the pulse under the forefinger." The pulse at the back indicates the pulse at the Cubit or the pulse under the ring-finger.

2. Syndrome at the Exterior: Syndrome with symptoms and signs such as headache, fever, sensitivity to wind and cold, etc. See Chapter I (Initial Yang Syndrome) of *Shanghan Lun*.

CLAUSE 1-10

Question: It is written in the Classic: "The exuberant Yang prevails and moves about alone." Could you explain the meaning?

Master: This is because when the exuberant Yang prevails, there will be no Yin, and Yang moves alone. So it is called "*Jue Yang* (1)."

NOTES

1. *Jue Yang*: *Jue* means the abnormal ascent of Yang Vital Energy. When Yang is too excessive to control itself, it ascends abnormally. (01-13)

Commentary: Under normal conditions, Yin and Yang are in a state of relative equilibrium. Under such condition, Yin is the ground of Yang. When Yin is exhausted violently, Yang Vital Energy will have no base and ascend vigorously, causing "the exuberant Yang to prevail and move about alone" (*Jue Yang du xing*). In a clinical situation, symptoms of the exuberant Yang of the Liver ascending abnormally would include flushed face, vertigo, or in severe cases, the patient's losing his footing. (02-5)

CLAUSE 1-11

Question: The pulse under the fore-finger is deep (1), gigantic (grand) and slippery. Deep pulse indicates a syndrome of an excessive nature. A slippery pulse reveals the existence of the Vital Energy. When the Excess and the Vital Energy intermingle, conflict with each other, and then invade the Viscera, the case will be fatal. This is called "*Cu Jue*" (2). When they invade the Bowels, the case will not be serious. Could Master explain this?

Master: Symptoms and signs of blue-purple lips and sensitivity to cold are indications of the invasion of pathogenetic factor into the Viscera, which is fatal. When the patient feels no uneasiness and perspires spontaneously, it is a case of pathogenetic factor invading the Bowels. Such cases are easy to cure.

NOTES

1. For different pulses, see Appendix I.

2. *Cu Jue*: Syncope, sudden loss of consciousness. Symptoms and signs include vertigo and dimness in vision, a feeling of heaviness in the head and weakness in the legs. The patient may suddenly fall to the ground with aphasia; this is caused by the abnormal ascent of the Vital Energy and the Blood into the head. (01-14)

CLAUSE 1-12

Question: The pulse suddenly disappears. When the syndrome invades the Viscera, death results. But the case will not be fatal if it invades the Bowels. Why?

Master: This is true of all diseases. Take *Jinyinchuang*, a form of skin sore, as an example. When it develops from the mouth to the extremities, it is curable. But when it spreads from the extremities to the mouth, it will be a fatal case. Syndrome at the Exterior indicates a curable case; syndrome invading the Interior will be fatal.

Commentary: Clauses 1-11 and 1-12 discuss different pulses. Pulse in Clause 1-11 is deep, gigantic and slippery. But pulse in this clause disappears. The Master tells us that regardless of which pulse may appear, the principle of "syndrome invading the Viscera is fatal; syndrome invading the Bowels is curable" is a fixed principle. This clause restates the following:

Syndrome invading Viscera— serious case;

Syndrome invading Bowels— easy to cure;

Syndrome transmitted from Exterior to Interior— difficult to cure;

Syndrome transmitted from Interior to Exterior— easy to cure.

(02-8)

CLAUSE 1-13

Question: What are the eighteen diseases of a Yang nature (1)?

Master: Headache, pains in the neck, waist, spine, arm, and referred pain in the foot.

Question: And the eighteen diseases of a Yin nature (2)?

Master: Cough, asthma, tachypnea, nausea, difficulty in swallowing, abdominal distention, intestinal gurgling (borborygmus), heart-stroke, or contraction of limbs. Each of the Five Viscera is subject to eighteen diseases, or ninety in total. Each of the Six Bowels is subject to eighteen diseases, which makes one hundred and eight in total (3). Besides, they are five factors causing fatigue or overstrain (*wu lao*) (4), seven types of injury (*qi shang*) (5), six types of exhaustion (*liu ji*) (6) and thirty-six gynecological diseases.

NOTES

1. Diseases of a Yang nature: Diseases located in the Exterior or in the Channels and Collaterals. (01-16)

2. Diseases of a Yin nature: Diseases located in the Viscera and Bowels. (01-16)

3. "Each of the Six Bowels is subject to eighteen diseases, which makes one hundred and eight in total" : This translation is based on *Jinkui E*, p. 15. According to *Comprehension of Synopsis*, p. 9, the sentence shoud read: "Each of the six climatic pathogenetic factors, Wind, Cold, Summer-heat, Humidity, Dryness and Fire, are subject to eighteen diseases...."

4. Five factors causing fatigue or overstrain (*wu lao*): a) Five consumptive diseases: consumption of the Lung, the Liver, the Heart, the Spleen and the Kidney. (*Common Terms of Traditional Chinese Medicine in English*, p. 395); b) Fatigue or strain caused by mental over-exertion, anxiety, melancholy, mental and physical fatigue. (01-16)

5. Seven types of injury (*qi shang*): Over-eating will injurè the Spleen; excessive rage will injure the Liver; over-exertion in lifting something heavy or sitting on damp ground will injure the Kidney; exposure to cold weather and intake of cold liquids will injure the Lung; too much melancholy and spiritual exertion will injure the Heart; exposure to wind, rain, cold and heat will injure the physical appearance; great rage and terror will bring about mental strain.

6. Six types of exhaustion (*liu ji*): Exhaustion of the Vital Energy, the Blood, tendons, bones, muscles and Essence of Life (fundamental substance which maintains the body function).

Pathogenetic factors of a clear and light nature will invade the upper part of the human body; pathogenetic factors of a heavy and turbid nature will invade the lower part of the human body. The six climatic pathogenetic factors will invade the Exterior and the seven emotional factors (1) will harm the Interior. Intemperance in eating will cause indigestion. Each of the five pathogenetic factors (2) has its own way of invading the body. Pathogenetic Wind will invade the human body in the morning, while pathogenetic Cold will invade it in the evening. Humidity will find its way into human body from the lower part, while fog will invade the upper part. Pathogenetic Wind causes the pulse to float, pathogenetic Cold accelerates the pulse. Fog injures the skin and *Couli* (see Clause 1-2). Humidity flows in the joints. Intemperance in eating will damage the Spleen and the Stomach. Excessive Cold will injure the Channels while excessive Heat will injure the Collaterals.

NOTES

1. Seven emotional factors (*qi qing*): Joy, anger, melancholy, anxiety, sorrow, fear and fright.

2. Five pathogenetic factors here include: Wind, Cold, Humidity, fog, intemperance in eating. (01-9)

CLAUSE 1-14

Question: There are some cases when Exterior syndromes should be given priority in treating an urgent case, and others when Interior syndromes should be given priority. Could you explain this?

Master: When a purgative is adopted, the patient will suffer continuous diarrhea containing undigested food (1), and general aching (2). In such cases, the Interior syndrome should be considered urgent. Or when the patient has normal stool with general aching, the Exterior syndrome can be treated first.

NOTES

1. Diarrhea containing undigested food (*xia li qing gu*): Watery diarrhea results from pathogenetic Cold or indigestion, the stool being watery and mixed with undigested food with little fecal smell. (08-447)

2. General aching, and body pain: Exterior syndrome. Diarrhea containing undigested food is a manifestation of an Interior syndrome.

Commentary: This clause is similar to Clause 91 in *Shanghan Lun*.

CLAUSE 1-15

When a patient with a chronic disease is affected by a new disease (1), the new disease should be given priority in treatment, after which the chronic disease can be treated.

NOTES

1. New disease (*cu bing*): Sudden attack of a serious illness; first seizure of a disease.

Commentary: Chronic disease cannot be cured within a short time, while a new disease can be treated easily as it has not penetrated deep into the Interior. Generally speaking, patients with chronic diseases lack Body Resistance, permitting pathogenetic factors to invade the Interior in a short period of time. If timely treatment is not directed at the new disease, it will aggravate and complicate the chronic disease. (02-9)

CLAUSE 1-16

Master: Diseases of the Five Viscera have their respective healthful and harmful foods. When a patient eats food he likes, he is likely to recover quickly. Or, on the other hand, when he is given food he dislikes, his disease will be aggravated. If a patient expresses a desire for food he usually dislikes, he is likely to contract a fever.

Commentary: In consideration of the specific physiological characteristics of the Five Viscera, attention should be given to the treatment of diseases of specific Viscus. For example, for Liver disease with deficient Yin, sour foods would be suitable, since they would act as an astringent for a case of Liver disease with stagnation of the Vital Energy, pungent foods would have a dispersing function. As the Heart controls Blood circulation, Heart disease will bring excessive Heat to the Blood. In such cases, the patient should not eat hot food or wear heavy clothing. As the Lung dominates the Vital Energy, when it is affected, the Vital Energy will be in a deficient state. For such a case, the patient should not be served cold food or wear light clothing. In accordance with what is healthful and harmful to the diseases of the Five Viscera, proper drugs should be administered, and proper nursing care provided. When the patient suddenly expresses a desire for food that he usually dislikes, it shows that the pathogenetic factor has altered the innate likes and dislikes of the affected Viscus. If such food is served, it will cause the pathogenetic factor to go rampant and most likely bring on a fever. (02-9)

CLAUSE 1-17

While the disease is affecting the Viscera, attacking or purgative therapy (1) is appropriate only when corresponding symptoms and signs are observed. For example, if the patient is thirsty for water, Decoction of Polyporus Umbellatus (2) can be administered. Similar treatment can be applied for all other cases.

NOTES

1. Attacking or purgative therapy (*gong xia fa*): Administering medicines (usually purgatives or laxatives) to counteract invading pathogenetic factors or loosen the bowels when there is constipation.

2. Decoction of Polyporus Umbellatus (*Zhuling Tang*): See Clause 13-14.

CHAPTER II

ON PULSE, SYMPTOM COMPLEX AND TREATMENT OF *JING*,* HUMIDITY** AND *YE**** DISEASES

CLAUSE 2-1

Initial Yang syndrome (1): Syndrome with symptoms and signs of fever, no perspiration, but aversion to cold is termed *Gang Jing* (2).

NOTES

1. Initial Yang syndrome (*Tai yang bing*): See *Shanghan Lun*, Chapter I.

2. *Gang Jing*: Initial Yang syndrome with Exterior Excess. See *Shanghan Lun*, Clause 35.

CLAUSE 2-2

Initial Yang syndrome: Syndrome with symptoms and signs of

**Jing*, convulsive diseases, or spasmodic symptoms: Febrile disease with such symptoms as opisthotonus, convulsions, trismus, etc. Either climatic or endogenous pathogenetic factors may cause *Jing* diseases. Most of the *Jing* diseases discussed in this chapter are caused by climatic (exogenous) pathogenetic factors. (02-12)

**Humidity (*Shi*): Disease of muscle and joints with symptoms and signs of fever, heaviness in movement, arthralgia and irritability. It can be divided into Interior Humidity and Exterior Humidity. Pathogenetic Humidity is always combined with pathogenetic Wind, Cold and Heat, causing different complications. In this chapter, diseases of the Exterior Humidity and its complications are discussed. (02-12)

****Ye*: Heatstroke, a syndrome with symptoms and signs of fever, spontaneous perspiration, thirst, irritability, red urine, Deficiency of Vital Energy and feeble pulse. It always appears with pathogenetic Cold and Humidity, resulting in different complications, thus the heatstroke discussed here differs from sunstroke or heatstroke in modern medicine. As *Jing*, *Shi* (Humidity) and *Ye* diseases are all caused by exogenous pathogenetic factors beginning from the Initial Yang Channel, they are included in the same chapter. (02-12) fever and perspiration, but with no aversion to cold, is termed *Rou Jing* (1).

NOTES

1. *Rou Jing*: Initial Yang syndrome with Exterior Deficiency. See *Shanghan Lun*, Clause 12.

CLAUSE 2-3

Initial Yang syndrome with fever and deep and slender pulse is termed *Jing* disease, and is difficult to cure (1).

NOTES

1. This clause describes the *Jing* disease according to the condition of the pulse. Initial Yang syndrome with fever is a case of Exterior syndrome of a Yang nature. The pulse should be floating. Even if it turns into a *Jing* disease, pulse should remain tight and tense with strong pulsations (pulse in Yang nature). In this case, the pulse is deep and slender, an indication of a Deficiency in the internal Vital Energy confronting a strong exogenous pathogenetic factor. In such cases, when drugs are used to disperse the pathogenetic factor, they will further weaken the Body Resistance; if tonic is adopted, pathogenetic factor will remain in place and be harder to disperse; such a case will be difficult to cure. This is true of all other diseases when pulse and symptoms do not agree with each other— a manifestation of a strong pathogenetic factor confronting deficient Body Resistance. (02-13)

CLAUSE 2-4

Initial Yang syndrome: Profuse perspiration will cause a *Jing* disease (1).

NOTES

1. Initial Yang syndrome requires perspiration, but not profuse perspiration. In Clause 12 of *Shanghan Lun*, the text states that after administering Decoction of Ramulus Cinnamomi, "cover the patient with a quilt for two hours to induce perspiration. A light sweat all over the body is suitable. If the sweat is too watery, it will not be of any benefit to the patient." In this case, profuse perspiration has caused the exhaustion of Yin and evanescence of Yang, resulting in a *Jing* disease. (01-25)

CASES

Case 1 (65-40):

Doctor Xue Lizhai treated a woman suffering from Yin-deficiency with itching over the body. When the patient was treated by another doctor, drugs aimed at dispersing pathogenetic Wind (understood as the cause of itching) were administered. She began to have trismus and convulsion with grand and speedy pulse at the bar position (under the doctor's middle-finger). Doctor Xue commented: This is a case caused by the excessive Fire over the deficient Blood of the Liver Channel, which should be treated as follows: nourish the Yin Blood and curb the Fire arising from the Liver.

Prescription:

Radix Paeoniae
Rhizoma Rehmanniae Praeparata
Radix Angelicae Sinensis
Rhizoma Ligustici Chuanxiong
Radix Ophiopogonis
Fructus Schisandrae
Ramulus Uncariae cum Uncis

CLAUSE 2-5

Using purgative for a syndrome caused by pathogenetic Wind will result in a *Jing* disease. If diaphoresis is adopted as a further treatment, the patient will suffer contraction of the extremities (1).

NOTES

1. When there are no visible symptoms and signs of Interior syndrome in a case of Exterior syndrome, no purgative should be adopted. Using one is a malpractice. Use of a purgative will hurt the Yin, causing a *Jing* disease, as tendons and Channels are denied their nourishment of Yin. If diaphoresis is adopted as a further treatment to hurt the Yang, it will result in contraction of the extremities, as the deficient Yang loses its normal function of warming and mobilizing the tendons. (01-25)

CLAUSE 2-6

Diaphoresis should not be applied for patients with skin sores, even if he had body pain. If applied, the patient will suffer spasms (contraction of extremities). (1)

NOTES

1. This clause also appears in *Shanghan Lun*, Clause 85.

CLAUSE 2-7

Jing diseases have the following symptoms and signs: Fever throughout the body with cold feet; rigid neck; aversion to cold; fever in head with flushed face and red eyes; shaking of head; sudden trismus and opisthotonus. If diaphoresis is adopted in such cases, Cold and Humidity will intermingle bringing about a greater Deficiency in the Exterior. The patient will develop an even greater aversion to cold (1). After adoption of diaphoresis, the pulse resembles a snake (2).

NOTES

1. When diaphoresis is adopted, exogenous pathogenetic Cold will intermingle with the sweat (Humidity). Since Exterior Body Resistance has been weakened by perspiration, the patient develops an even worse aversion to cold. (01-20)

2. After adoption of diaphoresis, pulse will change from a normal tight pulse, characteristic of *Jing* disease, to one with a feeling resembling the crawling of a snake. (01-20)

Commentary: According to *Treatise on Febrile Diseases Caused by Cold with Annotations by Cheng Wuji* and *The Pulse Classic* by Wang Shuhe, the last two sentences are not included in the original text. (02-12)

In *Jinjian*, this clause appears at the beginning of the chapter, as the author thought this offered the most detailed description of *Jing* disease. (01-20)

CLAUSE 2-8

When a patient suffering from a *Jing* disease suddenly feels abdominal distention, he is about to recover (1). If the pulse remains the same but then turns into hidden-tight, the disease is not subsiding.

NOTES

1. According to some annotators, abdominal distention is either the resto-

ration of Body Resistance and Body Fluid, or a sign that the syndrome is moving into the Bowels, from where it will find its way out. But in clinical observation, this is rarely seen. For this reason, other annotators considered this clause redundant. (01-20)

CLAUSE 2-9

Pulse of a *Jing* disease: When pressed, it is tense and tight with full pulsation from Inch to Cubit (1).

NOTES

1. From the pulse under the first finger to the pulse under the ring-finger. This means the pulse under all three fingers is tense and tight. "When pressed" suggests that when pulse is pressed deeply, the pulse is not only tense and tight but also deep and hidden. (02-13)

CLAUSE 2-10

Jing disease: The case will be difficult to treat if the patient has skin sores caused by moxibustion (1).

NOTES

1. Sores and carbuncles discharging bloody pus will exhaust the patient's Body Fluid, making the case difficult to treat. (01-21)

CLAUSE 2-11

Initial Yang syndrome with all corresponding symptoms and signs (1) and a rigid feeling throughout the body (neck and back) but with deep and slow pulse (2) is a *Jing* disease. Decoction of Radix Trichosanthis and Ramulus Cinnamomi can be prescribed as a remedy.

NOTES

1. Corresponding symptoms and signs include headache, rigid neck, fever, perspiration, aversion to cold, etc. See *Shanghan Lun*, Chapter I. (01-21)

2. The deep and slow pulse here is not an indication of Interior Cold, but a manifestation of insufficient Body Fluid.

Decoction of Radix Trichosanthis and Ramulus Cinnamomi (*Gualou Guizhi Tang*):

Radix Trichosanthis	2 *liang**
Ramulus Cinnamomi	3 *liang*
Radix Paeoniae	3 *liang*
Radix Glycyrrhizae	2 *liang*
Rhizoma Zingiberis Recens	3 *liang*
Fructus Ziziphi Jujubae	12 *pcs.*

Stew the drugs in nine *sheng* of water until three *sheng* remain. Serve the lukewarm decoction in three doses to induce a light sweat. If there is no sweat, hot porridge can be served to improve the effect of the decoction.

*Dosages varied in ancient times. According to *Explanation of Treatise on Febrile Diseases Caused by Cold*, p. 8, one Eastern Han *liang* is equivalent to 6.96 grams, or 13.92 grams according to *Concise Dictionary of Chinese Medicine*, p. 1009

Chinese measurements varied widely throughout history. In Han Dynasty, 6 *zhu* = 1 *fen*, 4 *fen* = 1 *liang* and thus 24 *zhu* = 1 *liang*. The precise weight or volume of the ingredients of any prescription must be determined on the basis of clinical experience. According to *Comprehension of Treatise on Febrile Diseases Caused by Cold* edited by the Institute of Chinese Medicine of Chengdu, p. 30, weights and volumes in this book can be understood as follows:

In the Book	*Present Practice*
1 *liang*	1 *qian* (3 grams)
1 *sheng* (weight)	6 *qian* to 1 *liang* (18-30 grams)
1 *sheng* (volume)	60-80 milliliters
1 *fangcunbi*	2-3 *qian* (6-9 grams)
1 foot	1 *liang* (30 grams)
as big as an egg	1.5 *liang* (45 grams)

The following two contemporary prescriptions for Decoction of Ramulus Cinnamomi may serve as a reference:

	In the first prescription	*In the second prescription*
Ramulus Cinnamomi	9 grams	9 grams
Radix Paeoniae Alba	9 grams	9 grams
Radix Glycyrrhizae Praeparata	3 grams	6 grams
Rhizoma Zingiberis Recens	9 grams	6 grams

Fructus Ziziphi Jujubae	7 pcs.	4 pcs.

— *Selected Readings of Treatise on Febrile Disease Caused by Cold*, p. 10, Science and Technology Press, Shanghai, 1979

Explanation of the Prescription: Initial Yang syndrome with aversion to cold and perspiration normally has a floating and moderate pulse. But pulse in this case is deep and slow, indicating exhaustion of the Body Fluid, which will cut off normal nourishment to tendons and Channels. The circulation of Nutrient Essence (*Ying*) and the Vital Resistance (defensive energy, *Wei*) become abnormal, causing a case of *Rou Jing* (see Clause 2-2). The deep-slow pulse mentioned in this clause must be deep-slow and tense-tight, differing from the deep-slow pulse which reflects the Interior Deficiency and Cold. Radix Trichosanthis is used to nourish the Body Fluid. Decoction of Ramulus Cinnamomi (see *Shanghan Lun*, Clause 12) will dispel the pathogenetic factors from the muscles, so that tendons and Channels can be nourished and contraction eased. (02-13)

CASES

Case 1 (52-649):

Pan, 53, first treatment on December 23, 1981.

The patient had suffered from Sheehan's disease for more than ten years. In the previous few days, she had a stiff, painful neck and back due to exposure to wind. Diaphoresis had been given. Profuse perspiration resulted, but the pain and stiffness did not subside. The patient had no aversion to cold or fever. Pulse was slender and weak and the tongue was coated and red.

Diagnosis: This case is caused by invasion of pathogenetic Wind to the Initial Yang Channel (see *Shanghan Lun*). Diaphoresis was given to induce profuse perspiration but failed to bring out the pathogenetic Wind. Body Fluid was badly consumed.

Prescription: Decoction of Radix Trichosanthis and Ramulus Cinnamomi adding Radix Puerariae was given:

Radix Trichosanthis	12 grams
Ramulus Cinnamomi	6 grams
Radix Paeoniae Alba	10 grams
Radix Puerariae	15 grams
Rhizoma Zingiberis Recens	10 grams
Fructus Ziziphi Jujubae	4 pcs.
Radix Glycyrrhizae	6 grams

After two doses of the above decoction, the syndrome was relieved.

Case 2 (65-48):

Ding, 6 months, first treatment: early summer 1931.

Symptoms: Fever, perspiration, thirst, staring, stiff neck, opisthotonos, contracture of extremities, coldness of finger tips, thin, yellow tongue coating.

Diagnosis: Invasion of pathogenetic humidity-wind to Initial Yang Channel, resulting in deficiency of Exterior and exhaustion of Body Fluid.

Treatment: To harmonize the Yin and Yang, nourish the Nutrient Essence.

Prescription: Decoction of Radix Trichosanthis and Ramulus Cinnamomi:

Radix Trichosanthis	6 grams
Ramulus Cinnamomi	5 grams
Radix Paeoniae Alba	3 grams
Radix Glycyrrhizae	2.4 grams
Rhizoma Zingiberis Recens	2 slices
Fructus Ziziphi Jujubae	2 pcs.

After three doses of decoction, symptoms subsided. In the next treatment, the following was prescribed:

Radix Angelicae Sinensis	3 grams
Radix Rehmanniae	6 grams
Radix Paeoniae Alba	3 grams
Radix Trichosanthis	6 grams
Bulbus Fritillariae Cirhosae	3 grams
Radix Gentianae Macrophyllae	3 grams
Caulis Lonicerae	6 grams

The syndrome was relieved after four doses.

CLAUSE 2-12

Initial Yang syndrome: *Gang Jing* (1) disease will appear when the following symptoms and signs are observed: No perspiration, but with little urination (2), sensation of gas rushing up towards the thorax, and trismus with aphasia. Decoction of Radix Puerariae will be a curative. (3)

NOTES

1. *Gang Jing*: See Clause 2-1.
2. No perspiration but with little urination: Under normal conditions, pers-

perspiration is accompanied by little urination. When there is no perspiration, there is usually ample urination. But in this case, there is no perspiration but little urination as well. (01-22)

3. Wu Qian: This clause discusses a *Gang Jing* disease at the Exterior. Symptoms of Initial Yang syndrome are headache, rigid neck, fever, etc. When there is no sweat, it is a case of febrile disease caused by Cold. In such cases, urination should be plentiful. But why is there little urination in this case? This is caused by excessive pathogenetic Cold which has an astringent element. The feeling of gas rushing up towards the thorax is a manifestation of the abnormal ascent of excessive pathogenetic Cold. Trismus with aphasia is also caused by excessive pathogenetic Cold. Febrile disease caused by Cold with such acute manifestations will lead to a *Gang Jing* disease.

Decoction of Radix Puerariae is used to deal with syndromes of both Initial Yang and Greater Yang Channels. This is a common way of treating a *Gang Jing* disease without perspiration. (05-464)

Decoction of Radix Puerariae
(*Gegen Tang*):

Radix Puerariae	4 *liang*
Herba Ephedrae	3 *liang*
Ramulus Cinnamomi	2 *liang*
Radix Paeoniae	2 *liang*
Radix Glycyrrhizae Praeparata	2 *liang*
Rhizoma Zingiberis Recens	3 *liang*
Fructus Ziziphi Jujubae	12 pcs.

(This prescription also appears in *Shanghan Lun*, Clause 31.)

Chop up the drugs. Stew Radix Puerariae in one *dou* of water until eight *sheng* remain. Skim off foam and add remaining ingredients, stewing it until three *sheng* remain. Filter the decoction and serve one *sheng* of the lukewarm decoction per dose. Cover the patient to induce a light sweat; no need to take porridge. Treatment should be identical to that when Decoction of Ramulus Cinnamomi is prescribed.

Explanation of the Prescription: This decoction is composed of Decoction of Ramulus Cinnamomi adding Radix Puerariae and Herba Ephedrae. Decoction of Ramulus Cinnamomi is used to dispel the pathogenetic factor from the muscles. As a stiff back is a sign of a *Gang Jing* disease, Radix Puerariae is added. Herba Ephedrae is used to induce perspiration. (01-22)

CLAUSE 2-13

Decoction of Greater *Chengqi* can be prescribed for a *Jing* disease (according to another edition, for a *Gang Jing* disease) when the following symptoms and signs are observed: Fullness in the chest, trismus, serious opisthotonus that prevent the patient from lying flat on bed, with contraction of legs and grinding of teeth. (1)

NOTES

1. Wu Qian: This clause discusses treatment of a *Jing* disease when pathogenetic factor has invaded the Interior. All the symptoms and signs mentioned in this clause indicate excessive Heat of Greater Yang Channel heating the tendons. When tendons are heated in such a way, symptoms and signs of trismus, opisthotonus, contraction of legs and grinding of teeth will appear. Decoction of Greater *Chengqi* can be prescribed to purge the Heat, but not the Excess, of Greater Yang Channel. When text states the decoction "can be prescribed," this means the doctor should be cautious in his diagnosis. (05-464)

Decoction of Greater *Chengqi*
(*Da Chengqi Tang*):

Radix et Rhizoma Rhei (steeped in wine)	4 *liang*
Cortex Magnoliae Officinalis Praeparata	0.5 *jin**
Fructus Aurantii Immaturus	5 *pcs.*
Natrii Sulfas	3 *ge***

(This prescription also appears in *Shanghan Lun*, Clause 208.)

Stew Cortex Magnoliae Officinalis and Fructus Aurantii Immaturus in one *dou* of water until five *sheng* remain. Remove dregs and add Radix et Rhizoma Rhei. Stew until two *sheng* remain. Filter the decoction and add Natrii Sulfas, stew until it dissolves. Serve lukewarm decoction in two doses. When loose stool appears, stop taking the decoction.

*Jin: One Eastern Han jin is equivalent to 7.13 liang (356.5 grams).
— *Concise Dictionary of Chinese Medicine*, p. 1009
**Ge: 1 sheng= 10 ge, also see Notes under Clause 2-26.

Explanation of the Prescription: Opisthotonus, contraction of legs, grinding of teeth, etc., indicate a serious *Jing* disease. Decoction of Greater *Chengqi* is adopted in emergencies to purge the pathogenetic factors and rescue the Yin. This decoction is useful for excessive cases of Greater Yang Channel with dried feces. (01-23)

Commentary: The three prescriptions in this chapter are for treating *Jing* diseases: Decoction of Radix Trichosanthis and Ramulus Cinnamomi for *Rou Jing* disease (with symptoms of perspiration); Decoction of Radix Puerariae for *Gang Jing* disease (without perspiration); Decoction of Greater *Chengqi* for *Jing* disease caused by formation of dried feces. These prescriptions deal with the secondary aspects, as they are urgent cases. These prescriptions will not cure the principal aspects of the disease. (01-23)

CLAUSE 2-14

Initial Yang syndrome: Rheumatic arthritis due to Humidity (*Shibi*) (1) can be diagnosed when the following symptoms and signs are observed: Arthralgia, restlessness, pulse *deep and slender* (according to another edition, pulse is *moderate*). When symptoms of dysuria and smooth stool are observed, diuretic should be prescribed. (2)

NOTES

1. *Shibi*, rheumatic or rheumatoid arthritis due to pathogenetic Humidity, marked by swelling of joints with localized pain.

2. Yu Chang: In *Shibi*, rheumatic arthritis due to Humidity, pathogenetic Humidity hampers the normal flow of Yang Vital Energy. When diuretic is taken, Yang Vital Energy will resume its normal circulation, expelling the pathogenetic Humidity from the joints. When symptoms of rheumatic arthritis do not subside after use of diuretic, the Yang Vital Energy, hampered by pathogenetic Humidity, has lost its normal function of circulating outwardly. The corresponding symptoms and signs are sweating on head, preference for heavy clothing and warm environment. In such cases, diaphoresis can be

adopted to bring about a light perspiration, to activate Yang Vital Energy and restore it to its normal condition.

CLAUSE 2-15

Humidity diseases exhibit symptoms and signs of general aching (according to another edition, general aching and restlessness), fever, and "fumigated yellow" complexion (1).

NOTES

1. You Yi: With excessive pathogenetic Humidity at the Exterior, Yang Vital Energy must be stagnant at the Interior. Excessive pathogenetic Humidity at the Exterior will cause general aching, while stagnant Yang Vital Energy at the Interior will cause fever. Then Humidity and Heat will intermingle and turn the skin "fumigated yellow," as if it were being fumigated by smoke. This dark yellow complexion is an indication of the stagnant pathogenetic Humidity. In cases of Jaundice in Heat and excessive nature, complexion will be bright yellow. See Chapter XV.

CLAUSE 2-16

The patient who is suffering from chronic disease caused by pathogenetic Humidity will sweat only on head, have a stiff back, prefer heavy clothing and warm environment (he prefers to remain near a fire). When purgative is given too early, nausea will occur. There will also be symptoms and signs of fullness in the chest, or dysuria (according to another edition, normal urination). When a thick coating appears on the tongue, it can be diagnosed as pathogenetic Heat in the Elixir Field (1) and pathogenetic Cold in the chest. The patient is thirsty but cannot drink (2), so he suffers from a parched mouth.

NOTES

1. Elixir Field, *Dantian*: This may refer to a) the region three inches below the umbilicus, believed by the Taoists to be the seat of the womb of the female and semen of the male; b) body region upon which the will is focused while practicing breathing exercise: the lower Elixir Field (region below the umbilicus), the middle Elixir Field (the pectoral region) and the upper Elixir Field (region between the eyebrows). In this clause, the lower Elixir Field is indicated. (08-377)

2. When the patient has excessive pathogenetic Heat in the Lower Portion

of Body Cavity (the Elixir Field mentioned in the text), he will develop a strong thirst for water. This is a spontaneous physiological reaction which represents an attempt at self-rescue. But the pathogenetic Cold in the Upper Portion of Body Cavity (the chest, as mentioned in the text) will reject the water (both water and pathogenetic Cold are of a Yin nature). So the patient is thirsty but cannot drink, hence he feels parched sensation in his mouth and tongue. (01-24)

Wu Qian: The patient who suffers a chronic disease caused by pathogenetic Humidity sweats only on his head. This is a case of Humidity at the Upper Portion of Body Cavity and Heat at the Lower Portion. It is not the excessive Interior Heat of the Greater Yang Channel that ascends and causes perspiration. A stiff back is caused by an influx of pathogenetic Humidity. The reason why the patient prefers to wear heavy clothing and seek a warm environment is because when pathogenetic Humidity is excessive, it will sometimes give the patient aversion to cold. This differs from the aversion to cold in febrile diseases caused by Cold. If it is mistaken as a case of Heat caused by Interior Humidity of the Greater Yang Channel and a purgative is prescribed, pathogenetic Humidity will turn into Cold and ascend to the chest, causing a sensation of fullness. When the pathogenetic factor invades the Middle Portion of Body Cavity, the Stomach function will be damaged, causing nausea. Or it may invade the Lower Portion of Body Cavity, hampering the normal functioning of the Vital Energy in the Urinary Bladder, resulting in dysuria. The thick white slippery coating on the tongue is a manifestation of descending pathogenetic Heat into the Elixir Field, which results from the malpractice of using purgatives. (05-469)

CLAUSE 2-17

The malpractice of prescribing purgatives for a patient who suffers from a Humidity disease will end in death when the following symptoms and signs are observed: Sweating on forehead, slight wheezing (1), incontinence of urination (2). Case will also be fatal when continuous diarrhea is observed.

NOTES

1. Sweat on forehead and slight wheezing indicate abnormal evanescence of Yang Vital Energy. (01-25)

2. Incontinence of urination indicates downward evasion of Yin Vital Essence. (01-25)

Zhao Liang: Malpractice of prescribing purgatives brings about an adverse case with upward evanescence of Yang Vital Energy and downward evanescence of Yin Vital Essence. Sweating on forehead and slight wheezing indicate evanescence of Yang; incontinence of urination and continuous diarrhea foretell the evanescence of Yin. Separation of Yin and Yang indicates a fatal case, leading to the following conclusion: With symptoms and signs of sweating on forehead and slight wheezing caused by incorrect adoption of purgatives, if there is no incontinence of urination or continuous diarrhea, Yin Vital Essence still continues to act as a substantial base of Yang Vital Energy. If, on the other hand, there are no symptoms and signs of sweating on the forehead and slight wheezing, but incontinence of urination and continuous diarrhea are present, Yin can still find its root in Yang. Neither case will be fatal, as Yin and Yang are not separated yet. Treatment can be determined according to specific cases. (05-470)

Li Weixi: Text (Clause 2-14) states diuretic can be prescribed for Humidity diseases. In that case, the pathogenetic Humidity stagnates in the Interior with dysuria, and diuretic is adopted to ease the urination. This case is one of Interior Deficiency and incontinence of urination. When Body Fluid is totally exhausted, case will be fatal. (05-470)

CLAUSE 2-18

When pathogenetic Wind and Humidity intermingle and struggle against each other, the patient will suffer from general aches. Correct therapy is to disperse pathogenetic factors through diaphoresis. On a raining day, the doctor says, "Diaphoresis will do." But after attempting diaphoresis, the syndrome does not subside. Why does this happen?

Master: This must be a case of diaphoresis inducing profuse perspiration. Profuse perspiration will dispel pathogenetic Wind, but not the Humidity, the syndrome remains. To disperse the Wind and Humidity simultaneously, only a light perspiration should be induced (1).

NOTES

1. As a general rule, pathogenetic Wind and Humidity will first invade the Exterior and skin, remaining in muscle and *Couli* (see Clause 1-2), flowing through joints and causing stagnation of the Vital Resistance (defensive energy, *Wei*). This results in general body aches. A diaphoretic will disperse pathogenetic factors at this time. When it is raining, the climatic Humidity factor is more intense, and diaphoretic is needed. However, physical characteristics of Wind and Humidity should be taken into consideration: Pathogenetic Wind is of a Yang nature and easily dispersed from the Exterior; pathogenetic Humidity, of a Yin nature, dull and sticky, is not easily dispersed. When profuse perspiration is induced, Wind evanesces immediately, leaving Humidity unchecked.

Syndrome is still present and Yang Vital Resistance is also hurt. Thus, correct therapy is to disperse both pathogenetic Wind and Humidity by inducing light perspiration. This is an effective treatment for Wind-Humidity syndrome.(02-16)

CLAUSE 2-19

Pathogenetic Cold-Humidity factors in the head will cause the following symptoms and signs in a patient suffering from Humidity disease: General aches, fever, sallow facial complexion, wheezing, headache with stuffy nose, restlessness, with huge pulse, normal appetite and harmony of abdomen (digestive tract is normal). Stuffy nose is caused by the pathogenetic Cold-Humidity in head. Drugs (1) can be taken through the nasal cavity to dispel the syndrome (2).

NOTES

1. No prescription is given in the original text.

2. Different annotators suggest the following prescriptions:

a) Powder of Pedicelus Melo (*Guadi San*) can be taken through the nasal cavity to release the pathogenetic Cold-Humidity;

b) Drugs with a pungent and fragrant odor can be used as olfactory agents;

c) Prescribe Powder of Flos Magnoliae (*Xinyi San*), a prescription from *Standards for Diagnosis and Treatments* (*Zheng Zhi Zhun Sheng*) by Wang Kentang:

Powder of Flos Magnoliae
(*Xinyi San*):

Flos Magnoliae
Herba Asari
Rhizoma Ligustici
Radix Angelicae Dahuricae
Rhizoma Ligustici Chuanxiong
Rhizoma Cimicifugae
Radix Ledebouriellae
Radix Glycyrrhizae
Caulis Akebiae
Fructus Xanthii

Remark: According to *The Pulse Classic*, the original text of this clause reads: "Pathogenetic Cold-Humidity factors resting in the head will cause the following symptoms and signs in a patient suffering from wheezing: Headache with stuffy nose, restlessness, with huge pulse, normal appetite and harmony of abdomen (digestive tract is normal). Stuffy nose is caused by pathogenetic Cold-Humidity in the head. Drugs can be taken through the nasal cavity to dispel the syndrome.'' (01-25)

CLAUSE 2-20

Decoction of Herba Ephedrae adding Rhizoma Atractylodis Macrocephalae can be adopted as a diaphoretic for a patient suffering from Humidity disease with general aching and restlessness. Prescribing such a diaphoretic is suitable. Fire therapy (1) should never be used in such cases.

NOTES

1. Fire therapy: therapies such as scorching (to induce perspiration by scorching the patient) or warming needles (acupuncture with needles warmed by burning moxa stick). (01-26)

Decoction of Herba Ephedrae adding Rhizoma Atractylodis Macrocephalae (*Mahuang Jia Zhu Tang*):

Herba Ephedrae	3 *liang*
Ramulus Cinnamomi	2 *liang*
Radix Glycyrrhizae Praeparata	2 *liang*
Semen Armeniacae Amarum	70 pcs.
Rhizoma Atractylodis Macrocephalae	4 *liang*

Stew Herba Ephedrae in nine *sheng* of water until seven *sheng* remain. Skim off foam and add other drugs. Stew until two and a half *sheng* remain. Filter the decoction. Serve eight-*ge* lukewarm decoction per dose and cover the patient to induce light perspiration.

Explanation of the Prescription: Zhao Liang: Intermingling of Cold and Humidity will make the patient feel a general aching. According to principle, diaphoresis can be adopted when there is a fever and Exterior Excess.* With no fever (as in this case), diagnosis is that Yang Vital Energy is in a deficient state. If diaphoresis is adopted, Exterior Deficiency** will result. Although "restlessness" is the only symptom mentioned in the clause, it can be inferred that "restlessness" arises from a fever. Diaphoresis is adopted to induce light perspiration, since Humidity cannot be dispersed by profuse perspiration.*** Thus Decoction of Herba Ephedrae is used to treat the Cold, and Rhizoma Atractylodis Macrocephalae is added to disperse Humidity. (05-468)

Yu Chang: When Herba Ephedrae is combined with Rhizoma Atractylodis Macrocephalae, it will only induce a light perspiration (function of inducing perspiration is restricted). When Herba Ephedrae is combined with Rhizoma Atractylodis Macrocephalae, it will reinforce the function of dispersing Humidity from both the Exterior and the Interior.

*Exterior Excess (*Biao Shi*): Excessiveness in the Exterior, an Exterior symptom complex in which the external part of the body is attacked by exogenous pathogenetic factors, yet the patient's vital function is undamaged; characteristic symptoms are headache, general aching, no sweating, floating and forceful (excessive) pulse, etc. (08-370)

**Exterior Deficiency (*Biao Xu*): Deficiency in the Exterior, an Exterior symptom complex marked by lowered superficial resistance. Symptoms are spontaneous sweating, sensitivity to wind and floating, moderate and feeble pulse, etc. (08-370)

***See Clause 2-18.

CASES

Case 1 (65-64):

Mr. Huang, in his thirties, was overweight and suffered from Humidity syndrome. When exposed to cold, he got sick and had been treated by several doctors. Finally the patient went to Doctor Zhao Shouzhen, who examined him and found he was having pain and soreness all over the body, difficultly moving his extremities, anorexia, tastelessness, reluctance to speak, moderate pulse on the right wrist and tense pulse on the left wrist, white and greasy tongue coating. This is a case of body pain caused by Humidity.

Prescription: Decoction of Herba Ephedrae adding Rhizoma Atractylodis Macrocephalae.

Herba Ephedrae	2.4 grams
Ramulus Cinnamomi	2.1 grams
Semen Armeniacae Amarum	4.5 grams
Radix Glycyrrhizae Praeparata	1.5 grams
Rhizoma Atractylodis	3 grams

After two doses of decoction, the syndrome was gone.

Case 2 (46-36):

Mr. Chen, 46, was caught in the rain after perspiring profusely. Being attacked by Humidity (rain) and Cold, he had fever and chill, with a severe headache; a feeling of heaviness all over the body without perspiration. Tongue coating was thin and white, with tight-tense pulse.

Diagnosis: Pathogenetic Cold resting at the Exterior and Humidity remained in the muscle.

Treatment: Disperse Exterior syndrome and pathogenetic Cold, induce perspiration to drive out the Humidity factor.

Prescription: Decoction of Herba Ephedrae adding Rhizoma Atractylodis Macrocephalae.

Herba Ephedrae	3 grams
Semen Armeniacae Amarum	9 grams
Ramulus Cinnamomi	10 grams
Radix Glycyrrhizae	3 grams
Rhizoma Atractylodis Macrocephalae	10 grams

After two doses of decoction, fever and chill, heaviness all over body and headache were gone. The patient still had no appetite and felt a general lassitude. Three doses of the following prescription were given to clear away the remaining trouble:

Radix Ginseng
Rhizoma Atractylodis Macrocephalae
Poria
Radix Glycyrrhizae
Pericarpium Citri Reticulatae
Rhizoma Zingiberis Recens
Fructus Ziziphi Jujubae

Case 3 (52-709): Dropsy on Legs

Ms. Hu, 54, farmer, first treatment on August 26, 1981. Four or five days prior to consultation with the doctor, she had a cold, followed by shortness of breath, chest pain and palpitation, heaviness and dropsy in legs and anorexia. Sleep was good. Constipation was reported. Menstruation had ceased for four years. Tongue proper was pink with tip red. Tongue coating seen only around the edges was greasy. Pulse was tight-slippery.

Diagnosis: Exterior syndrome had introduced pathogenetic Humidity among the muscle, which should be dispersed.

Prescription: Decoction of Herba Ephedrae adding Rhizoma Atractylodis

Macrocephalae.

Herba Ephedrae	6 grams
Ramulus Cinnamomi	10 grams
Semen Armeniacae Amarum	9 grams
Radix Glycyrrhizae	6 grams
Rhizoma Atractylodis Macrocephalae	30 grams

Eight doses were given. The patient reported subsidence of symptoms. Eight more doses of the prescription were given to guarantee full recovery.

CLAUSE 2-21

Symptoms of general aches and fever that become aggravated in the afternoon (1) indicate a Wind-Humidity disease caused by exposure to wind when the patient is sweating all over or by remaining in a cold spot for long periods on a hot day. Decoction of Herba Ephedrae, Semen Armeniacae Amarum, Semen Coicis and Radix Glycyrrhizae may be prescribed.

NOTES

1. In the afternoon: Original text is "*Ribusuo*," the period from 3 to 5 p.m. (01-26)

Decoction of Herba Ephedrae, Semen Armeniacae Amarum, Semen Coicis and Radix Glycyrrhizae (*Mahuang Xingren Yiyi Gancao Tang*):

Herba Ephedrae	0.5 *liang*
Radix Glycyrrhizae Praeparata	1 *liang*
Semen Coicis	0.5 *liang*
Semen Armeniacae Amarum	10 pcs.

Chop up the drugs. Allow four *qianbi* for each dose. Stew the drugs in one and a half cups of water until eight *fen* remain. Filter the decoction and serve warm to induce a light perspiration. Keep the patient away from wind.

Explanation of the Prescription: Herba Ephedrae and Semen Armeniacae Amarum ventilate and smooth the Lung to disperse pathogenetic Wind. Semen Coicis and Radix Glycyrrhizae tonify Spleen and Stomach to dispel pathogenetic Humidity. This prescription treats both the Exterior and the Interior syndrome, dispersing Wind and Humidity simultaneously. (01-27)

Commentary: Clauses 2-20 and 2-21 both deal with Humidity disease. Note the following comparisons:

	Clause 2-20	*Clause 2-21*
Syndrome:	General aching, high fever	General aching, low fever becomes aggravated in the afternoon
Pathology:	Exterior syndrome caused by Cold-Humidity	Exterior syndrome caused by Wind-Humidity
Therapy:	Disperse pathogenetic factors with warm and pungent ingredients	Disperse pathogenetic factors with cool and pungent ingredients

CASES

Case 1 (64-98):

Li, 11, first treatment on November 14, 1978. The boy was caught in the rain ten days ago and had been suffering from a cold, with pain over lower extremities that made him difficult to walk.

Examination: Pulse was floating-tense, slightly speedy; with tongue coating thin, white and greasy, and red tongue proper. Temperature in the afternoon was 38°C. Rosy cheeks, slight dropsy over both knees with local hot feeling.

Diagnosis: Pathogenetic Wind-Humidity was invading the joints causing obstruction of normal physiological function.

Treatment: Disperse Wind and Humidity, activate blood circulation to facilitate normal supply to the collaterals.

Prescription: Decoction of Herba Ephedrae, Semen Armeniacae Amarum, Semen Coicis and Radix Glycyrrhizae.

Herba Ephedrae	10 grams
Semen Armeniacae Amarum	10 grams
Semen Coicis	20 grams

Fructus Chaenomelis	10 grams
Radix Achyranthis Bidentatae	10 grams
Caulis Spatholobi	20 grams
Radix Glycyrrhizae	3 grams

Second treatment on November 10: After six doses of the decoction, pain reduced. All other symptoms were subsiding. He began to walk normally, but the syndrome was not completely gone. The patient was instructed to continue the medicament.

Third treatment on November 16: Five doses were given. Syndrome was almost gone. Treatment continues for consolidation, pills (*Jin Ji Hu Wan**) were given for thirty days. Dosage: Ten pills per dose, three times a day. One month later, syndrome was gone.

**Jin Ji Hu Wan*: Rhizoma Cibotii, Fructus Rosae Laevigatae, Caulis Spatholobi, Radix Kadsurae Coccineae.

Case 2 (48-89):

Mr. Zhang, 24, farmer. In early summer when it was cold, cloudy and raining, he worked in the fields. After perspiring, he was caught in the wind and rain. Urticaria appeared over the body, the upper extremities being worst. There was a slight fever, with aversion to wind. Pulse was floating, tongue coating was thin and white. Benadryl had been used, but did not seem to help.

Diagnosis: This syndrome was caused by the invasion of pathogenetic Wind and Humidity resting at the Exterior and muscle. While movement of the Yang Vital Energy was obstructed, Nutrient Essence was put into disorder. Urticaria was a reflection of the pathological change.

Treatment: Induce perspiration and disperse the Wind-Humidity.

Prescription: Decoction of Herba Ephedrae, Semen Armeniacae Amarum, Semen Coicis and Radix Glycyrrhizae with additions:

Herba Ephedrae	5 grams
Semen Coicis	9 grams
Radix Glycyrrhizae	3 grams
Periostracum Cicadae	9 grams
Bombyx Batryticatus	9 grams

Three doses of the above decoction cured the patient.

CLAUSE 2-22

Decoction of Radix Stephaniae Tetrandrae and Radix Astragali Hedysari may be prescribed for Wind-Humidity disease with floating pulse, heaviness in movement, perspiration and sensitivity to wind.

Decoction of Radix Stephaniae Tetrandrae and
Radix Astragali Hedysari*
(*Fangji Huangqi Tang*):

Radix Stephaniae Tetrandrae	1 *liang*
Radix Astragali Hedysari	1 *liang* 1 *fen*
Radix Glycyrrhizae Praeparata	0.5 *liang*
Rhizoma Atractylodis Macrocephalae	7.5 *qian*

Chop up the drugs. Five *qianbi* per dose. Stew in one and a half cups water with four pieces of Rhizoma Zingiberis Recens and one piece of Fructus Ziziphi Jujubae until eight *fen* remain. Filter the decoction and serve warm. A second dose can be served after a long interval.

*Dosage in this prescription is not identical possibly due to copying mistakes. According to *Prescriptions Worth a Thousand Gold (Qianjin Yaofang*, hereinafter *Qianjin*) by Sun Simiao, following prescription should be taken as the original prescription:

Radix Stephaniae Tetrandrae	4 *liang*
Radix Glycyrrhizae	2 *liang*
Radix Astragali Hedysari	5 *liang*
Rhizoma Zingiberis Recens	3 *liang*
Rhizoma Atractylodis Macrocephalae	3 *liang*
Fructus Ziziphi Jujubae	12 pcs.

Additions and Subtractions:

1) If the symptoms include wheezing, add one half *liang* Herba Ephedrae;

2) For discomfort in the Stomach, add three *fen* Radix Paeoniae;

3) For feeling of abnormal gas ascending, add three *fen* Ramulus Cinnamomi;

4) For chronic Cold syndrome in the Lower Portion of Body Cavity, add three *fen* Herba Asari.

After taking the decoction, the patient should feel "worms-crawling under the skin" and icy cold at lower lumbar region. Have the patient sit on quilt and wrap another quilt around his waist to induce a sweat. Light sweat signifies the patient is recovering.

Explanation of the Prescription: You Yi: When pathogenetic Wind-Humidity is at the Exterior, correct therapy is to disperse syndrome by perspiration. But in this case, the patient perspires before diaphoretic is given. This indicates Exterior Deficiency, rendering diaphoresis inapplicable. In this prescription, Herba Ephedrae is not used to disperse syndrome from the skin, but Radix Stephaniae Tetrandrae is used to dispel pathogenetic factors from the muscle. After taking the decoction, the patient feels "worms-crawling under the skin" and icy cold at lower lumbar region, indicating the down-flowing of pathogenetic Humidity. Radix Astragali Hedysari, Rhizoma Atractylodis Macrocephalae and Radix Glycyrrhizae are used to reinforce Yang Vital Energy and are active in dispersing the pathogenetic Humidity. (05-471)

CASES

Case 1 (65-67):

Ms. He, 27, was suffering from chronic rheumatic arthritis with difficulty in moving the body, plenty of sweat, lassitude over the extremities. Pain in the upper limbs was more severe than in lower limbs, both were more painful when it was cloudy and rainy. Pulse was soft, floating and strengthless, and tongue was pale with white coating.

Diagnosis: Syndrome was caused by the encroachment of pathogenetic Wind and Humidity at the Exterior with weak Body Resistance. Normal circulation in the Channels and Collaterals was obstructed, resulting in pain.

Prescription: Decoction of Radix Stephaniae Tetrandrae and Radix Astragali Hedysari with additions:

Radix Stephaniae Tetrandrae	10 grams
Radix Astragali Hedysari	12 grams
Radix Glycyrrhizae	4 grams
Rhizoma Atractylodis	10 grams
Rhizoma Zingiberis Recens	3 slices
Fructus Ziziphi Jujubae	3 pcs.
Ramulus Cinnamomi	6 grams
Radix Clematidis	3 grams

Ten doses were given. Pain subsided greatly, heaviness and frequent sweat disappeared. Another five doses were given to completely cure the ailment.

Case 2 (64-100):

Mr. Tian, 50, had been suffering from pain in both legs for six months, which was more severe on cloudy and rainy days. His legs felt heavy and numb and the lower legs were puffy. When the syndrome was worst, he had difficulty walking. Other symptoms included: scanty urination, pale tongue with white and greasy coating, deficient, huge and speedy pulse. Several treatments of Chinese medicine and prednisone had not helped.

Prescription: Decoction of Radix Stephaniae Tetrandrae and Radix Astragali Hedysari with additions:

Radix Stephaniae Tetrandrae
Radix Astragali Hedysari
Radix Glycyrrhizae Praeparata
Rhizoma Atractylodis Macrocephalae
Poria
Semen Coicis
Ramulus Cinnamomi

Four doses were prescribed. Symptoms subsided after decoctions were used. Puffiness reduced significantly. Urination returned to normal. After another four doses, the syndrome was gone.

Case 3 (49-307):

Mr. Li, 40, suffered from rheumatic pain for two years. Pain and soreness in the extremities and joints were aggravated on cloudy and rainy days. In recent week, the patient had a cold and was treated with drugs to reduce fever. Pain over joints became worse. Other symptoms were: spontaneous perspiration, aversion to wind, shortness of breath, floating and hesitant pulse and white-greasy tongue coating.

Diagnosis: Syndrome was caused by the invasion of Cold-Humidity factor causing the obstruction of normal circulation when Body Resistance was in a deficient state.

Treatment: Decoction of Radix Stephaniae Tetrandrae and Radix Astragali Hedysari was given to reinforce the Vital Energy, stabilize the Exterior defense and remove the Humidity. The decoction worked as expected.

Case 4 (46-39):

Wang, 25, female, suffered from rheumatic pain for more than a month, with swollen, aching knees and elbows. After treatment with penicillin, Vitamin B_1 and aspirin, the pain was reduced, but there was profuse perspiration, a feeling of heaviness, aversion to cold, white-slippery tongue coating, and floatingulse.

Diagnosis: This syndrome was caused by profuse perspiration that had driven out the pathogenetic Wind but failed to disperse the pathogenetic Humidity when Body Resistance was deficient.

Treatment: Enhance the Body Resistance and stabilize the Exterior defense, disperse the Humidity to facilitate normal circulation.

Prescription: Decoction of Radix Stephaniae Tetrandrae and Radix Astragali Hedysari:

Radix Stephaniae Tetrandrae	12 grams
Rhizoma Atractylodis Macrocephalae	10 grams
Radix Astragali Hedysari	15 grams
Radix Glycyrrhizae	3 grams
Rhizoma Zingiberis Recens	3 slices
Fructus Ziziphi Jujubae	1 pc.
Radix Ledebouriellae	10 grams
Ramulus Cinnamomi	6 grams
Radix Paeoniae Alba (prepared with wine)	10 grams

Five doses cured the ailment.

CLAUSE 2-23*

Febrile disease caused by Cold, eight to nine days: When Wind and Humidity factors conflict (1), the patient will suffer acute body pain, and moving around will be difficult. If the patient is not nauseous or thirsty and has floating-deficient and hesitant pulse, Decoction of Ramulus Cinnamomi and Radix Aconiti Praeparata can be a curative.

If there is constipation and normal urination, Decoction subtracting Ramulus Cinnamomi adding Rhizoma Atractylodis Macrocephalae can be given.

*This clause also appears in Clause 174 of *Shanghan Lun*.

NOTES

1. Wind and Humidity are both pathogenetic factors. When they invade the muscles, tendons or bones, the Body Resistance conflicts with them. This will bring about a series of symptoms described in the clause. (04-110)

Cheng Lin: Pathogenetic Wind causes acute body pain, Humidity makes it difficult for the patient to move around. As Wind and Humidity conflict between *Ying* (Nutrient Essence) and *Wei* (Body Resistance) with no relation to to the Interior, there is no nausea or thirst. Floating pulse indicates Wind while hesitant pulse indicates Humidity. As pulse is close to deficient type, Decoction of Ramulus Cinnamomi and Radix Aconiti Praeparata may be given to warm the Channels and Collaterals and disperse Wind-Humidity. When there is constipation and normal urination, Ramulus Cinnamomi is inappropriate as it may cause perspiration (perspiration will further exhaust the Body Fluid and thus worsen constipation). Rhizoma Atractylodis Macrocephalae is added to eliminate Humidity from the muscle. (05-473)

Decoction of Ramulus Cinnamomi and Radix Aconiti Praeparata (*Guizhi Fuzi Tang*):

Ramulus Cinnamomi	4 *liang*
Radix Aconiti Praeparata	3 pcs.
Radix Glycyrrhizae Praeparata	2 *liang*
Rhizoma Zingiberis Recens	3 *liang*
Fructus Ziziphi Jujubae	12 pcs.

Stew the drugs in six *sheng* of water until two *sheng* remain. Filter the decoction and serve in three doses.

Decoction of Rhizoma Atractylodis Macrocephalae and Radix Aconiti Praeparata*
(*Baizhu Fuzi Tang*):

Rhizoma Atractylodis Macrocephalae	2 *liang*
Radix Aconiti Praeparata	1.5 pcs.
Radix Glycyrrhizae Praeparata	1 *liang*
Rhizoma Zingiberis Recens	1 *liang*
Fructus Ziziphi Jujubae	6 pcs.

Stew the drugs in three *sheng* of water until one *sheng* remains. Filter the decoction and serve in three doses. After taking first dose, the patient will have a sensation of numbness. After half a day, give the second dose. After taking three doses, the patient will feel dizzy; this is a normal reaction. When Radix Aconiti Praeparata and Rhizoma Atractylodis Macrocephalae move under skin to disperse Water-Humidity, dizziness occurs before pathogenetic factors are dispersed.

*This decoction is listed as Decoction subtracting Ramulus Cinnamomi adding Rhizoma Atractylodis Macrocephalae in *Shanghan Lun*.

Explanation of the Prescriptions: The two decoctions above cure the syndrome caused by Wind-Humidity. The first decoction is Decoction of Ramulus Cinnamomi subtracting Radix Paeoniae and adding Radix Aconiti Praeparata, and aims at dispersing Wind and Humidity. Ramulus Cinnamomi and Radix Glycyrrhizae, pungent and sweet, disperse the Wind from the Exterior. Radix Aconiti Praeparata, pungent and hot, disperses the Humidity in the Channels and Collaterals and eases pain. Rhizoma Zingiberis Recens and Fructus Ziziphi Jujubae harmonize the *Ying* and *Wei*.

The second decoction is Decoction of Ramulus Cinnamomi and Radix Aconiti Praeparata adding Rhizoma Atractylodis Macrocephalae; it aims at tonifying the Stomach to eliminate Humidity. Radix Aconiti Praeparata, pungent and hot, warms the Channels and Collaterals. Rhizoma Atractylodis Macrocephalae, sweet and warm, tonifies the Spleen. When Radix Aconiti Praeparata and Rhizoma Atractylodis Macrocephalae are used in the same prescription, they are highly effective in curing syndrome caused by Wind and Humidity. Radix Glycyrrhizae, Rhizoma Zingiberis Recens and Fructus Ziziphi Jujubae, pungent and sweet, aid in dispersing and easing the syndrome. (04-110)

CLAUSE 2-24*

Conflicting Wind and Humidity factors cause acute pain in joints which impairs movement of joints due to serious referred pain. The pain is aggravated if pressure is applied. The patient is short of breath, perspires, avoids wind, is reluctant to remove clothing, suffers from dysuria and a slight swelling of the body. Decoction of Radix Glycyrrhizae and Radix Aconiti Praeparata can be prescribed.

*This clause also appears in *Shanghan Lun*, Clause 175.

Decoction of Radix Glycyrrhizae and Radix Aconiti Praeparata (*Gancao Fuzi Tang*):

Radix Glycyrrhizae Praeparata 2 *liang*

Radix Aconiti Praeparata	2 pcs.
Rhizoma Atractylodis Macrocephalae	2 *liang*
Ramulus Cinnamomi	4 *liang*

Stew the above drugs in six *sheng* of water until three *sheng* remain. Filter the decoction and give three doses per day of one *sheng* each. After the first dose, there will be a slight perspiration and syndrome will disappear. The patient has a good appetite. When perspiration stops, the patient will feel restless again. Give another five *ge* of the decoction. If one *sheng* appears to be too much for initial dose, reduce to six to seven *ge*.

Explanation of the Prescription: In this decoction, Radix Atractylodis Macrocephalae and Radix Aconiti Praeparata are used to warm the Channels and Collaterals and dispel Humidity. Ramulus Cinnamomi, pungent and warm, when used combined with Radix Aconiti Praeparata and Rhizoma Atractylodis Macrocephalae, has the function of warming the Interior Yang Vital Energy and dispersing the Wind. As pathogenetic factors have penetrated deep into the joints, Wind should be dispersed gradually. Otherwise, Wind will be dispersed but Humidity will remain as a sequela. Thus Radix Glycyrrhizae is used to retard action of the decoction. (04-111)

CLAUSE 2-25

Initial Yang syndrome caused by *Ye* (heatstroke): the patient has both fever and aversion to cold, heaviness of movement and general aching, with pulse tight, slender, void and slow. After passing urine, the patient feels cold as if his hair were standing on end. He also feels cold in the extremities. If he does any work, fever will be aggravated. When he opens his mouth (1), his front teeth appear parched. When sweating is induced, aversion to cold will be aggravated. If warming needles are given, fever will intensify. If purgatives are adopted repeatedly, serious strangury will result.

NOTES

1. When he opens his mouth: The patient is suffering from interior Humidity-

Heat and an unpleasant feeling that causes tachypnea, he will open his mouth. (02-21)

Commentary: No therapy is given in this clause. Later scholars gave prescriptions for treating such diseases. Li Gao and Wang Mengying both prescribed Decoction of *Qingshu Yiqi* as follows:

Li Gao in his *Treatise on Spleen and Stomach (Pi Wei Lun)* recorded Decoction of *Qingshu Yiqi* with the following ingredients:

Radix Astragali
Rhizoma Atractylodis
Rhizoma Cimicifugae
Radix Ginseng
Rhizoma Atractylodis Macrocephalae
Pericarpium Citri Reticulatae
Medicated Leaven
Rhizoma Alismatis
Radix Ophiopogonis
Radix Angelicae Sinensis
Radix Glycyrrhizae Praeparata
Cortex Phellodendri
Radix Puerariae
Pericarpium Citri Reticulatae Viride
Fructus Schisandrae

Wang Mengying in his *Compendium of Seasonal Febrile Diseases (Wen Re Jing Wei)* recorded the prescription with the following ingredients:

Radix Panacis Quinquefolii
Exocarpium Citrulli
Petiolus Nelumbinis
Rhizoma Coptidis
Herba Dendrobii
Radix Ophiopogonis
Folium Bambusae (or Herba Lophatheri)
Rhizoma Anemarrhenae
Radix Glycyrrhizae
Semen Oryzae Nonglutinosae

CASES

Case 1 (65-77): Syndrome Caused by Summer-heat Complicated by Humidity

Duan, 20, female, first treatment on July 10, 1970. The patient had suffered for five days when she consulted the doctor on this hot summer day.

Examination: She had the feeling that her head was wrapped with something, chest and epigastric fullness and distention, anorexia, heaviness and lassitude, aversion to cold, with sporadic perspiration. She had a dry mouth but could drink only a little water, and parched, red lips. Urine was scanty, yellowish and turbid. Stool was not smooth. Pulse was slender and speedy. Tongue was red, with tongue proper swollen, covered with greasy coating. Diaphoretics, sulfanilamide, antibiotics and Powder of Flos Lonicerae and Fructus Forsythiae (*Yin Qiao San*) had been used, but did not help.

Diagnosis: The syndrome occurred in hot summer when it was also raining. It was caused by invasion of Summer-heat and Humidity.

Treatment: Summer-heat and Humidity should be dispersed simultaneously. A combination of Decoction of *Baihu* and Powder of *Liu Yi* (*Baihu Tang* and *Liu Yi San*) was prescribed as follows:

Rhizoma Anemarrhenae	10 grams
Gypsum Fibrosum	24 grams
Radix Glycyrrhizae Praeparata	6 grams
Talcum	15 grams
Herba Eupatorii	12 grams
Herba Agastachis	9 grams
Flos Lonicerae	18 grams
Flos Chrysanthemi	9 grams

Only one dose of the above decoction alleviated the ailment.

CLAUSE 2-26

Initial Yang syndrome caused by heatstroke is a case of *Ye*. Decoction of *Baihu* adding Radix Ginseng can be adopted when the following symptoms and signs are observed: perspiration, aversion to cold (1), fever and thirst.

NOTES

1. Aversion to cold is not caused by either the Exterior syndrome of the Initial Yang Channel or by the Interior Deficiency of the Yang Vital Energy. It is due to the dispersal of the excessive Interior Heat that has penetrated the *Couli* on the skin. (01-30)

Decoction of *Baihu* adding Radix Ginseng*
(*Baihu Jia Renshen Tang*):

Rhizoma Anemarrhenae	6 *liang*
Gypsum Fibrosum	1 *jin***
Radix Glycyrrhizae	2 *liang*
Semen Oryzae Nonglutinosae	6 *ge*
Radix Ginseng	3 *liang*

Stew the drugs in one *dou* of water until Semen Oryzae Nonglutinosae is thoroughly cooked. Filter the decoction and serve one *sheng* of lukewarm decoction per dose three times per day.

*This prescription also appears in *Shanghan Lun*, Clause 26.
**The following ancient system may be taken as a reference:

Weight	*Volume*
1 *jin* = 16 *liang*	1 *hu* = 10 *dou*
1 *liang* = 4 *fen*	1 *dou* = 10 *sheng*
1 *fen* = 6 *zhu*	1 *sheng* = 10 *ge*

CLAUSE 2-27

Initial Yang syndrome caused by *Ye* (heatstroke) has the following symptoms and signs when caused by exposure to cold water in summer: fever, general aching and heaviness, with feeble and weak pulse. Such symptoms are caused by the circulation of pathogenetic Water under the skin. Decoction of Pedicellus Melo can be prescribed.

Decoction of Pedicellus Melo
(*Yi Wu Guadi Tang*):

Pedicellus Melo	20 pcs.

Stew the drug in one *sheng* of water until five *ge* remain. Filter the decoction and take all at once.

CHAPTER III

ON PULSE, SYMPTOM COMPLEX AND TREATMENT OF BULBUS LILII SYNDROME,* *HUHUO* SYNDROME** AND *YINYANGDU* SYNDROME***

CLAUSE 3-1

Classic states: The hundred Channels originate from one root (1). Any one of them may cause a Bulbus Lilii syndrome. Symptoms and signs of the syndrome may include: The patient wants to eat, but is reluctant to swallow food and unwilling to speak. Or he prefers to lie in bed, yet cannot lie quietly due to restlessness. He may want to walk about, but soon becomes tired. Now and then he may enjoy eating certain delicacies, but at other times he cannot even tolerate the smell of food. He may feel either cold or hot, but without fever or chill. He also has a bitter taste in his mouth and passes reddish urine. No drugs appear able to cure the syndrome. After taking medicine, acute vomiting and diarrhea may occur. The disease "haunts" the patient, and though his appearance is normal, he is actually suffering. His pulse is somewhat speedy. If the patient has a headache while he is passing urine, he may recover within sixty days. If he has no headache but feels chills when passing urine, he is likely to recover within forty days. If he feels comfortable after urination but has a slight sensation of vertigo, he can recover within twenty days. Symptoms and signs of the Bulbus

*Bulbus Lilii syndrome (*Baihe bing*): Psychic depression. Bulbus Lilii syndrome is named after its curative which has Bulbus Lilii as its main ingredient. This syndrome may occur after febrile diseases or periods of mental depression. Its symptoms and signs generally include mental distress and confusion, abnormal eating and irregular movements. (02-24)

***Huhuo* syndrome: Syndrome characterized by ulceration of throat, anus and external genitals.

*** *Yinyangdu* syndrome: An acute disease with symptoms of skin rash and pharyngalgia.

Lilii syndrome may appear before the onset of the disease, or from four or five to twenty days or a month after the onset. Treatment should be given according to the specific case (2).

NOTES

1. *Wu Qian*: The hundred Channels originate from one root: This includes the whole body. Channels can be considered as a single entity or as one hundred Channels. The text states that Bulbus Lilii syndrome is caused by the Channels, which include twelve Channels and three hundred and sixty-five Collaterals. After febrile disease caused by Cold subsides, pathogenetic Heat remains in the body, affecting the normal functioning of the hundred Channels. When the patient suffers from emotional distress or depression, he is subject to Bulbus Lilii syndrome, affecting both the mind and body. (05-478)

2. Bulbus Lilii syndrome is caused by Interior Heat of the Heart, and the Lung in Yin and deficient nature. Therapy replenishes Yin and removes endogenous pathogenetic Heat. Diaphoretics, emetics and purgatives are all prohibited, as these will further consume the Yin Vital Essence and Body Fluid. (02-24)

CLAUSE 3-2

When Bulbus Lilii syndrome occurs after the adoption of diaphoretic, Decoction of Bulbus Lilii and Rhizoma Anemarrhenae can be used as a curative.

Decoction of Bulbus Lilii and Rhizoma Anemarrhenae
(*Baihe Zhimu Tang*):

Bulbus Lilii (break open)	7 pcs.
Rhizoma Anemarrhenae	3 *liang*

Wash Bulbus Lilii and soak in water overnight. When white foam appears, remove drug and place in two *sheng* of spring water. Stew until one *sheng* remains. Filter the decoction. Stew Rhizoma Anemarrhenae separately in two *sheng* of spring water until one *sheng* remains. Filter the decoction. Combine decoctions and stew until one and a half *sheng* remain. Serve lukewarm decoction in two doses.

CASES

Case 1 (65-86): Bulbus Lilii Syndrome, Case Reported in Journal of *Fujian Chinese Medicine and Pharmacology*, 10:44, 1958

Mr. Lin, in his twenties. At the end of summer, the patient suffered from a febrile disease similar to typhoid fever. He was attended by his family for about a month and feeling better although he had not cousulted a doctor. He always felt thirsty, had reddish urine and poor appetite. One day, he suddenly wept profusely, followed by insanity, delirium, and excessive anger. At times he sang with a beautiful voice, at other times he sat quietly, as if he was an idiot. Often he would tear his clothing. These attacks were frequent. After ten days of attacks, he had constipation and unconsciousness. Pulse was speedy-deficient. Tongue was red and parched.

Diagnosis: Bulbus Lilii syndrome.

Prescription:

Bulbus Lilii	18 grams
Rhizoma Anemarrhenae	9 grams
Radix Rehmanniae	24 grams
Radix Ophiopogonis	24 grams
Radix Scrophulariae	18 grams
Talcum	18 grams
Folium Bambusae	9 grams
Concha Ostreae	15 grams
Radix Trichosanthis	15 grams
Concha Haliotidis	12 grams
Rhizoma Polyganati Odorati	9 grams

Stew the above decoction to get two decoctions and mix them for use in three servings. Serve every four hours, finish one dose within twenty-four hours. Another decoction was made to quench thirst: Stew of equal doses of Rhizoma Phragimitis (fresh), Semen Coicis, Radix Trichosanthis and crystal sugar was given for three consecutive days.

Second treatment on the fourth day: All symptoms were gone except for a slight cough and constipation. Still no appetite. The following prescription (*Yi Wei Tang* with additions) was given:

Bulbus Lilii	9 grams
Radix Glehniae	9 grams
Radix Ophiopogonis	15 grams
Radix Rehmanniae	15 grams
Rhizoma Polygonati Odorati	9 grams
Herba Dendrobii	9 grams

When the decoction is ready to serve, add 30 grams of honey, serve in two servings. After taking the decoction, pieces of hard feces were defecated three times in the same day. The syndrome was completely gone.

Case 2 (64-123): Case Recorded in Journal of *Jiangxi Chinese and Western Medicine*, 12:14, 1960

Wang, female, 13, a student, was frightened while watching an autopsy operation. On her way to the restroom, she fainted and fell, and was sent to a hospital. The examination did not show anything wrong, but her neck could not support her head in an upright position and the head turned involuntarily. She could not speak. Sedatives had been used to no avail. The patient turned to a doctor of Chinese medicine.

Dagnosis: Pulse was floating-speedy, there was no tongue coating. No other diseases were reported. Bulbus Lilii syndrome was suspected.

Prescription:

Bulbus Lilii	7 pcs.
Rhizoma Anemarrhenae	4.5 grams

After taking one dose of the above decoction, the patient's neck could support the head and the head did not turn as frequent. She had a sense of pain and still could not speak.

Second treatment: Another dose of the same decoction was given. After she could keep her head upright and the head remained steady. She began to ask for water and drank.

Third treatment: The following prescription was given:

Fructus Trichosanthis	9 grams
Concha Ostreae	9 grams

She recovered after this.

Case 3 (52-509):

Male patient, 19, first treatment on February 11, 1965. The patient felt a foreign object in his throat one week after he returned from traveling. He tried to swallow or bring it out, but there was actually nothing there. The patient had anorexia, insomnia and experienced pain while urinating. He also had headache, tastelessness, stuffy feeling in ears and dim vision. He lost response to outside stimulus. Urine was brown, tongue free from coating, tip red. Pulse was tight and slippery. Routine urine exam did not show anything wrong. Drugs to clear Interior Heat were given, but did not relieve the symptoms.

Diagnosis: This was a syndrome with ascent of deficient fire. The overall fire was deficient, throat was not moistened, so feeling of a foreign object occurred. Other symptoms came from this pathological condition.

Treatment: To nourish the Yin and bring down the pathogenetic fire by prescribing Decoction of Bulbus Lilii combining Decoction of Semen Ziziphi Spinosae as follows:

Bulbus Lilii	30 grams
Rhizoma Anemarrhenae	10 grams
Radix Rehmanniae	30 grams
Talcum	18 grams
Rhizoma Ligustici Chuanxiong	4.5 grams
Poria cum Ligno Hospite (prepared with Cinnabaris)	10 grams
Rhizoma Acori Graminei	9 grams
Semen Ziziphi Spinosae Praeparata	18 grams

Three doses were given, one dose served per day. Syndrome subsided. Another three doses were given, one every other day. Full recovery resulted. On August 30 the next year, when the doctor visited the patient, no recurrence was reported.

CLAUSE 3-3

When Bulbus Lilii syndrome occurs after giving purgative, Decoction of Talcum and Ochra Haematitum can be used.

Decoction of Talcum and Ochra Haematitum
(*Huashi Daizhe Tang*):

Bulbus Lilii (break open)	7 pcs.
Talcum (break open, wrap in silk)	3 *liang*
Ochra Haematitum (size of a bullet*)	1 pc.

Wash Bulbus Lilii and soak in water overnight. When white foam appears, remove drug and place in two *sheng* of spring water. Stew until one *sheng* remains. Filter the decoction. Stew Talcum and Ochra Haematitum in two *sheng* of spring water until one *sheng* remains. Filter the decoction. Combine two decoctions and stew until one and a half *sheng* remain. Serve the decoction warm.

*Size of an egg yolk.

CASES

Case 1 (65-87) Bulbus Lilii Syndrome, Case Recorded in Journal of *Fujian Chinese Medicine and Pharmacology*, 10:43, 1958

Lin, female, in her thirties, contracted febrile disease in hot summer and was treated by a doctor of Western medicine. After recovering from the ailment, she began to feel lassitude and depression. A few days later, she got very excited, became over-sensitive and skeptical.

Examination: The patient had thirst, scanty urine in reddish color, constipation, headache, palpitation and irritation, dim vision, preference to quiet environment, anorexia, insanity that made her talk, weep and laugh. Body temperature was 37.3 ℃. Pulse was speedy and soft, with parched lips, red tongue and parched feeling in mouth. She was in bed with depressed mentality and malnourished.

Diagnosis: Bulbus Lilii syndrome, treated by adoption of decoction based on Decoction of Talcum and Ochra Haematitum.

Prescription:

Bulbus Lilii	15 grams
Talcum	18 grams
Radix Rehmanniae	24 grams
Radix Polygonati	9 grams
Radix Ophiopogonis	15 grams
Concha Haliotidis	9 grams
Semen Coicis	15 grams

Stew the above drugs to make two decoctions. Mix them and serve in three equal doses. Serve every three hours and finish three doses within twenty-four hours. Another decoction was given repeatedly, made of Semen Coicis, Rhizoma Phragmitis and Radix Trichosanthis. After the patient finished the first serving, vomiting was induced. Medication continued when she felt thirsty. No more vomiting occurred.

Second treatment: The next day when the patient consulted the doctor, she looked better and reported a significant improvement. In the second prescription, dosage was reduced with the following alterations:

Subtract: Talcum, Radix Rehmanniae and Concha Haliotidis.

Add: Fructus Oryzae Germinatus and Rhizoma Dioscoreae.

One dose was served per day, for three consecutive days. The patient was able to walk by herself. Nourishing food like milk and Powder of Bulbus Lilii were given for a full recovery.

CLAUSE 3-4

The following prescription is suitable for Bulbus Lilii syndrome which appears after emetics are given.

Decoction of Bulbus Lilii and Egg Yolk
(*Baihe Jizi Tang*):

Bulbus Lilii (break open)	7 pcs.
Egg yolk	1 pc.

Wash Bulbus Lilii, soak in water overnight. When white foam appears, remove the drug and place in two *sheng* of spring water. Stew until one *sheng* remains. Filter the decoction. Add egg yolk to the decoction and stir until blended in. Stew the decoction again until five *fen* remain. Serve the decoction warm.

Commentary: The three prescriptions above are curatives for cases resulting from incorrect treatment of Bulbus Lilii syndrome. After prescribing diaphoretic for Bulbus Lilii syndrome which has exhausted Body Fluid and caused pathogenetic Dryness, Decoction of Bulbus Lilii and Rhizoma Anemarrhenae can be used. After giving purgative for Bulbus Lilii syndrome which has caused diarrhea, Decoction of Talcum and Ochra Haemetitum can be used to stop the diarrhea. Decoction of Bulbus Lilii and Egg Yolk cures the syndrome of Interior Deficiency after emetic is wrongly used to treat Bulbus Lilii syndrome.

CASES

Case 1 (51-84): Case Recorded in Journal of *New Medicine and Pharmacology*, 2:13, 1974

Mr. Wang, 44, suffered from cirrhosis complicated with Cruveilhier-Baumgarten syndrome after contracting hepatitis. When ascitic fluid occurred for the second time, it remained for nine months. The patient was hospitalized on September 4, 1970. After a combination treatment, ascitic fluid disappeared. On January 21, 1971, the patient began to talk loudly and laugh profusely and later developed insanity. Both Chinese and Western medicines were given, but did not seem to help.

Diagnosis: Insanity, which was aggravated in the afternoon, red tongue and deficient pulse. This was a Bulbus Lilii syndrome.

Prescription (Feb. 1):

Bulbus Lilii	30 grams
Egg yolk	1 pc.

One dose was served each day.

On February 2, the patient felt better. The next day he returned to normal. Another two doses of Decoction of Bulbus Lilii and Egg Yolk were served.

Second treatment: Decoction of Bulbus Lilii and Radix Rehmanniae was prescribed:

Bulbus Lilii	30 grams
Radix Rehmanniae	15 grams

The patient was in stable condition, on March 21, 1971, when he left the hospital. In June 1972, he was still in good health.

CLAUSE 3-5

If no emetic, purgative or diaphoretic has been prescribed for Bulbus Lilii syndrome, yet symptoms and signs of Bulbus Lilii syndrome are still present, Decoction of Bulbus Lilii and Radix Rehmanniae will be effective in curing the case.

Decoction of Bulbus Lilii and Radix Rehmanniae
(*Baihe Dihuang Tang*):

Bulbus Lilii (break open)	7 pcs.
Juice of Radix Rehmanniae	1 *sheng*

Wash Bulbus Lilii, soak in water overnight. When white foam appears, remove the drug and place in two *sheng* of spring water. Stew until one *sheng* remains. Filter the decoction and add juice of Radix Rehmanniae. Stew the decoction again until one and a half *sheng* remain. Serve the warm decoction in two doses. When cure is effected, stop taking the medicine. Feces will be black as lacquer.* (01-35)

Explanation of the Prescription: Bulbus Lilii and spring water, combined with juice of Radix Rehmanniae, nourish the Blood and the Yin, eliminate pathogenetic Heat. (01-36)

Commentary: This prescription is effective for cases when pathogenetic Heat remains after certain infectious diseases subside. According to clinical observation, it is an effective treatment for neuroses caused by Interior pathogenetic Heat in deficient and Yin nature of the Heart and the Lung. The text states, "When the cure is effected, stop taking the medicine." This is because juice of Radix Rehmanniae, which is of Cold nature, is taken in quantity and may cause diarrhea. When the medicine is effective, the remainder need not be taken. (02-25)

*Due to juice of Radix Rehmanniae.

CASES

Case 1 (65-90): Prolonged Bulbus Lilii Syndrome

Xu, 42, female, first treatment on May 10, 1974.

Symptoms: The patient was suffering from vertigo, amnesia, trance, preference to quiet environment. Appetite was variable. When she was walking, she might collapse, legs unable to support her. One or two hours later, she would return to normal. There was slight fever and chill. Repeated treatments and frequent doctor visits had made her lose confidence, as the syndrome was no better. She had not worked for eleven years.

Diagnosis: Pulse was slender-speedy and weak when pressed hard. Tongue was pale pink with thin and white coating, complexion pale. It was a Bulbus Lilii syndrome.

Prescription: Decoction of Bulbus Lilii and Radix Rehmanniae with additions. Six doses were given.

Bulbus Lilii	18 grams
Radix Rehmanniae	15 grams
Poria	12 grams
Radix Ophiopogonis	9 grams
Radix Pseudo Stellariae	9 grams
Rhizoma Acori Graminei	9 grams

Second treatment on May 18: After taking decoctions, the patient was feeling better. The same prescription was given with addition of fifteen grams of Radix Salviae Miltiorrhizae. Thirty doses were taken. The patient felt that eighty percent of the symptoms had disappeared. Diet was controlled for a period of time, followed by a good recovery.

Case 2 (51-81):

Mr. Zeng, 56. The patient had mental depression and trance for many years. He consulted many doctors but could not get relief.

Symptoms: Palpitation and irritation, absent-mindedness, depression, temper, and tired easily. He had bitterness in mouth, thirst, brown urine, purple-red tongue with little coating. Pulse was tight and slightly speedy. The body was covered with sores and ulcers.

Diagnosis: This syndrome was caused by excessive Interior Heat that had hurt the Yin in the Heart and the Lung, a typical Bulbus Lilii syndrome.

Prescription:

Bulbus Lilii
Radix Rehmanniae
Rhizoma Anemarrhenae
Talcum

After ten doses of the decoction were consumed, the symptoms subsided. Skin sores and ulcers remained.

Second treatment: Original recipe adding Flos Lonicerae (intending to detoxicate the sores and ulcers).

Third treatment: Before one course of medication was finished, the patient reported severe vomiting and loose bowels. Reason: Flos Lonicerae was a drug of cold nature, which was not good for Bulbus Lilii syndrome as it was harmful to the Stomach. The patient was instructed to use the first prescription without Flos Lonicerae. He took twenty doses and strength returned. Skin sores and ulcers disappeared.

Case 3 (48-418): Insomnia

Zhang, 34, female, first treatment on April 21, 1974. After the patient recovered from a severe cold, with high fever, she suffered from vertigo, headache, trance, insomnia, serious fatigue, mental depression and no appetite.

Examination: Symptoms and signs: bitterness in mouth, brown urine, tongue covered with thin and white coating, tip of tongue red. Pulse was slightly tight-speedy.

Diagnosis: After contraction of febrile disease, the remaining pathogenetic Heat was hurting the Yin in the Heart and the Lung.

Treatment: Decoction of Bulbus Lilii was used to clear the remaining Heat and moisten the Heart and the Lung.

Prescription:

Bulbus Lilii	30 grams
Radix Rehmanniae	6 grams
Rhizoma Anemarrhenae	9 grams

Talcum	9 grams
Caulis Polygoni Multiflori	30 grams
Concha Ostreae	30 grams

Five doses were consumed. The patient reported some improvement.

Second treatment: Fifteen doses of the original decoction were administered, which succeeded in restoring the patient's health.

Six months later the patient reported that she was enjoying good health.

Case 4 (48-418): Vegetative Nerve Functional Disturbance

Yang, 54, female.

Symptoms: Vertigo, distended feeling in the eyes, insomnia, Heat rushing to face, followed by perspiration. Other symptoms: parched feeling in mouth but reluctance to drink, constipation, tongue covered with little coating and tip of tongue red. Pulse was slender-speedy.

Diagnosis: Rampage of ascending Fire in Yin nature.

Prescription: Decoction of Bulbus Lilii with additions.

Bulbus Lilii	15 grams
Radix Rehmanniae	15 grams
Rhizoma Anemarrhenae	9 grams
Radix Glycyrrhizae	6 grams
Fructus Tritici	30 grams
Fructus Ziziphi Jujubae	5 pcs.
Folium Mori	10 grams

Six doses of the above decoction cured the problem.

CLAUSE 3-6

When Bulbus Lilii syndrome lasts for an entire month, the patient will become thirsty. Washing Therapy of Bulbus Lilii can be adopted.

Washing Therapy of Bulbus Lilii
(*Baihe Xifang*):

Soak one *sheng* of Bulbus Lilii in one *dou* of water overnight.

Wash the patient with the solution.* Feed the patient boiled wheat cakes. Do not add salt or Semen Sojae Praeparatum to the food.

Explanation of the Prescription: Bulbus Lilii is cool in nature. When such decoction is used to wash a patient, it has the function of ventilating and smoothing the Lung Vital Energy. In this way, pathogenetic Heat in the Lung can be dispersed.

*Wash the patient with the solution: It should be understood as "after boiling the water (with Bulbus Lilii), wash the patient when decoction is lukewarm." (1-36)

CLAUSE 3-7

If the syndrome (described in Clause 3-6) remains after the adoption of Washing Therapy, Powder of Radix Trichosanthis and Concha Ostreae can be given.

Powder of Radix Trichosanthis and Concha Ostreae
(*Gualou Muli San*):

Radix Trichosanthis
Concha Ostreae

Grind the drugs in equal amounts into powder. Take one *fangcunbi* (1 gram) of the powder with water three times a day.

Explanation of the Prescription: This prescription is a subsidiary treatment for Bulbus Lilii syndrome when Washing Therapy is adopted. Radix Trichosanthis moistens the Dryness and produces Body Fluid. Concha Ostreae eliminates the pathogenetic Heat in deficient nature and eases restlessness. (01-37)

CASES

Case 1 (64-131): Case Recorded in Journal of *Traditional Chinese Medicine*, 11:21, 1965

Mr. Chen, 50, had been sick for a long time.

Examination: Complexion was yellow with rosy cheeks and slightly dropsy face. Other symptoms: bad breath, restlessness, chills and fevers, constipation, urine brown and red, with urodynia. Temperature was always 37.8 ℃ in the morning and 39 ℃ in the afternoon. This syndrome was caused by deficient Yin, which should be treated by Decoction of Fu Mai (*Fu Mai Tang*, or *Zhi Gancao Tang*):

Radix Glycyrrhizae Praeparata
Rhizoma Zingiberis Recens

Radix Ginseng
Radix Rehmanniae
Ramulus Cinnamomi
Colla Corii Asini
Radix Ophiopogonis
Fructus Cannabis
Fructus Ziziphi Jujubae

After three doses of the above decoction, fever subsided and constipation no longer existed. The patient was well during the day but had delirium and insomnia at night.

Second treatment: Decoction of Bulbus Lilii and Radix Rehmanniae was given:

Bulbus Lilii	4 *liang*
Radix Rehmanniae	8 *qian*
Egg yolk	1 pc.

One dose every day continued for ten days. The patient had no more delirium and could sleep four to five hours at night. But the patient was thirsty. This was caused by exhaustion of Body Fluid due to excessive heat.

Third treatment: Decoction of Fructus Trichosanthis and Concha Ostreae was prescribed:

Bulbus Lilii	4 *liang*
Radix Rehmanniae	8 *qian*
Egg yolk	1 pc.
Radix Trichosanthis	4 *qian*
Concha Ostreae	6 *qian*

Thirst disappeared after three doses of the decoction. All other symptoms subsided. Urine was still in brown color and urination difficult. Dropsy appeared at both legs.

Fourth treatment: Eight *qian* of Talcum added to the above decoction served in two doses. Urination returned to normal.

Fifth treatment: The following prescription was given as a harmonization:

Bulbus Lilii	8 *qian*
Radix Rehmanniae	6 *qian*
Radix Scrophulariae	4 *qian*
Plastrum Testudinis	6 *qian*
Carapax Trionycis	5 *qian*
Egg yolk	1 pc.

After eight doses, the patient was well. Six months later no recurrence was reported.

Case 2 (46-56):

Xie, 23, female, suffered from neurosis.

Examination: The patient reported frequent headache, insomnia, dim vision, parched and bitter feeling in mouth, hot feeling of hands and feet, sporadic poor appetite, preceded menstrual cycle with small quantity of discharge, scanty and reddish urine and constipation. When asked about other symptoms, the patient could not give a clear answer. Nutrition average, normal complexion, tongue moist free from coating, with red edge and tip were diagnosed. Pulse was tight-slender and speedy. The syndrome had lasted more than a year.

Diagnosis: Seemed to be Bulbus Lilii syndrome, which should be treated by Decoction of Bulbus Lilii to clear the Heat and tranquilize the spirit, nourish the Yin in the Lung and Heart. Combination of Decoction of Bulbus Lilii and Radix Rehmanniae, Decoction of Bulbus Lilii and Rhizoma Anemarrhenae, Decoction of Fructus Trichosanthis and Concha Ostreae, and Decoction of Bulbus Lilii and Talcum was prescribed:

Bulbus Lilii	23 grams
Radix Rehmanniae	15 grams
Rhizoma Anemarrhenae	10 grams
Talcum	10 grams
Radix Trichosanthis	12 grams
Concha Ostreae	20 grams
Fructus Tritici	15 grams
Radix Paeoniae Alba	10 grams
Radix Glycyrrhizae Praeparata	6 grams
Fructus Ziziphi Jujubae	3 pcs.

Ten doses of the above decoction were given. Parched and bitter feeling in mouth were gone and urination returned to normal.

Second treatment: Twenty doses of the decoction with alterations were given:

Subtract:

Rhizoma Anemarrhenae
Talcum
Radix Trichosanthis

Add:

Radix Glehniae	15 grams
Radix Ophiopogonis	10 grams
Semen Ziziphi Spinosae	10 grams

Colla Corii Asini	10 grams
Egg yolk	2 pcs.

Then a full recovery was resulted.

CLAUSE 3-8

When fever (1) accompanies the symptoms of Bulbus Lilii syndrome, Powder of Bulbus Lilii and Talcum can be adopted (2).

NOTES

1. According to another edition, "*fever*" should read "*fever and chill.*"
2. As stated in Clause 3-1, symptoms and signs of Bulbus Lilii syndrome include, "the patient may feel either cold or hot, but without fever or chill." But this clause states, "fever accompanies the symptoms." From this we can infer that the Interior pathogenetic Heat is rampant. Thus Powder of Bulbus Lilii and Talcum is adopted to eliminate the Heat. (01-37)

Powder of Bulbus Lilii and Talcum
(*Baihe Huashi San*):

Bulbus Lilii Praeparata	1 *liang*
Talcum	3 *liang*

Pound the drugs into powder. Take one *fangcunbi* (1 gram) with water, three times a day. When slight diarrhea appears, stop taking the drug, as Heat has been eliminated.

Explanation of the Prescription: Talcum, sweet and cold, helps ease urination. Pathogenetic Heat is released with urine. Bulbus Lilii aids Talcum in eliminating Heat. (01-37)

CLAUSE 3-9

Bulbus Lilii syndrome of a Yin nature should be treated with Yang; Bulbus Lilii syndrome of a Yang nature should be treated with Yin. When syndrome of a Yang nature is observed, it is incorrect to attack the Yin. Prescribing a diaphoretic will result in malpractice. When syndrome of a Yin nature appears, attacking the Yang is also an incorrect treatment: If a purgative is adopted, this is also a malpractice (1).

NOTES

1. It is difficult to understand this clause without consideration of the clauses preceding and following it. It can be understood as follows: Bulbus Lilii syndrome with symptoms of Interior pathogenetic Heat (of a Yin nature) can be treated with Washing Therapy (treat with Yang). Bulbus Lilii syndrome with fever (Exterior syndrome, of a Yang nature) should be treated with drugs which moisten the Yin (treat with Yin). When Bulbus Lilii syndrome with Exterior syndrome (of a Yang nature) is treated with a purgative (which attacks the Yin) and then with a diaphoretic, this is a malpractice. When Bulbus Lilii syndrome with Interior syndrome (of a Yin nature) is treated with a diaphoretic (which attacks the Yang) and then with a purgative, this is also incorrect. (01-37)

CLAUSE 3-10

Symptoms and signs of *Huhuo* syndrome are similar to those of febrile diseases caused by Cold. The patient is reluctant to speak and tends to sleep. But he cannot shut his eyes when he feels restless. When ulceration appears in the throat, this is a *Huo* syndrome; when ulceration appears on external genitals, it is a *Hu* syndrome. Decoction of Radix Glycyrrhizae *Xiexin* can be adopted when the following symptoms and signs are observed: reluctance to eat, aversion to food odors, facial complexion occasionally red, sometimes black or pale. When ulceration appears in throat, the patient's voice becomes hoarse.

Decoction of Radix Glycyrrhizae *Xiexin**
(*Gancao Xiexin Tang*):

Radix Glycyrrhizae	4 *liang*
Radix Scutellariae	3 *liang*
Radix Ginseng	3 *liang*
Rhizoma Zingiberis	3 *liang*
Rhizoma Coptidis	1 *liang*
Fructus Ziziphi Jujubae	12 pcs.
Rhizoma Pinelliae	0.5 *jin*

Stew the drugs in one *dou* of water until six *sheng* remain. Filter the decoction and stew again. Serve one *sheng* lukewarm decoction per dose three times a day.

*This prescription also appears in *Shanghan Lun*, Clause 158.

CASES

Case 1 (64-139): Oculo-oro-genital Syndrome (Behcet's Syndrome), Case Recorded in *Clinical Experience of Dr. Zhao Xiwu*, p. 99

Guo, 36, female. Ulcer had appeared in oral cavity and vulva for more than six months. Examination in a hospital proved an oculo-oro-genital syndrome. Hormone was used, but did not help. After examination, the doctor diagnosed *Huhuo* syndrome.

Treatment: Decoction of Radix Glycyrrhizae *Xiexin* with additions was prescribed as follows:

Radix Glycyrrhizae	30 grams
Radix Codonopsis Pilosulae	18 grams
Rhizoma Zingiberis Recens	6 grams
Rhizoma Zingiberis	3 grams
Rhizoma Pinelliae	12 grams
Rhizoma Coptidis	6 grams
Radix Scutellariae	9 grams
Fructus Ziziphi Jujubae	7 pcs.
Radix Rehmanniae	30 grams

Twelve doses of the decoction were given. The following decoction for external use to wash genitals was prescribed:

Radix Glycyrrhizae	12 grams
Radix Sophorae Flavescentis	12 grams

Four doses of the decoction were served.

Second treatment: When the patient finished all the drugs the ulcer in oral cavity and vulva was almost gone. Fourteen doses of the decoction for oral administration and four doses of the decoction for external use were given. Full recovery was reported.

Case 2 (46-59): Oculo-oro-genital Syndrome

Mu, 30, female, was suffering from *Huhuo* syndrome. She had ulcer and pain in oral cavity and ulcer in vagina and vulva. The syndrome had lasted for more than a year. It was an oculo-oro-genital syndrome.

Treatment: Decoction of Radix Glycyrrhizae *Xiexin* was prescribed as follows:

Radix Glycyrrhizae	15 grams
Radix Codonopsis Pilosulae	10 grams
Radix Scutellariae	10 grams
Rhizoma Coptidis	5 grams
Rhizoma Pinelliae Praeparata	10 grams
Fructus Ziziphi Jujubae	3 pcs.

Drugs for external use: Powder of *Xilei San* was used to treat the oral cavity ulcer; Decoction of Radix Sophorae Flavescentis was used to wash the affected part in the pudendum.

Treatment lasted almost six months, and the syndrome was gone.

Case 3 (65-97): Ulcer in Oral Cavity, Case Recorded in Journal of *Zhejiang Chinese Medicine*, 11-12:515, 1980

Mr. Chen, 48, first treatment on January 4, 1973. Ulcer in oral cavity and on tongue for twenty days. Pulse was speedy, urine brown. Two doses of powder of *Daochi San* were given, but did not cure ulcer. Then powder of *Liangge San* was prescribed. The syndrome was gone after two doses. Fifteen days later the syndrome recurred. Tongue was red-purple, with purulent ulcer at the rim. Later, ulcer also appeared on lips. The patient could not eat anything salty. He could eat only cool porridge, and liked to hold water in mouth but could not swallow it.

Treatment: Decoction of Radix Glycyrrhizae *Xiexin* was given:

Radix Glycyrrhizae Praeparata	12 grams
Rhizoma Zingiberis	5 grams
Rhizoma Pinelliae	9 grams
Radix Scutellariae	9 grams
Radix Codonopsis Pilosulae	9 grams
Rhizoma Coptidis	6 grams
Fructus Ziziphi Jujubae	6 pcs.

After two doses of the decoction, ulcer subsided. Another two doses were given to complete cure.

CLAUSE 3-11

When ulceration appears on external genitals, the patient has a parched feeling in his throat. Decoction of Radix Sophorae Flavescentis can be used in Washing Therapy.

Decoction of Radix Sophorae Flavescentis
(*Kushen Tang*):

Radix Sophorae Flavescentis	0.5 *jin*
Cortex Sophorae	4 *liang*
Herba Agrimoniae	4 *liang*

Stew the drugs in five *dou* of water until three and a half *sheng* remain. Wash the diseased area.

Commentary: Jinjian, p. 484, gives the following prescription:

Decoction of Radix Sophorae Flavescentis
(*Kushen Tang*):

Radix Sophorae Flavescentis	1 *sheng*

Stew the drug in one *dou* of water until seven *sheng* remain. Fumigate and wash the diseased area three times a day.

CLAUSE 3-12

When ulceration appears on the anus, Fumigating Therapy of Realgar can be adopted.

Fumigating Therapy of Realgar
(*Xionghuang Xun Fang*):

Pound Realgar into powder. Spread powder on inner surfaces of two round tiles and place together to make a tube. Scorch the tiles and fumigate the anus.

CLAUSE 3-13

The patient has no fever, but is somewhat restless with speedy pulse. He is reluctant to speak and prefers to lie in bed. Sweating is also present. For the first three or four days, his eyes are as red as those of turtle dove. By the seventh or eighth day, his canthi turn black (1). If the patient has a good appetite, pus will form (2).

The following medicament will provide a cure.

NOTES

1. According to another edition, "black and yellow."

2. When pus forms, pathogenetic Heat concentrates on the ulcer, so the Liver and the Stomach are in harmony. Thus the patient has a good appetite. (01-40)

Powder of Radix Angelicae Sinensis and Semen Phaseoli (*Chixiaodou Danggui San*):

Semen Phaseoli (soak in water until it sprouts, dry it in the open air)	3 *sheng*
Radix Angelicae Sinensis	3 *liang*

Pound the drugs into powder. Take one *fangcunbi* with *jiangshui* water* three times a day.

**Jiangshui* water: Soak well-cooked Semen Setariae (a kind of millet) in cold water for five or six days until foam appears. This is *jiangshui* water.

Explanation of the Prescription: Semen Phaseoli has the function of eliminating pathogenetic Heat, dispersing ulcer and extravasating blood. Radix Angelicae Sinensis eliminates blood stasis and promotes tissue regeneration: *Jiangshui* water, cool in quality, harmonizes Viscera and Bowels. (01-41)

CASES

Case 1 (52-543):

Li, 34, female, first treatment on October 13, 1981. The patient suffered from hemorrhoids and habitual constipation. Ten days ago, when the patient had a cold, blood was seen in stool with anal pain. Pulse was slender-speedy. Tongue was red with coating. At the root of the tongue, there was a yellow and greasy thin coating.

Diagnosis: The patient had deficient Yin and insufficient Body Fluid with Interior pathogenetic Humidity-Heat which was descending to the intestine, causing trouble.

Treatment: Powder of Radix Angelicae Sinensis and Semen Phaseoli with additions was prescribed as below:

Semen Phaseoli	15 grams

Radix Angelicae Sinensis	18 grams
Fructus Sophorae	10 grams
Radix Sophorae Flavescentis	9 grams
Cortex Phellodendri	9 grams
Radix Scutellariae	9 grams
Radix Scrophulariae	15 grams
Radix Rehmanniae	18 grams
Radix Sanguisorbae (fried)	10 grams
Radix et Rhizoma Rhei (prepared with wine)	6 grams
Cortex Moutan Radicis	15 grams
Semen Trichosanthis	15 grams

After three doses of the decoction, blood in stool and anal pain subsided. Stool was smooth.

Second treatment: The decoction was given for the second treatment with the alterations:

Subtract: Radix et Rhizoma Rhei.

Add: Herba Cistanchis, Radix Polygoni Multiflori.

Increase dosage of Radix Angelicae Sinensis, Cortex Phellodendri, Fructus Sophorae.

Twelve doses of the decoction cured the ailment.

Case 2 (64-146): Case Recorded in Journal of *Shandong Chinese Medicine*, 3:23, 1983

Liu, 25, male, first treatment on January 21, 1980. The patient began to have puffy eyelids and itching on penis in October 1979. Later, he developed an ulcer on his tongue. In January 1980, he had ulcer on penis. Other accompanying symptoms were general lassitude and fatigue, slight fever and yellow urine. Pulse was tight-slender and slightly speedy.

Diagnosis: Syndrome was caused by Humidity-Heat factors.

Treatment: Powder of Radix Angelicae Sinensis and Semen Phaseoli with additions was prescribed:

Radix Angelicae Sinensis	15 grams
Semen Phaseoli	30 grams
Rhizoma Cimicifugae	12 grams
Radix Rehmanniae	15 grams
Caulis Akebiae	6 grams
Folium Bambusae	12 grams
Radix Glycyrrhizae	3 grams
Fructus Gardeniae	9 grams

Seven doses of the decoction brought the patient relief, all symptoms subsided. Another six doses were given to complete the treatment.

CLAUSE 3-14

Yangdu syndrome has the following symptoms and signs: Erythema on the face as bright as brocade designs, pharyngalgia, spittle with bloody pus. If discovered within five days, syndrome is curable; after seven days, syndrome is difficult to cure (1). Decoction of Rhizoma Cimicifugae and Carapax Trionycis is an effective cure.

NOTES

1. Within five days pathogenetic factor has not penetrated very deep into the body. After seven days, pathogenetic factor is too deep to be dispersed. This is difficult to cure. (01-41)

CLAUSE 3-15

Yindu syndrome has the following symptoms and signs: Bluish facial complexion, pharyngalgia, and general aching as if the patient were suffering a severe beating with sticks. Within five days, syndrome is still curable; after seven days, it is difficult to cure. Decoction of Rhizoma Cimicifugae and Carapax Trionycis subtracting Pericarpium Zanthoxyli and Realgar can be prescribed.

Decoction of Rhizoma Cimicifugae and Carapax Trionycis (*Shengma Biejia Tang*):

Rhizoma Cimicifugae	2 *liang*
Radix Angelicae Sinenis	1 *liang*
Pericarpium Zanthoxyli Praeparata	1 *liang*
Radix Glycyrrhizae	2 *liang*
Carapax Trionycis Praeparata (thumb-size)	1 pc.
Realgar	0.5 *liang*

Stew the drugs in four *sheng* of water until one *sheng* remains. Serve the decoction in one dose. For the aged and the young, serve in two doses. Cover the patient to induce a sweat.

Explanation of the Prescription: Treatment of *Yinyangdu* syndrome should concentrate on detoxication and promotion of normal Blood flow. Rhizoma Cimicifugae and Radix Glycyrrhizae both function as an antidote. Carapax Trionycis and Radix Angelicae Sinensis remove the blood stasis and promote the normal Blood flow.

Commentary: The Yin and Yang in *Yindu* and *Yangdu* syndromes are not Cold and Heat, Interior and Exterior in the normal sense. Red facial complexion can be considered an accumulation of pathogenetic Heat, and is termed *Yangdu* (pathogenesis of a Yang nature). A bluish facial complexion is termed *Yindu* (pathogenesis of a Yin nature). The pathology of these syndrome is the accumulation of pathogenesis in the Blood. (01-42)

CASES

Case 1 (64-150):

Sainan, female, suffered from scarlet fever in March 1956. At the onset, the patient had chills and fever, sore throat and lymphadenectasis. Tongue was covered with thin, white coating. Pulse was floating-speedy. Laboratory tests showed that it was scarlet fever.

Treatment: Decoction of Radix Cimicifugae and Carapax Trionycis was prescribed as follows:

Radix Cimicifugae	3 grams
Carapax Trionycis	10 grams
Radix Angelicae Sinensis	3 grams
Flos Lonicerae	10 grams
Fructus Forsythiae	10 grams
Fructus Arctii	10 grams
Radix Rehmanniae	12 grams
Cortex Moutan Radicis	10 grams
Radix Paeoniae Rubra	6 grams
Radix Platycodi	3 grams
Radix Glycyrrhizae	3 grams

Three doses were given. Skin rash appeared over the four extremities.
Second treatment: The above prescription was given with alterations:
Subtract: Radix Cimicifugae, Radix Angelicae Sinensis, Radix Platycodi.
Add: Radix Scrophulariae, Radix Ophiopogonis, Folium Isatidis.
Skin rash disappeared and the syndrome was gone after three doses.

Case 2 (65-104): *Yindu* Syndrome (Lupus Erythematosus), Case Recorded in Journal of *Guangxi Chinese Medicine*, 6:11, 1981

Gu, 43, female, suffered from subacute lupus erythematosus for more than two months with fever. Prednisone had been prescribed. Fever subsided, but skin erythema remained. Puffiness appeared on face and lower extremities. Soreness and pain occurred in all joints. Sore throat, scanty urine were reported. Pulse was slender-speedy, tongue red, covered with white coating.

Diagnosis: Pathogenetic Heat remained in the Blood. Water could not circulate normally due to deficiency of Kidney function.

Treatment: Decoction of Radix Cimicifugae and Carapax Trionycis was prescribed to clear the Heat, detoxicate the pathological condition, tonify the Kidney to facilitate Water circulation.

Prescription:

Radix Cimicifugae	15 grams
Carapax Trionycis (stewed for a longer time)	20 grams
Radix Angelicae Sinensis	6 grams
Cortex Moutan Radicis	10 grams
Rhizoma Rehmanniae Praeparata	20 grams
Radix Aconiti Praeparata	3 grams
Radix Achyranthis Bidentatae	12 grams
Semen Plantaginis	10 grams
Nidus Vespae	6 grams
Periostracum Serpentis	5 grams
Rhizoma Smilacis Glabrae	20 grams

Twenty doses of the decoction were served. All symptoms subsided.

Second treatment: Twenty doses of the decoction with alterations were given:

Subtract: Semen Plantaginis, Radix Moutan Radicis.

Add: One gram of Realgar.

Increase dosage of Radix Aconiti Praeparata to six grams.

CHAPTER IV

ON PULSE, SYMPTOM COMPLEX AND TREATMENT OF MALARIA

CLAUSE 4-1

Master says: Pulse of a patient with Malaria* is always tight. Tight-speedy pulse indicates a syndrome of Heat nature. Tight-slow pulse indicates a case of Cold nature. Cases with tight-small-tense pulse (1) can be cured with purgative. Tight-slow pulse responds well to drugs with warming agents. Cases with tight-tense pulse (2) can be treated with diaphoretic or acupuncture and moxibustion therapy. Emetic can be given when pulse is floating-huge (3). Tight-speedy pulse indicates evanescence of pathogenetic factors (4). A suitable diet is a proper treatment. (5)

*Malaria (*Nuebing*) in TCM is not totally equivalent to malaria in modern medicine.

NOTES

1. Wu Qian: "Tight-small-tense pulse" should be "tight-deep-tense." Purgative is thus a reasonable treatment. (05-487)

2. Wu Qian: "Tight-tense pulse" should be "tight-floating-tense." Diaphoretic can be adopted.

3. Wu Qian: "Floating-huge" pulse should be "tight-slippery-huge." Emetic can be adopted.

4. This sentence is translated according to *Jinkui E*. According to *Jinkui S*, the sentence should read: Tight-speedy pulse indicates fever caused by pathogenetic Wind.

5. Explanation of the clause by Wu Qian: Malaria is caused by an intermingling of pathogenetic Heat and Cold. It can appear in all three Yang and three Yin Channels. As the pathogenetic factors lie between the Interior and the Exterior (half-Exterior and half-Interior), it is a syndrome classified as belonging to the Lesser Yang Channel. Thus the pulse is always tight. (See Chapter on Lesser Yang syndrome in *Shanghan Lun*). For Lesser Yang syndrome of febrile diseases caused by Cold, diaphoretics, emetics and purgatives are all prohibited. Since Malaria is also part of the Lesser Yang syndrome, why can

diaphoretics, emetics and purgatives be adopted, as the text says? Because Malaria is classified as a "miscellaneous disease." At the onset of Malaria, the pulse is tight-deep-tense, indicating an Interior excessive syndrome. Thus a purgative can be adopted to eliminate the Interior Excess. When the pulse is tight-slow, it is a case of Cold nature, and drugs with a warm quality can be given to eliminate the Cold. When the pulse is floating-huge, it indicates the existence of an Exterior syndrome, and a diaphoretic can be adopted. A tight-slippery-huge pulse indicates stagnation of Fluid (Fluid-retention). Thus an emetic can be adopted. Tight-slippery pulse indicates pathogenetic Wind and Heat. Thus febrifugal therapy can be adopted. When the Malaria has lasted for a long period, the above therapies are inappropriate. A suitable diet and proper care should be provided to the patient, since at the initial stage of the disease, treatment aims to disperse the pathogenetic factors. For chronic diseases, priority should be given to building up Body Resistance. (05-487)

CLAUSE 4-2

If Malaria begins to attack on the first day of the month, it should subside on the fifteenth day. If it does not subside, it will disappear at the end of the month. If it does not subside, can Master explain why?

Master: This is due to the formation of *Zhengjia* (1). The syndrome is called Malaria with splenomegaly. Treatment must be given immediately. Pills of Carapax Trionycis will provide a cure.

NOTES

1. *Zhengjia*: A solid mass in the abdomen with a fixed shape and localized pain is called *Zheng*; that with neither fixed shape nor localized pain is called *Jia*.

Pills of Carapax Trionycis
(*Biejia Jian Wan*):

Carapax Trionycis Praeparata	12 *fen*
Rhizoma Belamcandae (burned)	12 *fen*
Radix Scutellariae	3 *fen*
Radix Bupleuri	6 *fen*
Armadillidium Vulgare (stewed)	3 *fen*
Rhizoma Zingiberis	3 *fen*
Radix et Rhizoma Rhei	3 *fen*
Radix Paeoniae	5 *fen*

Ramulus Cinnamomi	3 *fen*
Semen Lepidii seu Descurainiae (stewed)	1 *fen*
Folium Pyrrosiae	3 *fen*
Cortex Magnoliae Officinalis	3 *fen*
Cortex Moutan Radicis	5 *fen*
Herba Dianthi	2 *fen*
Flos Campsis	3 *fen*
Rhizoma Pinelliae	1 *fen*
Radix Ginseng	1 *fen*
Eupolyphaga seu Steleophaga (stewed)	5 *fen*
Colla Corii Asini Praeparata	3 *fen*
Nidus Vespae Praeparata	4 *fen*
*Chixiao** (Niter)	12 *fen*
Catharsius Molossus (or Dung Beetle, stewed)	6 *fen*
Semen Persicae	2 *fen*

**Chixiao* is identical to *Xiaoshi*, or Niter.

Pound the drugs into powder. Remove one *dou* of ash from furnace and soak in one *hu* and five *dou* of rice wine. Place Carapax Trionycis in the wine when half consumed.* Stew until decoction is as thick as glue. Add remaining drugs to the decoction and stew. Make pills the size of Chinese parasol seeds. Give seven pills per dose before meals three times a day.

Explanation of the Prescription: This is a prescription for eliminating the solid mass formed by the intermingling of pathogenetic Cold, Heat, Humidity and phlegm with the Vital Energy and the Blood. The ingredients perform the function of elimination and tonification, and can cure Malaria with splenomegaly. When taken over a long period of time, tonics should be given simultaneously to protect Blood and Vital Energy, since pills may weaken Body Resistance, especially in patients with weak constitutions. (02-35)

*This is obscure. According to *Qianjin*, this should read: "Soak ash in the wine, then filter the decoction."

CASES

Case 1 (65-109): Malaria with Splenomegaly, Case Recorded in Journal of *Jiangxi Chinese Medicine*, 11:27, 1960

Zhao, 21, first treatment on July 15, 1959. The patient had Malaria six years ago. After the syndrome was gone, there appeared at the side of the umbilicus a hard mass, which was growing and tenderness.

Other symptoms: Ascites, poor appetite, constipation, scanty urine of yellow color, yellow complexion, yellow and thin tongue coating, tight-slender and mighty pulse.

Diagnosis: This case was caused by checking the Liver Vital Energy over the Spleen with stagnation of the Blood and Vital Energy, resulting in the formation of a hard mass.

Treatment: Promote normal flow of Liver Vital Energy, replenish the Spleen and disperse the stagnation and mass.

Prescription:

Semen Myristicae Praeparata
Massa Fermentata (fried)
Rhizoma Cyperi
Poria Rubra
Pericarpium Citri Reticulatae
Pericarpium Citri Reticulatae Viride
Fructus Citri
Herba Artemisiae Scopariae
Fructus Aurantii
Endothelium Corneum Gigeriae Galli
Rhizoma Atractylodis
Radix Aucklandiae
Cortex Magnoliae Officinalis
Radix et Rhizoma Rhei
Radix et Rhizoma Rhei Praeparata

The above decoction was given daily, with alterations according to pathological changes. A week later, the patient had normal stool and urination, improved appetite and reduced hard mass. Yellow coating on the tongue disappeared.

Decoction was served a total of eighteen times. Pills of Carapax Trionycis were given, eighteen grams per day.

After administration of pills, mass and ascites disappeared.

Case 2 (64-159):

Guo, 52, female, suffered from splenomegaly for four to five years. Five years ago, the patient experienced chills and fevers. The diagnosis was Malaria.

After repeated treatment Malaria subsided, but a low fever remained. The patient was examined six months later and found to have splenomegaly of two to three cm. In recent years, although various treatments had been administered, the syndrome was worse. The patient became emaciated, with irregular fever and anemia. Abdomen was swollen, with distention and pain, aggravated in the afternoon. Anorexia, indigestion, chest distress, dyspnea, dropsy in lower extremities appeared. Pulse was speedy but weak, tongue was swollen with teeth prints.

Diagnosis: This was a syndrome of Malaria with splenomegaly, which should be treated with Pills of Carapax Trionycis.

Two pills, of ten grams, were served daily. After a period of medicament, the syndrome was relieved. Pills were given for a longer period. Dietary care was given and full recovery resulted.

Case 3 (964-160): Case Recorded in Journal of *Zhejiang Chinese Medicine*, 4:153, 1957

Chen, 45, female, first treatment on June 27, 1956. The patient had a hard mass in the abdomen with distention and sporadic pain, more than a year. Appetite was poor. She was a farmer and often worked in water. After eating, she often had a distended abdomen. Abdominal pain was also experienced now and then. Stool might occur three to six times a day, accompanied by tenesmus, and was mixed with bloody pus. The patient had lassitude and could work less and less.

Treatment: Pills of Carapax Trionycis started on June 28, taken a month. The patient recovered and was released.

CLAUSE 4-3

Master: When Yin (1) is isolated and exhausted, Yang Vital Energy will be unrestrained and cause a fever with restlessness and irritation, accompanied by heat in hands and feet and nausea. This is termed *Dannue* (2), or Malaria with fever but without chills, a syndrome caused by an accumulation of pathogenetic factors in the epigastrium and the muscles. This will consume the muscles and make the patient thin and weak.

NOTES

1. Yin here means the Body Fluid; Yang the pathogenetic Heat. (01-45)
2. *Dannue*: Malaria with high fever.

CLAUSE 4-4

Symptoms and signs of *Wennue* (febrile Malaria) generally include fever without chills (1), normal pulse condition (2), arthralgia with restlessness (3) and occasional nausea. Decoction of *Baihu* adding Ramulus Cinnamomi will cure the syndrome.

NOTES

1. According to clinical observation, symptoms of *Wennue* are more fever with less chills. Symptoms of *Dannue* are fever without chills. Thus some annotators believe the original text "fever without chills" should read "fever prevails first, followed by chills." (01-46)

2. Normal pulse should be understood as a pulse that is not tight. But according to other annotators, the pulse should conform with the syndrome, and be tight-speedy or grand-speedy. Versions vary. (02-33)

3. Arthralgia with restlessness indicates a severe case caused by uncontrolled pathogenetic factors. (01-46)

Decoction of *Baihu* adding Ramulus Cinnamomi
(*Baihu Jia Guizhi Tang*):

Rhizoma Anemarrhenae	6 *liang*
Gypsum Fibrosum	1 *jin*
Radix Glycyrrhizae Praeparata	2 *liang*
Semen Oryzae Nonglutinosae	2 *ge*
Ramulus Cinnamomi	3 *liang*

Pound the drugs. Divide into five *qian* doses. Stew each dose in one and a half cups of water until eight *fen* remain. Filter the decoction and serve warm. When perspiration is induced, syndrome disappears as well.

Explanation of the Prescription: Wennue is characterized by initial prevalence of fever followed by chill, or more fever and less chill. Thus Decoction of *Baihu* is adopted to eliminate the Interior Heat and Ramulus Cinnamomi is added to disperse Exterior Cold. (01-46)

CASES

Case 1 (46-70):

Tan, 31, was suffering from *Wennue*. At the beginning, the patient had a chill, followed by high fever, headache, flushed face, pain over the body, and vomiting. Symptoms lasted as long as eight hours then a profuse perspiration reduced the fever. The patient felt thirsty and drank cold water. Urine was scanty and reddish. Tongue was red, free from coating. Pulse was tight-huge-speedy.

Diagnosis: This condition resulted from prevalence of Yang Vital Energy accompanied by deficient Yin.

Treatment: Decoction of *Baihu* adding Ramulus Cinnamomi was prescribed with the following ingredients:

Gypsum Fibrosum	15 grams
Rhizoma Anemarrhenae	10 grams
Semen Oryzae Nonglutinosae	10 grams
Radix Glycyrrhizae	5 grams
Ramulus Cinnamomi (without bark)	5 grams
Radix Trichosanthis	15 grams
Concha Ostreae	30 grams

Three doses of the decoction were served, bringing relief. Syndrome was still there.

Second treatment: Five doses of *Qing Zhong Qu Nue Yin* (Decoction to Clear Interior Heat and Disperse Malaria), with the following drugs:

Radix Polygoni Multiflori
Radix Codonopsis Pilosulae
Radix Bupleuri
Radix Trichosanthis
Rhizoma Anemarrhenae
Radix Dichroae (prepared with vinegar)
Radix Glycyrrhizae

The decoction worked as anticipated.

Case 2 (51-102):

A lady was suffering from Malaria, had repeated nausea and was unable to eat. When food was taken, she would vomit. When Malaria attacked, she had chills, high fever and repeated vomiting which could be relieved with cold water. This was a typical Decoction of *Baihu* adding Ramulus Cinnamomi syndrome. The decoction was served warm, intending to cure simultaneous shivering of cold, fever, and profuse perspiration. The syndrome was cured.

Case 3 (48-248):

Mr. Wang, 32, was usually strong. A few days ago he began to have chills and fever with soreness of the extremities. Two days later his knees were red, swollen, with pain and hot feeling. The problem became more serious at dusk. Other symptoms were: difficulty in moving his legs, fever, aversion to cold, thirst for water. Pulse was floating-speedy. Tongue was covered with yellow coating.

Diagnosis: Syndrome was intermingling of pathogenetic Humidity-Wind-Heat.

Treatment should clear Heat, disperse Wind and Humidity.

Prescription: Decoction of *Baihu* adding Ramulus Cinnamomi with alterations.

Gypsum Fibrosum	30 grams
Rhizoma Anemarrhenae	9 grams
Radix Glycyrrhizae	3 grams
Semen Oryzae Nonglutinosae	15 grams
Ramulus Cinnamomi	4.5 grams
Caulis Lonicerae	30 grams
Excrementum Bombycis	9 grams
Radix Stephaniae Tetrandrae	9 grams
Ramulus Mori	a foot long

Three doses of the decoction were adopted. All symptoms subsided. Another five doses of the decoction were given to complete the treatment.

Case 4 (48-250):

Mr. Chen, 24, was suffering from Malaria in early summer. Four days before he consulted the doctor, Malaria attacked before noon and lasted till dusk. At the onset, there was an aversion to cold, followed by high fever, headache, thirst, soreness in joints, nausea and vomit of bitter and yellow fluid. Although there was a high fever, there appeared only slight perspiration. Tongue was covered with dry, white and slightly yellow coating. Pulse was tight-speedy.

Diagnosis: *Wennue* syndrome, which should be treated by Decoction of *Baihu* adding Ramulus Cinnamomi and Herba Artemisiae Chinghao.

Prescription:

Gypsum Fibrosum	60 grams
Rhizoma Anemarrhenae	9 grams
Radix Glycyrrhizae	3 grams
Semen Oryzae Nonglutinosae	15 grams
Ramulus Cinnamomi	4.5 grams
Herba Artemisiae Chinghao Recens	90 grams

Three doses were given. Malaria subsided.

Second treatment: A decoction made of only one drug, Herba Artemisiae

Chinghao Recens, was given for three consecutive days. Syndrome was gone.

CLAUSE 4-5

Malaria of a Cold nature (1) is termed *Munue*. Powder of Ramulus et Folium Dichroae will provide a cure.

NOTES

1. Malaria of a Cold nature, or *Munue* (according to another edition, *Pinnue*) is caused by uncontrolled pathogenetic Malaria of a Yin and Cold nature, or Malaria manifested as sthenia of Yin-Cold. According to another version, Malaria of a Cold nature results when the Yang Vital Energy is obstructed by retention of phlegm, obstructing the normal flow of Yang Vital Energy to the Exterior. Thus chill will occur. (01-46)

Powder of Ramulus et Folium Dichroae
(*Shuqi San*):

Ramulus et Folium Dichroae (washed)
Muscovitum (burned for two days)
Os Draconis

Pound the drugs in equal quantities into powder. Take half *qianbi* of the powder with *jiangshui* water (see Clause 3-13) before Malaria attacks. In cases of *Wennue* (febrile Malaria), increase dosage of Ramulus et Folium Dichroae by half *fen*. Serve one *qianbi* before the onset of an attack.

Commentary: According to clinical observation, prescriptions with Ramulus et Folium Dichroae or Radix Dichroae as their main ingredients are effective for treating Malaria. The drug should be given the night before the onset of an attack, or a half day before. A second dose can be given two hours before the attack. When Ramulus et Folium Dichroae or Radix Dichroae is the only drug in a treatment, it is also effective in curing Malaria, but the drug may also function as an emetic. Recurrence may occur when the drug is not taken. Side effect may by reduced in the following ways:

1) Stew the drug with wine or parch it;

2) Add ingredients to harmonize Stomach Vital Energy and stop vomiting, such as Rhizoma Pinelliae or Pericarpium Citri

Reticulatae. (02-34)

CASES

Case 1 (46-71): *Munue* (Doctor: Ding Ganren)

A case of Malaria with aversion to cold but without fever. This was termed *Munue*, occurring every other day. The syndrome had lasted more than a month. The patient had profuse perspiration, anorexia, deep-slender-tight pulse. Tongue was covered with white thin and greasy coating on the edge and exfoliative fur in the center.

Diagnosis: The deficient condition of Yang Vital Energy, pathogenetic Humidity with phlegm remained in the Interior, causing the malfunction of the Spleen and Stomach.

Treatment: Reinforce the Yang to disperse the pathogenesis, harmonize the Interior to dissolve the Humidity.

Prescription:

Radix Codonopsis Pilosulae	3 *qian*
Radix Aconiti Praeparata	2 *qian*
Ramulus Cinnamomi	1 *qian*
Radix Bupleuri	1 *qian*
Pericarpium Citri Reticulatae	1 *qian*
Rhizoma Pinelliae (prepared with ginger)	3 *qian*
Poria	3 *qian*
Cornu Cervi Degelatinatum	3 *qian*
Fructus Tsaoko Praeparata	8 *fen*
Radix Glycyrrhizae Praeparata	5 *fen*
Rhizoma Zingiberis Recens	2 slices
Fructus Ziziphi Jujubae	4 pcs.

Appendix:

Prescriptions from *Medical Secrets of an Official* (*Waitai Miyao*, hereinafter *Waitai*):

Decoction of Concha Ostreae
(*Muli Tang*):

For treatment of *Munue*

Concha Ostreae (stewed)	4 *liang*
Herba Ephedrae	4 *liang*
Radix Glycyrrhizae	2 *liang*

Ramulus et Folium Dichroae	3 *liang*

Stew Herba Ephedrae and Ramulus et Folium Dichroae in eight *sheng* of water until six *sheng* remain. Skim off foam and add other drugs. Stew until two *sheng* remain. Serve one *sheng* of warm decoction per dose. If the patient vomits, stop the decoction.

Explanation of the Prescription: Powder of Ramulus et Folium Dichroae is suitable for Malaria with retention of phlegm and light Exterior Heat. Decoction of Concha Ostreae is suitable for Malaria with retention of phlegm and severe Exterior Heat. (01-47)

Decoction of Radix Bupleuri subtracting Rhizoma Pinelliae adding Radix Trichosanthis
(*Chaihu Qu Banxia Jia Gualougen Tang*):

Radix Bupleuri	8 *liang*
Radix Ginseng	3 *liang*
Radix Scutellariae	3 *liang*
Radix Glycyrrhizae	3 *liang*
Radix Trichosanthis	4 *liang*
Rhizoma Zingiberis Recens	2 *liang*
Fructus Ziziphi Jujubae	12 pcs.

Stew the drugs in one *dou* plus two *sheng* of water until six *sheng* remain. Filter the decoction and stew again until three *sheng* remain. Serve one *sheng* warm decoction per dose twice a day.

This decoction is good for Malaria with thirst and Malaria caused by over-exertion.

CASES

Case 1 (46-76):

Wu, 40, female, had been suffering from Malaria for more than six months. Every afternoon, she suffered from aversion to cold, followed by headache and fever, perspiration and thirst. Urine was scanty and brown in color. Tongue was red, covered with thin coating. Pulse was tight-slender-speedy. At the onset the patient had taken quinine and got relief. But the syndrome attacked again when she worked hard. Decoction of Radix Bupleuri subtracting Rhizoma Pinelliae adding Radix Trichosanthis was prescribed:

Radix Codonopsis Pilosulae	51 grams
Radix Bupleuri	10 grams
Radix Scutellariae	10 grams
Radix Trichosanthis	12 grams
Radix Glycyrrhizae	5 grams
Rhizoma Zingiberis Recens	3 slices
Fructus Ziziphi Jujubae	3 pcs.
Ramulus et Folium Dichroae (prepared with vinegar)	10 grams

Three doses were served. Malaria subsided.

Second treatment: Seven doses of the following decoction were given to complete the treatment:

Radix Gentianae Macrophyllae
Carapax Trionycis
Cortex Lycii Radicis
Radix Bupleuri
Herba Artemisiae Chinghao
Radix Angelicae Sinensis
Rhizoma Anemarrhenae
Fructus Mume
Radix Polygoni Multiflori
Radix Codonopsis Pilosulae
Radix Glycyrrhizae

Case 2 (52-672):

Mr. Liu, 43, driver, first treatment on November 15, 1981. The patient had been suffering from thirst for more than a month. Sometimes he might drink a full thermos of water. At first he thought it was due to long driving time. Later, he began to have vertigo, restlessness and a hot face as if he were drunk.

Examination: Glucose in urine (+), slight congestion in throat. Tongue was red, covered with white and slightly greasy coating. The patient reported having had a cold with dryness in throat and oral cavity, chills and fever, about a month ago. When the cold was gone, the parched feeling remained. Pulse was tight-slender and speedy, with the pulse at the position of left Bar on the wrist more so.

Diagnosis: Pathogenetic Wind-Heat resting at the Lesser Yang Channel with damaged Body Fluid.

Treatment: Decoction of Radix Bupleuri subtracting Rhizoma Pinelliae adding Radix Trichosanthis with additions prescribed as follows:

Radix Bupleuri	9 grams

Radix Pseudostellariae	30 grams
Radix Glycyrrhizae	9 grams
Cortex Phellodendri	9 grams
Gypsum Fibrosum	40 grams
Herba Dendrobii	9 grams
Radix Ophiopogonis	15 grams
Folium Bambusae	9 grams
Radix Trichosanthis	45 grams
Radix Thalictri	10 grams

Three doses of the decoction quenched the thirst considerably. Another six doses were served. Test for glucose in urine was negative. The other symptoms were gone. Pill of Six Drugs* and Pill of *Yu Quan*** were given to stabilize the condition.

*Made up of Rhizoma Rehmanniae Praeparata, Rhizoma Dioscoreae, Fructus Corni, Poria, Rhizoma Alismatis, Cortex Moutan Radicis.

**Made up of Gypsum Fibrosum, Radix Glycyrrhizae, etc.

Decoction of Radix Bupleuri, Ramulus Cinnamomi and Rhizoma Zingiberis (*Chaihu Gui Jiang Tang*):

Radix Bupleuri	0.5 *jin*
Ramulus Cinnamomi	3 *liang*
Rhizoma Zingiberis	2 *liang*
Radix Trichosanthis	4 *liang*
Radix Scutellariae	3 *liang*
Concha Ostreae (stewed)	3 *liang*
Radix Glycyrrhizae Praeparata	2 *liang*

Stew the drugs in one *dou* plus two *sheng* of water until six *sheng* remain. Filter the decoction until three *sheng* remain. Give three doses per day. After the first dose, the patient feels slightly restless. Second dose will induce perspiration and cure the syndrome.

This decoction is good for Malaria with aversion to cold and a slight fever or Malaria with aversion to cold but without fever. After taking the decoction, it worked wonders.

CASES

Case 1 (46-73):

Mr. Li, 45, was suffering from Malaria (*Pinnue*).

Symptoms: When the syndrome attacked, the patient shivered with cold. Even if covered with heavy quilts, shivering continued. The patient had headache, pain all over the body, nausea and vomiting and a pale face. The symptoms could last for five hours, then a fever and perspiration would relieve the ailment. Tongue was covered with white and slippery coating. Pulse was tight-slender-soft.

Diagnosis: The syndrome was caused by long-time invasion of pathogenetic Humidity-Cold, which should be dispersed.

Treatment: Powder of *Wu Ji San* was given, which reduced shivering:

Herba Ephedrae
Rhizoma Atractylodis
Radix Angelicae Dahuricae
Radix Paeoniae Alba
Radix Angelicae Sinensis
Rhizoma Ligustici Chuanxiong
Fructus Aurantii
Radix Platycodi
Cortex Cinnamomi
Poria
Radix Ginseng

Second treatment: Decoction of Radix Bupleuri, Ramulus Cinnamomi and Rhizoma Zingiberis was prescribed as follows:

Radix Bupleuri	10 grams
Radix Scutellariae (prepared with wine)	6 grams
Ramulus Cinnamomi	10 grams
Rhizoma Zingiberis	6 grams
Concha Ostreae	15 grams
Radix Glycyrrhizae	3 grams
Radix Trichosanthis	10 grams
Ramulus et Folium Dichroae (prepared with vinegar)	10 grams
Semen Arecae	10 grams
Fructus Tsaoko	5 grams

Three doses of the above decoction alleviated the Malaria.

Third treatment: Decoction of *Si Shou Yin* made up of the following ingredients was prescribed for a full recovery:

Radix Codonopsis Pilosulae
Rhizoma Atractylodis Macrocephalae
Rhizoma Pinelliae
Poria
Pericarpium Citri Reticulatae
Fructus Tsaoko
Fructus Mume
Radix Glycyrrhizae
Rhizoma Zingiberis
Fructus Ziziphi Jujubae

CHAPTER V

ON PULSE, SYMPTOM COMPLEX AND TREATMENT OF APOPLEXY AND ACUTE ARTHRITIS*

CLAUSE 5-1

Disease brought on by pathogenetic Wind will cause hemiplegia. When a patient cannot move one or both arms freely, it is a case of *Bi* syndrome (1) with feeble-speedy pulse caused by pathogenetic Wind.

NOTES

1. *Bi* syndrome: a) Obstruction of the Vital Energy and the Blood flow, causing pain; b) Pain and numbness due to exogenous pathogenetic factors (usually Wind, Cold and Humidity) being blocked in blood vessels or Channels; c) Rheumatic pain.

*In a broad sense, apoplexy (*Zhongfeng*) and acute arthritis (*Lijie*) belong to the category of diseases caused by pathogenetic Wind, and are discussed in the same chapter.

Apoplexy, or *Zhongfeng*, differs from the *Zhongfeng* in *Shanghan Lun*. In Clause 2 of *Shanghan Lun*, it is stated: "Initial Yang syndrome with symptoms and signs of fever, perspiration, chill and moderate pulse is termed febrile disease caused by Wind (*Zhongfeng*). The *Zhongfeng* discussed herein is equivalent to "apoplexy" in modern medicine, and belongs to the category of "miscellaneous diseases." Pathology of the disease is as follows: When a patient is weak and has poor Body Resistance, exposure to pathogenetic climate will induce the disease. Symptoms and signs generally include: sudden attack of syncope, followed by hemiplegia, distortion of the mouth and eyes. In serious cases, the patient enters a deep coma.

Acute arthritis, or *Lijie*, is also caused when a patient who is weak and deficient in Body Resistance is exposed to pathogenetic climate. Its main symptom is arthralgia in all the joints of the body. (02-37)

CLAUSE 5-2

Pulse at *Cunkou* (1) is floating-tense. Tense pulse indicates existence of pathogenetic Cold, floating pulse signifies a case of a deficient nature (2). Pathogenetic Cold will enter the body when it is in a deficient state. Pathogenetic Cold first rests on the skin. Floating pulse indicates Blood Deficiency with Channels and Collaterals void and defenseless, allowing pathogenetic factors to circulate throughout the body, sometimes on the left side, sometimes on the right. When either side of the body is affected, muscles and Channels become loose. By comparison, the side which is not affected seems tense, and distortion of the mouth and eyes takes place on this side, with hemiplegia. This is called "attraction of pathogens by the Body Resistance" (*Zhengqi Yixie*). When pathogens rest in Collaterals, numbness of the skin results. When pathogenetic factors enter the Channels, normal movement of the extremities is hampered. When Bowels are affected by the pathogenetic factors, the patient will not be able to recognize people around him. If Viscera are affected, aphasia and salivation will occur (3). *Houshi Heisan* (4) is a prescription effective for severe cases of apoplexy (5), with heaviness in the extremities and chills, as in a deficient case.

NOTES

1. *Cunkou*: Point on the wrist above the radial artery where pulse is felt.

2. The floating pulse mentioned here is floating when felt lightly and strengthless when felt deeply. It indicates a deficient state of the Vital Energy and the Blood. (01-50)

3. Early scholars explained the etiology of apoplexy as an invasion of exogenous pathogenetic Wind. But later scholars such as Liu Wansu (ca. 1120-1200), Li Gao (1180-1251), Zhu Zhenheng (1280-1358) and Zhang Jingyue (ca. 1563-1640) produced new theories of the etiology. Liu Wansu explained the causa morbi of apoplexy as pathogenetic Heat caused by the five abnormal expressions of emotions (anger, joy, contemplation, sadness and fear), rather than by exogenous pathogenetic Wind. Li Gao thought the disease resulted from an abnormality in the Vital Energy and a Deficiency of Interior Body Resistance. Zhu Zhenheng advocated the idea of a Deficiency of the Vital Energy and excessive phlegm and Humidity. Zhang Jingyue proposed that the disease was caused by the "collapse of Interior Vital Energy resulting from chronic consumption and disorder." (02-38)

4. *Houshi Heisan*: Literally "Black Powder made by Dr. Hou."

5. Severe cases of apoplexy: *Dafeng* or "severe Wind," are cases when a patient suddenly falls down and loses consciousness. This is caused by invasion of pathogenetic Wind into the Viscera and the Bowels. (01-51)

Black Powder of *Houshi*
(*Houshi Heisan*):

Flos Chrysanthemi	40 *fen*
Rhizoma Atractylodis Macrocephalae	10 *fen*
Herba Asari	3 *fen*
Poria	3 *fen*
Concha Ostreae	3 *fen*
Radix Platycodi	8 *fen*
Radix Ledebouriellae	10 *fen*
Radix Ginseng	3 *fen*
Alumen	3 *fen*
Radix Scutellariae	5 *fen*
Radix Angelicae Sinensis	3 *fen*
Rhizoma Zingiberis	3 *fen*
Rhizoma Ligustici Chuanxiong	3 *fen*
Ramulus Cinnamomi	3 *fen*

Pound the drugs into powder. Take one *fangcunbi* with wine per dose once a day. During the first twenty days, take with warm wine. Avoid eating fish, meat, garlic, and eat cold food when possible. Continue for sixty days. Drugs will accumulate in the abdomen. If hot meals are taken, drugs will not remain in the abdomen. Cold food can increase the efficacy of the drugs.

CASES

Case 1 (56-36):

Mr. Sun, 70, first treatment on April 6, 1950. One morning when the patient woke up, he was unable to move one side of his body. Besides the hemiplegia, he had chills and fever. The patient was conscious and spoke well. Tongue was red, covered with thin, white coating. Pulse was floating.

Diagnosis: This was apoplexy with hemiplegia as its main symptom.

Treatment: Decoction of *Xiao Xuming* was prescribed to disperse the Exterior syndrome:

Herba Ephedrae
Radix Stephaniae Tetrandrae
Radix Ginseng
Radix Scutellariae
Cortex Cinnamomi

Radix Glycyrrhizae
Radix Paeoniae Alba
Rhizoma Ligustici Chuanxiong
Semen Armeniacae Amarum
Radix Aconiti Praeparata
Radix Ledebouriellae
Rhizoma Zingiberis Recens

Second treatment: Black Powder of *Houshi* was prescribed as follows:

Flos Chrysanthemi	120 grams
Rhizoma Atractylodis Macrocephalae	30 grams
Radix Stephaniae Tetrandrae	30 grams
Radix Platycodi	24 grams
Radix Scutellariae	15 grams
Herba Asari	9 grams
Rhizoma Zingiberis	9 grams
Radix Codonopsis Pilosulae	9 grams
Radix Angelicae Sinensis	9 grams
Rhizoma Ligustici Chuanxiong	9 grams
Concha Ostreae	9 grams
Alumen	9 grams
Ramulus Cinnamomi	9 grams

Serve three grams of the powder each dose, wash it down with water, two times a day. In the first twenty days of treatment, serve the patient hot food. In the period of the second twenty days, serve lukewarm food. In the last twenty days, serve cold food. One course of treatment lasted sixty days. Fish, meat and garlic were prohibited.

In sixty days of treatment, the patient gradually gained strength in his upper and lower extremities. On the fiftieth day, he felt abdominal distention and anorexia, but continued treatment till the sixtieth day when he regained his strength and could walk by himself. Abdominal distention disappeared and appetite improved.

Case 2 (55-57):

Mr. Shang, 60, was of plump build. For ten years, he had suffered from hypertension, with blood pressure ranging between 190/220 mm.Hg. He had vertigo, numbness in extremities and difficulty in walking. In recent years, he had difficulty talking and akinesia.

Treatment: Black Powder of *Houshi* was given, twice a day. Blood pressure went down to 120/180 mm.Hg. The patient regained confidence and continued the medication, which held the blood pressure at 110/160 mm.Hg.

Case 3 (46-77):

Mr. Tan, 71, had hypertension for more than ten years. One night, while he was getting up for the restroom, he felt to the floor, losing consciousness. Hemiplegia occurred on the right extremities. There was phlegm and salivation. Pulse was tight-slippery, tongue was covered with yellow and greasy coating.

Diagnosis: This syndrome caused by the accumulation of pathogenetic Heat intermingled with phlegm gave rise to ascending pathogenetic Wind.

Treatment: Decoction of *Ditan* (Decoction for Clearing the Phlegm) was prescribed with alterations. Prescription was as follows:

Rhizoma Arisaematis Praeparatae
Poria
Pericarpium Citri Reticulatae
Rhizoma Acori Graminei
Caulis Bambusae in Taeniam
Radix Glycyrrhizae
Rhizoma Zingiberis Recens
Ramulus Uncariae cum Uncis
Flos Chrysanthemi
Radix Achyranthis Bidentatae
Lumbricus
Cornu Bubali

After five doses of the above decoction, the patient was spitting less phlegm and regained consciousness.

Second treatment: Five doses of the prescription, with a minor alteration, were given. Coating on the tongue subsided, indicating subsidence of the syndrome, and pulse became tight-moderate.

Third treatment: Black Powder of *Houshi* was prescribed. Prescription was written out in the following way:

Radix Codonopsis Pilosulae	10 grams
Rhizoma Atractylodis Macrocephalae	10 grams
Poria	10 grams
Radix Angelicae Sinensis	10 grams
Rhizoma Ligustici Chuanxiong	3 grams
Flos Chrysanthemi	10 grams
Radix Scutellariae	6 grams
Radix Ledebouriellae	10 grams
Concha Ostreae	30 grams
Ramulus Uncariae cum Uncis	15 grams
Radix Paeoniae Alba	10 grams

Radix Achyranthis Bidentatae	12 grams
Cortex Eucommiae	12 grams
Ramulus Loranthi	15 grams

The above prescription was used as a decoction to be administered in a period of half a year. Then the patient resumed his ability and could speak normally.

CLAUSE 5-3

Pulse at *Cunkou* is slow-moderate. Slow pulse signifies Cold; moderate pulse indicates Deficiency. Moderate pulse in *Ying* (1) indicates loss of Blood. Moderate pulse in Vital Resistance (2) indicates disease caused by Wind (*Zhongfeng*). When pathogenetic factors invade the Channels, itch and rash will appear on the skin. With a Deficiency in the Heart Vital Energy (3), pathogenetic factor will penetrate into the Interior, causing a fullness in the chest and a shortness of breath. Decoction of *Fengyin* is a curative for apoplexy with epilepsy and spasms of a Heat nature.

NOTES

1. *Ying*: Nutrient Essence, or constructive energy, which moves through the conduits and nourishes all the organs. Thus moderate pulse in *Ying* means moderate-deep pulse.
2. Vital Resistance, or *Wei*, defensive energy, which moves outside the conduits, permeating the surface of the body and warding off exogenous pathogens. Thus moderate pulse in Vital Resistance means moderate-floating pulse.
3. Deficiency in Heart Vital Energy: Here it means Deficiency of Body Resistance. "Heart" sometimes means "Interior." (01-51)

Decoction of *Fengyin*
(*Fengyin Tang*):

Radix et Rhizoma Rhei	4 *liang*
Rhizoma Zingiberis	4 *liang*
Os Draconis	4 *liang*
Ramulus Cinnamomi	3 *liang*
Radix Glycyrrhizae	2 *liang*
Concha Ostreae	2 *liang*
Calcitum	6 *liang*

Talcum	6 *liang*
Halloysitum Rubrum	6 *liang*
Baishizhi (Kaolin)	6 *liang*
Fluoritum	6 *liang*
Gypsum Fibrosum	6 *liang*

Pound the drugs into powder. Pass through a coarse mesh screen and store in leather pouch. Stew "as much as can be pinched between three fingers" in three *sheng* of fresh spring water. Serve one *sheng* of warm decoction per dose.

CASES

Case 1 (65-130): Case Recorded in Journal of *Zhejiang Chinese Medicine*, 12:454, 1976

A boy of nine years suffered from epilepsy for several years. The ailment might attack several times within one day. Phenytoin sodium did not seem to help. When attacked, the boy would fall to the ground, and lose consciousness. Contracture occurred, with deviation of eyeballs, crying and profuse salivation. Lips were red, tongue dark-red. Constipation and scanty urine also resulted.

Treatment: Stew thirty grams of powder of Decoction of *Fengyin* and serve the same day. After ten days of the above drug, epilepsy was gone. Another thirty doses were given to complete the treatment.

Case 2 (46-79): (Doctor: Xiao Zhuoru)

Mr. Zhou, 30, was brought to the clinic for treatment of his apoplexy, which could attack at any time. When attacked, the patient had severe contracture of extremities, shaking of skin on cheeks and dim vision. After the seizure, the patient had vertigo and bitterness in mouth, numbness of hands and feet. The patient had a flushed face, tongue covered by thick yellow moist coating, and at tip of tongue a red spot. Pulse was tight-speedy.

Treatment: Decoction of *Fengyin* was prescribed. The doctor told the patient to stop the medicament when there was a loose bowel and the subsidence of apoplexy.

Two weeks later the patient reported that after having two doses of the decoction, he had a loose stool and the apoplexy subsided greatly. The syndrome attacked less frequently and less severely, but the patient was worried and asked for help.

Second treatment: Decoction of Rhizoma Coptidis and Colla Corii Asini was given as follows. After ten doses, the syndrome was gone.

Rhizoma Coptidis
Colla Corii Asini

Radix Paeoniae
Egg yolk
Radix Scutellariae

Case 3 (64-182): Case Recorded in Journal of *Zhejiang Chinese Medicine*, 3:117, 1982

Mr. Li, 47, first treatment on April 8, 1976. The patient had been suffering from headache and vertigo for about five years. In the five days before he came to consult the doctor, headache and vertigo were aggravated, with difficulty in moving the left side of body. He had to remain in bed. The diagnosis was hypertension, cerebrovascular spasm and cerebral hemorrhage.

Examination: The patient had a plump build. He was suffering occasional unconsciousness and irritation, flushed face, pink eyes, parched mouth and bad breath, hemiplegia on the left side and deviation of mouth to the right, no stool for seven days. Tongue was covered with gray-yellow and turbid coating. Pulse was tight-slippery and mighty. Blood pressure was 140/220 mm.Hg.

Diagnosis: Pathogenetic Wind had penetrated the Bowels, with Interior Excess. Heat and phlegm had hampered the orifices and Channels.

Treatment: Decoction of *Fengyin* was prescribed as follows:

Gypsum Fibrosum	30 grams
Radix et Rhizoma Rhei (soak in the already-stewed decoction)	9 grams
Natrii Sulfas Exsiccatus (soak in the already-stewed decoction)	9 grams
Flos Chrysanthemi	9 grams
Bombyx Batryticatus	9 grams
Lumbricus	9 grams
Fluoritum	15 grams
Os Draconis	15 grams
Concha Ostreae	15 grams
Ramulus Cinnamomi	4.5 grams
Concha Haliotidis	18 grams
Scorpio	3 grams

Two doses of the decoction were served. The patient returned to normal. Stool was smooth. Coating on tongue faded. Pulse was growing moderate. Blood pressure went down to 110/180 mm.Hg.

Decoction of *Fengyin* with alterations was given for thirty doses before final recovery.

Decoction of Radix Stephaniae Tetrandrae and Radix Rehmanniae (*Fangji Dihuang Tang*):

Radix Stephaniae Tetrandrae	1 *qian*
Ramulus Cinnamomi	3 *qian*
Radix Ledebouriellae	3 *qian*
Radix Glycyrrhizae	1 *qian*

Steep the drugs in a cup of wine overnight. Filter the decoction. Steam two *jin* of Radix Rehmanniae for as much time as it takes to cook one *dou* of rice. Extract juice of Radix Rehmanniae and store in brass container. Mix the two decoctions and serve in two doses.

CASES

Case 1 (52-534):

Xu, 6, female, had severe pain over her left knee on the night of October 2, 1979. Her parents thought this was due to a sprain.

The second night the girl cried again with pain over the joint. The knee was swollen and had local swelling. The patient could not stand walk. She was taken to the hospital for Western medicine treatment but it did not help. The diagnosis: infantile rheumatoid arthritis.

Diagnosis: This was an obstruction syndrome complicated with Yin Deficiency, treated by adoption of Decoction of Radix Stephaniae Tetrandrae and Radix Rehmanniae.

Prescription:

Radix Stephaniae Tetrandrae	6 grams
Radix Rehmanniae	10 grams
Ramulus Cinnamomi	6 grams
Radix Ledebouriellae	6 grams
Radix Glycyrrhizae	5 grams
Ramulus Mori	9 grams
Caulis Lonicerae	9 grams
Fructus Chaenomelis	9 grams
Caulis Sinomenii	9 grams
Caulis Piperis Futokadsurae	6 grams
Radix Achyranthis Bidentatae	6 grams
Radix Angelicae Sinensis	9 grams

Twenty doses of the decoction were served. Aspirin also given. After two months of treatment, pain was gone and swelling disappeared. No recurrence was reported in the following two years.

Case 2 (46-80):

Cui, 51, female, was suffering from chronic rheumatic arthritis. The patient was thin with pain in all joints. Finger distortion, condyle swelling and muscular atrophy of legs appeared. She stayed in bed all the time. Constipation was reported. Urination was normal. Tongue was pale, free from coating, pulse was tight-slender.

Diagnosis: A syndrome caused by the obstruction of Nutrient Essence when both the Liver and Kidney were deficient.

Treatment: Nourish the Blood to harmonize the Nutrient Essence, tonify the Liver and Kidney. This was a chronic disease, and treatment was directed to gradually recovery. Decoction of Radix Stephaniae Tetrandrae and Radix Rehmanniae was prescribed in the following way:

Radix Rehmanniae	30 grams
Radix Stephaniae Tetrandrae	10 grams
Ramulus Cinnamomi	10 grams
Radix Ledebouriellae	10 grams
Radix Glycyrrhizae	10 grams
Radix Angelicae Sinensis	10 grams
Rhizoma Ligustici Chuanxiong	3 grams
Radix Paeoniae Alba	10 grams
Rhizoma Dioscoreae Hypoglaucae	10 grams
Fructus Chaenomelis	6 grams
Semen Coicis	12 grams

Thirty doses were served. Pain and swelling subsided.

Second treatment: The prescription was alterated:

Subtract: Radix Stephaniae Tetrandrae and Semen Coicis.

Add: Lumbricus and Flos Carthami.

Thirty doses were given. The patient had a relief from the rheumatic pain.

Third treatment: The decoction prescribed in the second treatment was given, with the following alterations:

Subtract: Ramulus Cinnamomi and Radix Ledebouriellae.

Add: Radix Achyranthis and Ramulus Loranthi.

Another thirty doses were consumed, bringing patient easier movement of her joints.

Fourth treatment: Pills were made of the original prescription adding the following:

Radix Codonopsis Pilosulae

Cortex Eucommiae
Radix Dipsaci
Caulis Spatholobi

Pills were taken daily for about a year. The patient was instructed to walk by herself to help resume ability. Gradually she could walk normally.

Circular-rubbing Therapy for Head-wind
(*Toufeng Mo San*):

Radix Aconiti Praeparata	1 large piece
Sal (Salt)	equal weight

Pound the drugs into powder. After washing the head, rub the affected area in a circular motion with the drug until a cure is effected.*

*This therapy is efficacious for headache of the Yang deficient type.

CLAUSE 5-4

Pulse at *Cunkou* is deep-weak. Deep pulse indicates the disease is affecting the bones, and is also a manifestation of a Kidney disease. Weak pulse indicates disease in tendons, and is also a manifestation of a Liver disease. When the patient is immersed in water when sweating all over, the pathogenetic Water will affect his Heart (1). Acute arthritis will occur with yellowish sweat (2).

NOTES

1. Sweat is the Body Fluid of the Heart. Thus when sweat and pathogenetic Water combat each other, Heart function will be hampered. (01-53)
2. When the out-flow of sweat is obstructed by Water, sweat flows into the joints, causing arthritis and yellowish sweat. (01-53)

CLAUSE 5-5

Pulse at *Fuyang* (anterior tibial artery) is floating-slippery. Slippery pulse indicates Excess of Cereal Vital Energy (1). Floating pulse signifies spontaneous perspiration.

NOTES

1. Excess of Cereal Vital Energy: indigestion that will turn into Heat. Cereal Vital Energy: essential substance from cereals, or Vital Energy produced by the digestion of cereals.

CLAUSE 5-6

Pulse of *Shaoyin* (Lesser Yin pulse of malleolus artery) is floating-weak. Weak pulse indicates insufficiency of Blood (1). Floating pulse is an indication of pathogenetic Wind. When the deficient Blood is attacked by the Wind, there will be referred pain.

NOTES

1. Insufficiency of the Blood here means the deficient state of the Blood.

CASES

Case 1 (65-135): Case Recorded in Journal of *Zhejiang Chinese Medicine*, 2:53, 1980

Wang, 34, female, first treatment on September 10, 1970. The patient had suffered rheumatoid arthritis for five years with attacks from time to time. The previous year after giving birth to a baby, she was exposed to cold and wind, which caused chill and fever and pain in the extremities and joints. Accompanying symptoms included heaviness in extremities, pain and swollen joints that made her unable to move, flushed cheeks, emaciation, afternoon fever, thirst but unable to drink, palpitation and dyspnea.

Diagnosis: Yin was badly consumed by the disease that had lasted five years and the deficient and weak condition of both Vital Energy and Blood after childbirth. Channels and conduits in the extremities lost their normal nourishment. That explained the pathology of the arthritis and accompanying symptoms.

Prescription:

Semen Arecae
Fructus Aurantii Immaturus
Radix Aucklandiae
Pericarpium Citri Reticulatae
Poria
Radix Angelicae Sinensis
Radix Achyranthis Bidentatae
Scorpio
Zaocys
Radix Aconiti (stewed twenty minutes prior to other drugs)

Radix Aconiti Kusnezoffii (stewed twenty minutes prior to other drugs)
Radix Paeoniae Alba
Radix Gentianae Macrophyllae
Cortex Lycii Radicis
Radix Astragali Hedysari

Sixty doses were served, which brought the disease under control.

CLAUSE 5-7

The pulse of a patient with plump physique is hesitant and small. Other symptoms and signs include shortness of breath, spontaneous perspiration, and acute arthritis preventing patient from moving his extremities. This is caused by exposure to wind when the patient is sweating after drinking wine. (1)

NOTES

1. Cao Yingfu explained the pathology of the disease: People with plump physique are generally having floating-slippery and huge pulses as they are rich in Vital Energy and Blood. When hesitant and small pulses appear to such people, it can be inferred that it must be a condition of the rampant Humidity factor that is invading the Spleen, making the latter unable to exercise the normal circulation of Yang Vital Energy. Shortness of breath is resulted from the overdrinking of wine that has damaged the Lung Vital Energy. Spontaneous perspiration is an indication of the outgoing pathogenetic Wind which failed to bring with it the Cold and Humidity factors. When the patient is exposed again to pathogenetic Wind, all the pathogenetic factors such as Wind, Cold and Humidity will be forced to invade the joints, causing pain and other rheumatic troubles.

CLAUSE 5-8

Decoction of Ramulus Cinnamomi, Radix Paeoniae and Rhizoma Anemarrhenae is a curative for acute arthritis with the following symptoms and signs: Arthralgia in all joints of the extremities, thin and weak physique, severe swelling of feet (as if they are falling off the legs) (1), vertigo and shortness of breath, restlessness and nausea.

NOTES

1. The feet are swollen to the point that they resemble melons so ripe that

they are about to fall off from the vine. (01-54)

Decoction of Ramulus Cinnamomi, Radix Paeoniae and Rhizoma Anemarrhenae
(*Guizhi Shaoyao Zhimu Tang*):

Ramulus Cinnamomi	4 *liang*
Radix Paeoniae	3 *liang*
Rhizoma Anemarrhenae	4 *liang*
Herba Ephedrae	2 *liang*
Rhizoma Zingiberis Recens	5 *liang*
Rhizoma Atractylodis Macrocephalae	5 *liang*
Radix Glycyrrhizae	2 *liang*
Radix Ledebouriellae	4 *liang*
Radix Aconiti Praeparata	2 pcs.

Stew the drugs in seven *sheng* of water until two *sheng* remain. Serve seven *ge* of the warm decoction per dose three times a day.

Explanation of the Prescription: This prescription is effective for rheumatic and rheumatoid arthritis. Cure is obtained by dispersing pathogenetic Wind and Humidity, eliminating of pathogenetic Heat of a deficient nature and promoting tonification of the Blood. (02-40)

Action of the specific ingredients is as follows:

Ramulus Cinnamomi: smooths the circulation of the Vital Energy in the extremities;

Radix Paeoniae: analgesic;

Rhizoma Anemarrhenae: antioncotic;

Herba Ephedrae and Radix Ledebouriellae: disperse pathogenetic Wind;

Rhizoma Zingiberis Recens and Radix Aconiti Praeparata: disperse pathogenetic Cold;

Rhizoma Atractylodis Macrocephalae: drains the pathogenetic Humidity.

CASES

Case 1 (63-118):

Geng, first treatment on August 27. The patient was suffering from pain in the joints and feet, with a cold feeling in the tibia and fever at dusk. Pulse was deep-slippery. This was a case of *Lijie*. Decoction of Ramulus Cinnamomi, Radix Paeoniae and Rhizoma Anemarrhenae was prescribed:

Ramulus Cinnamomi	15 grams
Radix Paeoniae Alba	9 grams
Radix Paeoniae Rubra	9 grams
Radix Glycyrrhizae	9 grams
Herba Ephedrae	9 grams
Radix Aconiti Praeparata	15 grams
Rhizoma Atractylodis Macrocephalae	15 grams
Rhizoma Anemarrhenae	15 grams
Radix Ledebouriellae	15 grams
Rhizoma Zingiberis Recens	1 slice

Second treatment: After taking a few doses of the decoction, pain on legs subsided and fever was not as high. Pain and soreness in the extremities remained the same. The same decoction should be served with alterations as follows:

Ramulus Cinnamomi	15 grams
Radix Paeoniae Alba	15 grams
Radix Paeoniae Rubra	15 grams
Radix Glycyrrhizae	9 grams
Herba Ephedrae	12 grams
Rhizoma Atractylodis	15 grams
Rhizoma Atractylodis Macrocephalae	15 grams
Rhizoma Anemarrhenae	15 grams
Radix Ledebouriellae	15 grams
Rhizoma Zingiberis Recens	1 slice
Radix Aconiti Praeparata	9 grams

Case 2 (46-84):

Peng, 32, female, suffered from rheumatoid arthritis for about three years. She had pain over the joints and extremities, and finger distortion. Whenever the patient was exposed to cold and humid weather there was an attack. She had vertigo, shortness of breath and nausea. Tongue was covered with white and slippery coating. Pulse was soft-moderate.

Diagnosis: This syndrome was caused by the intermingling of pathogenetic Cold-Humidity-Wind factors, resulting in an obstruction syndrome.

Treatment: Decoction of Ramulus Cinnamomi, Radix Paeoniae and Rhizoma Anemarrhenae was prescribed to disperse the pathogenetic factors. The prescription was as follows:

Ramulus Cinnamomi	10 grams
Radix Paeoniae (prepared with wine)	10 grams
Rhizoma Anemarrhenae	6 grams
Herba Ephedrae	3 grams
Radix Ledebouriellae	10 grams
Rhizoma Atractylodis Macrocephalae	10 grams
Radix Aconiti Praeparata	10 grams
Radix Glycyrrhizae	3 grams
Rhizoma Zingiberis Recens	3 slices

Five doses were served, all symptoms subsided.

Second treatment: The following decoction was prescribed as a treatment to disperse the pathogenesis and establish Body Resistance:

Ramulus Cinnamomi
Radix Ledebouriellae
Radix Gentianae Macrophyllae
Radix Angelicae Pubescentis
Herba Asari
Poria
Radix Codonopsis Pilosulae
Radix Astragali Hedysari
Rhizoma Rehmanniae Praeparata
Radix Angelicae Sinensis
Radix Paeoniae Alba
Rhizoma Ligustici Chuanxiong
Cortex Eucommiae
Radix Dipsaci
Radix Achyranthis Bidentatae
Fructus Ziziphi Jujubae

Case 3 (51-126):

Mr. Zhou, 20, fell into the river while he was sweating on a cold day. He did not sense any uncomfortable feeling at the time. After a few days he began to have sore and numb feet, followed by swelling of knees and feet. It was difficult for him to move. His hands shook. Spermatorrhea occurred. He became emaciated and could not work, although he had been treated for the condition in the past three years.

Diagnosis: Pulse on left wrist was deep-weak and on right wrist was floating-soft. The sudden fall into cold water while he was perspiring made the Humidity factor (in the form of sweat) unable to ease as usual and returned to the muscle to invade the joints. Later he was exposed to wind which also intruded into the body mingling with the Humidity, causing trouble in the joints and tendons. At first the doctor thought, since the patient was having emission, it must be a case of deficient nature, which ought to be tonified. The tonifications made the case worse. Emission was caused by the invasion of pathogenetic Wind-Humidity to the Kidney. It was not the conventional Kidney Deficiency that caused emission in many cases. Therefore, it could be concluded that the syndrome was caused by invasion of Wind-Humidity factors, calling for the adoption of Decoction of Ramulus Cinnamomi, Radix Paeoniae and Rhizoma Anemarrhenae.

Prescription No. 1:

Ramulus Cinnamomi	12 grams
Radix Paeoniae Alba	9 grams
Rhizoma Anemarrhenae	12 grams
Rhizoma Atractylodis Macrocephalae	12 grams
Radix Aconiti (stewed prior to other drugs)	12 grams
Herba Ephedrae	6 grams
Radix Ledebouriellae	6 grams
Radix Glycyrrhizae	6 grams
Rhizoma Zingiberis Recens	15 grams

Prescription No. 2:

Radix Paeoniae Alba	18 grams
Radix Glycyrrhizae Praeparata	9 grams

Prescription No. 3 (for external use: grind the drugs into powder and blend with wine into paste):

Herba Ephedrae	30 grams
Lignum Pini Nodi	30 grams
Semen Sinapis Albae	30 grams

Serve the Prescription No. 1 for fifteen days, daily. Then serve one dose of Prescription No. 2. Apply Prescription No. 3 to the affected part. After treatments were adopted, the patient's feet could stretch straight. In the following fifteen days, same treatments were given. The patient could then stand on his feet. In the following month, he began to walk by himself. Fifteen days later, his hands no longer shook and emission stopped. He could walk normally. No recurrence was reported in twenty years.

CLAUSE 5-9

Consumption of too many sour foods will harm the tendons, and they will become loose; this is called *Xie* (disability). Consumption of too much salt will harm the bones, and they will become flaccid; this is called *Ku* (withering). When *Xie* (disability) and *Ku* (withering) occur at the same time, this is a case of *Duan Xie* (disability and withering, an incurable disease). When Nutrient Essence does not circulate smoothly, normal flow of Vital Resistance is also hampered. When normal circulation of Nutrient Essence and Body Resistance in the Three Portions of Body Cavity are obstructed, skin, muscle, fat and marrow are deprived of their nourishment. The patient becomes thin and weak, with swollen feet, yellowish sweat, and chill in shins. When the patient has a fever, it is a case of acute arthritis (*Lijie*).

CLAUSE 5-10

For acute arthritis (*Lijie*), with paralysis of the extremities and arthralgia, give Decoction of Rhizoma Aconiti.

Decoction of Rhizoma Aconiti
(*Wutou Tang*):

Cures arthralgia of the foot joints and paralysis*

Herba Ephedrae	3 *liang*
Radix Paeoniae	3 *liang*
Radix Astragali	3 *liang*
Radix Glycyrrhizae Praeparata	3 *liang*
Rhizoma Aconiti (chop up the drug, stew in two *sheng* of honey until one *sheng* remains, remove the drug)**	5 pcs.

Stew the first four drugs in three *sheng* of water until one *sheng* remains. Filter the decoction. Pour honey, in which Rhizoma Aconiti had been stewed, into the decoction and stew again. Serve seven *ge* for the first dose. If not efficacious, give the remainder.

* According to *jinjian*, this sentence is deleted.

**Why is Rhizoma Aconiti stewed in honey? When Rhizoma Aconiti is prepared this way, it will remain in the joints for a longer time, thus prolonging the duration of the effectiveness of the drug. (01-56)

Commentary: Rhizoma Aconiti is poisonous. When the following reactions occur, caution should be taken: numbness in lips, tongue and extremities and, in some cases, vertigo, vomiting and loose bowels. Toxicosis by Rhizoma Aconiti has the following symptoms: acceleration of respiration and heart beat, with intermittent pulsation or a comatose state. (02-41)

CASES

Case 1 (51-127):

Xu, 47, female, suffered from rheumatic arthritis for two years. Recently, she also suffered from hyperosteogeny of cervical spine.

Symptoms: Rigid neck and severe pain in elbow and shoulders (pain in left shoulder was worse). She could not button her clothes or comb her hair. The patient also had the feeling of cold wind. Tongue was pale, covered with white coating, thick in the center. Pulse was tense-tight and mighty.

Treatment: Decoction of Rhizoma Aconiti was prescribed as follows:

Rhizoma Aconiti	9 grams
Herba Ephedrae	9 grams
Radix Paeoniae Alba	15 grams
Radix Astragali Hedysari	15 grams
Radix Glycyrrhizae Praeparata	15 grams
Ramulus Mori	9 grams
Rhizoma Curcumae Longae	9 grams

Two doses were served. She began to move her extremities more easily and pain subsided. Three doses were served, which alleviated the syndrome. Further treatment was given for ten days to complete the treatment.

Case 2 (46-86):

Mr. Xu, 35, suffered from rheumatoid arthritis, accompanied by pain and cold feeling in joints hampering normal movement. Tongue was covered with thin white coating. Pulse was deep-slender. This syndrome was caused by excessive pathogenetic Cold. Decoction of Rhizoma Aconiti was prescribed:

Rhizoma Aconiti (stew in 30 grams of honey and blend the syrup into the already stewed decoction before service)	10 grams

Herba Ephedrae	3 grams
Radix Paeoniae	10 grams
Radix Astragali Hedysari	10 grams
Radix Glycyrrhizae	3 grams

After three doses were given, extremities became warm and pain subsided.

Second treatment: Same decoction with the following alterations:

Subtract: Herba Ephedrae.

Add: 10 grams of Ramulus Cinnamomi.

Three doses stopped the pain, but the patient could not move his extremities normally.

Third treatment: Decoction of Radix Angelicae Pubescentis and Ramulus Loranthi (*Du Huo Ji Sheng Tang*) was prescribed.

Prescription: Radix Angelicae Pubescentis; Remulus Loranthi; Radix Gentianae Macrophyllae; Radix Ledebouriellae; Herba Asari; Rhizoma Ligustici Chuanxiong; Radix Angelicae Sinensis; Radix Rehmanniae; Radix Paeoniae; Cortex Eucommiae; Radix Achyranthis Bidentatae; Radix Ginseng; Poria; Radix Glycyrrhizae.

Decoction of Alumen is an effective cure for cardiac beriberi.

Decoction of Alumen
(*Fanshi Tang*):

Alumen	2 *liang*

Stew Alumen in one *dou* five *sheng* of *jiangshui* water. Soak the affected feet in this solution.

Appendix:

Prescription from *Records of Present-day and Ancient Proven Prescriptions*:

Decoction of *Xuming*: Efficacious for apoplexy with the following symptoms and signs: difficulty in normal body movements, aphasia, pains in different parts of the body, contraction of extremities which hampers turning the body:

Decoction of *Xuming*
(*Xuming Tang*):

Herba Ephedrae	3 *liang*
Ramulus Cinnamomi	3 *liang*
Radix Angelicae Sinensis	3 *liang*
Radix Ginseng	3 *liang*
Gypsum Fibrosum	3 *liang*
Rhizoma Zingiberis	3 *liang*
Radix Glycyrrhizae	3 *liang*
Rhizoma Ligustici Chuanxiong	1 *liang*
Semen Armeniacae Amarum	40 pcs.

Stew drugs in one *dou* of water until four *sheng* remain. Give one *sheng* of warm decoction per dose. Cover the patient's waist with a thin quilt while he leans on a chair. A light perspiration signifies recovery. Further doses can be given if no perspiration is induced. Don't expose the patient to wind. No need to avoid particular foods. This decoction is also efficacious for patients who curl up in bed but do not sleep well, and who suffer from coughing and inspiratory dyspnea and facial swelling.

CASES

Case 1 (65-146):

A gentleman of seventy years suffered rigidity and pain over shoulders, back and sometimes arms. One day he had severe pain and rigidity in the right shoulder. He went to the doctor for a massage. While the doctor was massaging him, he suddenly had difficulty speaking and had hemiplegia on the right side of the body.

Diagnosis: The patient did not seem to suffer from any other disease as he could still eat normally. But pulse was grand and excessive.

Treatment: Decoction of *Xuming* was given. After taking the decoction, the patient resumed his speaking ability and hemiplegia subsided. After more decoctions were given, he was able to walk with a cane.

Case 2 (65-147):

A lady of plump build, 57, had apoplexy, fell to the ground and lost consciousness. She lay rigid, unable to speak, with clenched teeth. Pulse was floating-huge-slippery tight, more so on the right. Three grams of Powder of Radix Vertatrum Nigrum blended with powder of Moschus were blown into the nasal cavity, which revived the patient. She vomited phlegm. She could then move. Decoction of *Xuming* was served with a double dosage of Herba Ephedrae. Another dose was given after a short interval. The patient was covered with a quilt and perspiration induced, which enabled her to feel better. She could not move the right arm and leg, with logopathy.

Second treatment: Decoction of *Er Chen* with additions was prescribed:

Radix Pinelliae Praeparata
Pericarpium Citri Reticulatae
Poria
Radix Glycyrrhizae Praeparata
Fructus Mume
Rhizoma Ligustici Chuanxiong
Radix Angelicae Sinensis
Rhizoma seu Radix Noto-pterygii
Radix Ledebouriellae

Juice of ginger and Succus Bambusae were blended into the already-stewed decoction before serving. There was no stool for three or four days and the patient lost her speaking ability. A laxative was given. The patient passed away a few years later from another disease.

Prescription from *Qianjin*:

Decoction of *Sanhuang*: Efficacious for treating apoplexy with contraction of extremities, acute arthralgia in all the joints, restlessness, fever and irritation, aversion to cold and anorexia.

Decoction of *Sanhuang*
(*Sanhuang Tang*):

Herba Ephedrae	5 *fen*
Radix Angelicae Pubescentis	4 *fen*
Herba Asari	2 *fen*
Radix Astragali Hedysari	2 *fen*
Radix Scutellariae	3 *fen*

Stew the drugs in six *sheng* of water until two *sheng* remain. Serve the warm decoction in three doses. The first dose will induce a light perspiration. The second dose will bring on profuse perspiration.

Additions and Subtractions:

1. When symptom of heartburn is observed, add two *fen* of Radix et Rhizoma Rhei;

2. When symptom of abdominal distention is observed, add one piece of Fructus Aurantii Immaturus;

3. When symptom of inspiratory dyspnea is observed, add three *fen* of Radix Ginseng;

4. When palpitation is observed, add three *fen* of Concha Ostreae;

5. When symptom of thirst is observed, add three *fen* of Radix Trichosanthis;

6. When aversion to cold at the initial state of the disease is observed, add one piece of Radix Aconiti Praeparata.

CASES

Case 1 (65-148):

A gentleman was attacked by apoplexy. Symptoms: distortion of eyes and mouth, logopathy, salivation, hemiplegia and difficulty in moving the body.

Diagnosis: The patient was weak and exposed to harmful climatic factors. Over-indulgence in sex and wine worsened the syndrome.

A prescription based on Decoction of *Sanhuang* was given. Ingredients included:

Herba Ephedrae
Rhizoma seu Radix Noto-pterygii
Herba Asari
Radix Scutellariae
Radix Ginseng
Radix Ledebouriellae
Rhizoma Cimicifugae
Radix Platycodi
Gypsum Fibrosum
Herba Schizonepetae
Rhizoma Gastrodiae
Rhizoma Arisaematis
Herba Menthae
Radix Puerariae
Radix Paeoniae Rubra

Semen Armeniacae Amarum
Rhizoma Ligustici Chuanxiong
Radix Angelicae Sinensis
Rhizoma Atractylodis Macrocephalae
Fructus Gleditsiae Sinensis
Rhizoma Zingiberis Recens
Caulis Allii Fistulosi
Succus Bambusae (blend into the already-stewed decoction before serving)

Acupuncture points: Fengshi (GB 31), Baihui (DU 20) Quchi (LI 11), Huantiao (GB 30), Jianyu (LI 15), Zusanli (ST 36)

Prescription from *Prescriptions with Ready Efficacy*:

Decoction of Rhizoma Atractylodis Macrocephalae and Radix Aconiti Praeparata: Efficacious for curing Wind-deficient syndrome* with severe vertigo, anorexia and sense of heaviness in movement. This prescription tonifies the Interior Vital Energy, warms the muscle and strengthens the Essence and Vital Energy (*Jing Qi*).

Decoction of Rhizoma Atractylodis Macrocephalae and Radix Aconiti Praeparata (*Zhu Fu Tang*):

Rhizoma Atractylodis Macrocephalae	2 *liang*
Radix Aconiti Praeparata	1.5 pcs.
Radix Glycyrrhizae Praeparata	1 *liang*

Pound the drugs into powder. Stew five *qianbi* in one and a half cups of water with five slices of Rhizoma Zingiberis Recens and one piece of Fructus Ziziphi Jujubae until seven *fen* remain. Filter the decoction and serve warm.

*Wind-deficient syndrome, *Fengxu*, is caused by Deficiency of the Yang Vital Energy at the lower part of the body, which will allow pathogenetic Wind to enter the upper part of the body (the head). (01-57)

CASES

Case 1 (65-149): Case Recorded in Journal of *Liaoning Chinese Medicine*, 2:11, 1980

Wu, 43, female, was suffering from vertigo with repeated attacks. At onset of the disease, the patient could only lie in bed quietly. Whenever she moved, she had a feeling of sea sickness and could lose consciousness. One day while being examined on the diagnostic couch, the doctor accidentally struck the patient's pillow. She experienced severe vertigo and almost lost consciousness. The patient was of plump build and had aversion to cold. Her pulse was deep-feeble at the time of examination.

Diagnosis: This syndrome was caused by Deficiency of Yang in Spleen and Kidney.

Treatment: Decoction of Rhizoma Atractylodis Macrocephalae and Radix Aconiti Praeparata was prescribed:

Radix Aconiti Praeparata	15 grams
Rhizoma Atractylodis Macrocephalae	9 grams
Radix Glycyrrhizae Praeparata	6 grams

One dose of the decoction was served to observe the effect.

Second treatment: The first dose of the decoction worked. Three more doses of the decoction were given.

After that, vertigo subsided. Then Pills of Eight Ingredients (see the clause below) were given to complete the treatment.

Pills of Eight Ingredients:* Efficacious in treating abdominal disorders caused by upward invasion of beriberi.**

Pills of Eight Ingredients
(*Cuishi Bawei Wan*):

Radix Rehmanniae	8 *liang*
Fructus Corni	4 *liang*
Rhizoma Dioscoreae	4 *liang*
Rhizoma Alismatis	3 *liang*
Poria	3 *liang*
Cortex Moutan Radicis	3 *liang*
Ramulus Cinnamomi	1 *liang*
Radix Aconiti Praeparata	1 *liang*

Pound the drugs into powder. Make pills with honey (Mel) the size of Chinese parasol seeds. Take fifteen pills with wine per dose two times per day.

*The original text reads: Pills of Eight Ingredients of Dr. Cui (*Cuishi Bawei Wan*). According to some annotators, this prescription was originally found in a collection of prescriptions edited by Cui Zhiti. But this prescription was quoted from Zhang Zhongjing's treatise. Thus later scholars called this prescription "Pills of Kidney Vital Energy from *Jinkui*" (*Jinkui Shenqi Wan*). (01-58)

**For efficacy of the drug, see "Explanation of the Prescription."

Explanation of the Prescription: This prescription treats syndromes with Deficiency of both the Kidney Yang and Yin. Radix Aconiti Praeparata and Ramulus Cinnamomi (according to other annotators, Cortex Cinnamomi) tonify the Kidney Yang Vital Energy. The other six drugs tonify the Kidney Yin Vital Essence. Efficacy includes treatment of chronic nephritis, diabetes millitus, lumbago caused by Deficiency of the Kidney Vital Energy, impotence, and involuntary seminal discharge. It is also effective in treating beriberi caused by Deficiency of the Kidney Vital Energy. (01-58)

CASES

Case 1 (48-421): Case Recorded in *Cases of Dr. Pu Fuzhou*

Mr. Zhang, 86, first treatment on April 25, 1960.

Symptoms: Pain and soreness over back and lumbar region, cold legs, frequent and scanty urine, constipation, bitter and parched mouth, tongue pale and dry, free from coating. Pulse on the right wrist was grand but strengthless; pulse on the left was deep-slender and strengthless.

Diagnosis: Syndrome was caused by the Deficiency of both Yin and Yang, insufficient Water and Fire.

Treatment: Warm the Kidney Yang, moisten and nourish the Kidney Yin. Pills of Eight Ingredients were prescribed (in decoction form):

Rhizoma Rehmanniae Praeparata	9 grams
Poria	6 grams
Rhizoma Dioscoreae	6 grams
Cortex Eucommiae (prepared with salt water)	9 grams
Rhizoma Alismatis	4.5 grams
Radix Aconiti Praeparata	3 grams
Cortex Cinnamomi (prepared with salt water)	1.5 grams
Radix Achyranthis Bidentatae	6 grams
Fructus Psoraleae	9 grams
Honey (blend in the already stewed decoction before service)	30 grams

Second treatment: After three doses of decoction, all the symptoms subsided. Three additional doses were prescribed.

Third treatment: The patient received an examination by a Western physician diagnosed as suffering from hypertrophy of prostate. Accompanying symptoms were frequent urination, slight pain over lumbar region and general lassitude. Pills of Eight Ingredients were prescribed again (in pill form):

Rhizoma Rehmanniae Praeparata	90 grams
Fructus Corni	30 grams
Rhizoma Dioscoreae	60 grams
Rhizoma Alismatis	30 grams
Radix Aconiti Praeparata	30 grams
Cortex Cinnamomi	18 grams
Radix Achyranthis Bidentatae	30 grams
Fructus Psoraleae	60 grams
Semen Cuscutae	60 grams
Radix Morindae Officinalis	30 grams

Grind the above drugs into powder and blend with honey to make pills of nine grams each. Serve one pill every night. Every morning serve one spoonful syrup of mulberry fruit (Fructus Mori). Two doses of the pills (with syrup) were served in succession. The patient had recovery which lasted at least five years.

Case 2 (48-423): Diabetes Insipidus (Doctor: Zhang Dechao)

Mr. Xu, 32, suffered thirst and frequent urination for three years. He was diagnosed, in a hospital, as having diabetes insipidus. He drank five thermos of water and urinated more than twenty times within twenty-four hours. Urine was plenty and clear. He also had lumbago and weak knees. Pulse was slender-small and strengthless and pulse at Cubit position was too deep and slender to detect. Tongue was covered with pale, white, dry coating.

Diagnosis: Deficiency of Kidney made it difficult for the Body Fluid to ascend, causing thirst, and the Kidney lost control of Water circulation, causing frequent urination.

Treatment: Pills of Eight Ingredients were prescribed (in decoction form):

Radix Aconiti Praeparata	4.5 grams
Cortex Cinnamomi	2.4 grams
Rhizoma Rehmanniae Praeparata	15 grams
Rhizoma Dioscoreae	12 grams
Fructus Corni	9 grams
Poria	9 grams
Cortex Moutan Radicis	4.5 grams

Rhizoma Alismatis	9 grams
Semen Cuscutae	9 grams
Ootheca Mantidis	9 grams

Five doses were given. Symptoms subsided. One month of such treatment alleviated the ailment.

Case 3 (48-424): Sterility (Doctor: Yue Meizhong)

Mr. Pei in his twenties. His wife was infertile. When Mr. Pei had a semen examination, he was told that he had asthenospermia (insufficient sperm activity). Pulse on both Cubit positions was weak. No other diseases were found. Pills of Eight Ingredients were prescribed and the doctor told the patient to take them over a long period of time. Six months later the patient reported that his wife was pregnant. The couple had three children later.

Case 4 (48-425): Case Recorded in Journal of *Jiangsu Chinese Medicine*, Vol. 9, 1965

Mr. Liu, 43, was suffering from dropsy of head, face and extremities. Other symptoms: emission, impotence, soreness and coldness of waist and legs, disabled feet, diarrhea occurring at early morning, tongue swollen and tender. Pulse was deep-slow. The disease lasting more than fifty days was diagnosed as chronic nephritis.

Diagnosis: Edema of Yin nature, to be treated with Pills of Eight Ingredients as follows:

Poria	15 grams
Rhizoma Rehmanniae Praeparata	9 grams
Rhizoma Dioscoreae	9 grams
Fructus Corni	9 grams
Radix Aconiti Praeparata	15 grams
Cortex Cinnamomi	6 grams
Semen Plantaginis	6 grams
Cortex Moutan Radicis	6 grams
Rhizoma Zingiberis Praeparata	3 grams
Radix Achyranthis Bidentatae	9 grams

Sixteen doses were given. The syndrome was gone. Drugs harmonizing the Spleen and Stomach were given to complete the treatment.

Case 5 (48-425): Coughing and Asthma

Shen, 64, female, had vertigo and dim vision that kept her in bed. She coughed, panted and spat dense phlegm, had shortness of breath and chest distress. Other symptoms: No appetite, sporadic fever, trance, dry lips and oral cavity. Tongue was covered with white, dry coating. Pulse was soft-slender slippery.

Diagnosis: *Tanyin* Fluid-retention syndrome (see Chapter XII).

Treatment: Warm the Yang, disperse the retention and regulate the Vital Energy.

Prescription:

Radix Aconiti Praeparata	9 grams
Cortex Cinnamomi	3 grams
Fructus Corni	6 grams
Rhizoma Rehmanniae Praeparata	9 grams
Rhizoma Pinelliae (prepared with ginger)	9 grams
Cortex Mori Radicis	9 grams
Pericarpium Citri Reticulatae	6 grams
Semen Armeniacae Amarum	9 grams

In the first treatment two doses were given. Another six doses achieve a full recovery.

Case 6 (48-426): Case Recorded in Journal of *Jiangsu Medicine and Pharmacology*, Vol. 10, 1975

Ten cases of leukorrhea were cured by adoption of Pills of Eight Ingredients:

Prescription:

Radix Rehmanniae	12 grams
Rhizoma Dioscoreae	9 grams
Fructus Corni	9 grams
Rhizoma Alismatis	6 grams
Poria	9 grams
Cortex Moutan Radicis	6 grams
Cortex Cinnamomi	2.4 grams
Radix Aconiti Praeparata	6 grams
Herba Cistanchis	9 grams
Semen Cuscutae	9 grams
Rhizoma Cibotii	9 grams

All ten cases ended in recovery after eight doses of decoction. There was one of the cases:

Zhang, 42, married, suffered from leukorrhea for ten years. Recently, leukorrhea was profuse. Pulse was soft-slender, with Cubit position deep-slow. The patient had dark complexion and was emaciated. Tongue was pale, covered with thin coating. Stool was watery and urine clear. Pain and coldness in lower abdomen.

Diagnosis: Leukorrhea was caused by the Cold and deficient state of the Kidney, which should be warmed and tonified.

Prescription above was given.

Six doses were served at first. The syndrome was almost gone. Eight more doses, followed by Pills of Eight Ingredients for a month, brought full recovery.

Prescription from *Qianjin*:

Decoction of *Yuebei* adding Rhizoma Atractylodis Macrocephalae, efficacious for syndromes with the following symptoms and signs: Exhaustion of muscles,* fever with profuse perspiration which exhausts Body Fluid and opens the *Couli*, invasion of pathogenetic Wind, weakness in the feet.

Decoction of *Yuebei*** adding Rhizoma Atractylodis Macrocephalae (*Yuebei Jia Zhu Tang*):

Herba Ephedrae	6 *liang*
Gypsum Fibrosum	0.5 *jin*
Rhizoma Zingiberis Recens	3 *liang*
Radix Glycyrrhizae	2 *liang*
Rhizoma Atractylodis Macrocephalae	4 *liang*
Fructus Ziziphi Jujubae	15 pcs.

Stew Herba Ephedrae in six *sheng* of water. Filter the decoction and add other drugs. Stew again until three *sheng* remain. Serve the decoction warm in three doses. When the patient is sensitive to wind, add one piece of Radix Aconiti Praeparata.

*Exhaustion of muscles: Muscles are extraordinarily feeble.

**Decoction of *Yuebei*: See Clause 14-23.

CASES

Case 1 (65-151):

Mr. Chen, 25, tailor, treated by Dr. Zhao Shouzhen. Mr. Chen visited his relatives in the neighboring village the previous month and was caught in the rain on his way home. As soon as he got home, he changed the wet clothes. Three days later, he began to have fever, chill, headache, pain over the whole body, heaviness in moving. Diaphoretics were given, inducing slight perspiration. He stopped taking the medicine before a complete recovery. A few days later, he began to have dropsy over the whole body. Other symptoms: aversion to wind, difficulty in moving, parched feeling in mouth and tongue, floating-tense pulse.

Diagnosis: This was first caused by invasion of Cold-Humidity factors. After improper treatment, the Humidity was accumulated to evolve into Heat.

Treatment should be directed to disperse the Cold-Humidity by inducing a perspiration. Decoction of *Yuebei* adding Rhizoma Atractylodis Macrocephalae was the cure.

CHAPTER VI

ON PULSE, SYMPTOM COMPLEX AND TREATMENT OF ARTHRALGIA DUE TO STAGNATION OF BLOOD AND CONSUMPTIVE DISEASES

CLAUSE 6-1

Question: What is the cause of arthralgia due to stagnation of Blood (1)?

Master: Persons who live lives of leisure generally have weak bones and rich flesh and muscle. After working for a short period of time, they will feel tired and begin to sweat. When they lie in bed, they will toss and turn frequently. If they are exposed to a breeze at this time, they will suffer from arthralgia due to stagnation of Blood. The pulse will be feeble and hesitant and slender-tense at Inch and Bar (2). Acupuncture therapy can be adopted to stimulate Yang Vital Energy (3). When the tense pulse disappears and the pulse returns to normal, the patient is recovering.

NOTES

1. Arthralgia due to stagnation of Blood (*Xuebi*) as discussed in this chapter is a form of arthralgia which has as its main symptom local numbness in the extremities. It is caused by exposure to exogenous climatic factors when the patient is suffering from Deficiency in both the Vital Energy and the Blood. (02-44)

2. Feeble pulse indicates feeble Yang Vital Energy; hesitant pulse indicates stagnation of Blood; tense pulse indicates existence of pathogenetic Wind and Cold. Slender-tense pulse at Inch and Bar signifies that the pathogenetic factors have not penetrated deep into the Interior. (02-44)

3. Stagnation of Blood, the cause of arthralgia, is itself caused by stagnation and obstruction of Yang Vital Energy. Acupuncture therapy can be adopted to stimulate (harmonize) the Yang Vital Energy. When Yang Vital Energy is restored to normal circulation, the disease is cured. (02-44)

CLAUSE 6-2

Arthralgia due to stagnation of Blood with Deficiency in both Yin and Yang has the following symptoms and signs: Pulse feeble at Inch and Bar and slender-tense at Cubit. Exterior symptoms include local numbness and other manifestations of arthralgia due to pathogenetic Wind (1). Decoction of Five Drugs with Radix Astragali Hedysari and Ramulus Cinnamomi will provide a cure.

NOTES

1. Arthralgia due to pathogenetic Wind, *Fengbi*, is a form of arthralgia with symptoms of muscle numbness and pain. (01-61)

Decoction of Five Drugs with Radix Astragali Hedysari and Ramulus Cinnamomi (*Huangqi Guizhi Wu Wu Tang*):

Radix Astragali Hedysari	3 *liang*
Radix Paeoniae	3 *liang*
Ramulus Cinnamomi	3 *liang*
Rhizoma Zingiberis Recens	6 *liang*
Fructus Ziziphi Jujubae	12 pcs.

Stew drugs in six *sheng* of water until two *sheng* remain. Serve seven *ge* of lukewarm decoction per dose three times a day. (According to another edition, prescription includes Radix Ginseng).

Explanation of the Prescription: Zhou Yangjun: Radix Astragali Hedysari stabilizes the Vital Resistance. Radix Paeoniae tonifies the Yin Vital Essence. Ramulus Cinnamomi harmonizes the Nutrient Essence with the Vital Resistance by aiding the Interior Vital Energy in dispersing the pathogenetic factors. Rhizoma Zingiberis Recens is added to activate the Stomach Vital Energy. Fructus Ziziphi Jujubae tonifies the Spleen. (05-497)

Jinkui E: Radix Astragali Hedysari has the function of activating the Yang Vital Energy, eases Blood circulation and disperses numbness. Ramulus Cinnamomi and Radix Paeoniae promote Blood circulation and remove stasis. Rhizoma Zingiberis Recens and Fructus Ziziphi Jujubae harmonize the Nutrient Essence with the Vital Resistance. Since arthralgia due to stagnation of

Blood is an Exterior syndrome, a strong dose of Rhizoma Zingiberis Recens is given to activate the Vital Energy, enabling it to disperse the pathogenetic factors in the Exterior. When Vital Energy flows normally, the Blood will not stagnate, and the syndrome disappears. (01-61)

CASES

Case 1 (46-95): Periarthritis of Shoulder

Mr. Song, 52, suffered from periarthritis of the shoulder. There was distention and pain over the right shoulder and back, soreness and numbness of the right arm. Normal movement was hampered. Tongue was covered with thin, white coating. Pulse was moderate and weak.

Diagnosis: Syndrome caused by weakness and Deficiency of the Nutrient Essence and Body Resistance, and obstruction of normal flow of Vital Energy and Blood.

Treatment: Decoction of Five Drugs with Radix Astragali Hedysari and Ramulus Cinnamomi.

Prescription:

Radix Astragali Hedysari	15 grams
Ramulus Cinnamomi	10 grams
Radix Paeoniae Alba	10 grams
Rhizoma Zingiberis Recens	3 slices
Fructus Ziziphi Jujubae	3 pcs.
Rhizoma Curcumae Longae	5 grams

Five doses were given, accompanied by acupuncture therapy. Ache and distention subsided.

Second treatment: Ten doses of the same decoction (subtracting Rhizoma Curcumae Longae) were given to complete the treatment.

Case 2 (65-156):

A lady of thirty-eight suffered from numbness with pain in both arms. The ailment made her unable to sleep. Pulse was tense-slender and hesitant when pressed deeply. Tongue was pale, covered with white coating.

Diagnosis: Syndrome was caused when the patient was weak and exposed to climatic pathogenetic factors.

Treatment: Decoction of Five Drugs with Radix Astragali Hedysari and Ramulus Cinnamomi with additions was prescribed as follows:

Radix Astragali Hedysari	24 grams
Ramulus Cinnamomi	9 grams

Radix Paeoniae Alba	12 grams
Rhizoma Zingiberis Recens	12 grams
Fructus Ziziphi Jujubae	6 pcs.
Ramulus Mori	30 grams
Radix Gentianae Macrophyllae	9 grams
Radix Angelicae Sinensis	12 grams

Second treatment: Three doses relieved the condition. Seven more doses were given.

Third treatment: After second treatment, the syndrome was gone.

Fourth treatment: Six doses were given with alterations:

Add nine grams of Rhizoma Ligustici Chuanxiong.

Reduce dosage of Ramulus Cinnamomi to six grams.

In the following year, no recurrence was reported.

CLAUSE 6-3

A man (1) who looks healthy but has a huge pulse is suffering from a consumptive disease (general debility). When the pulse is extremely deficient, it also indicates a consumptive disease. (2)

NOTES

1. "Man" here indicates a male patient, as this chapter covers diseases which generally affect male patients.

2. This clause discusses the different pulses of consumptive diseases. Huge and extremely deficient pulses reflect the exhaustion and Deficiency of the Kidney. When Yin Vital Essence is insufficient, deficient Yang Vital Energy flows outward, a phenomenon reflected by a huge pulse, or huge-void pulse. While the Yang Congenital Vital Energy is deficient, this is reflected by an extremely deficient pulse, sometimes deep and slow, sometimes tense. (02-45)

CLAUSE 6-4

Pallid facial complexion in a male patient indicates thirst (1) and loss of Blood. When the patient suddenly feels like gasping and exhibits palpitations and a floating pulse, he is suffering from Interior Deficiency (2).

NOTES

1. Thirst caused by an insufficiency of Body Fluid. (01-62)

2. *Jinjian*, p. 499, states that the following clause "... and a floating

pulse, he is suffering from Interior Deficiency'' is a redundancy due to miscopying.

Commentary: Wu Qian: this clause states the cause of a pallid facial complexion. When a pallid facial complexion is not caused by epistaxis (loss of Blood), then it is a case of insufficiency of the Blood owing to a failure of reproducing the Blood. When it is caused by epistaxis, it is a case of loss of Blood. A pallid, lusterless facial complexion indicates an insufficiency of Blood. In such cases, thirst due to an insufficiency of the Body Fluid will result. Gasping occurs with a Deficiency in the Vital Energy; palpitations appear with a Deficiency of the Blood. (05-499)

CLAUSE 6-5

Consumptive diseases of male patients bear the following symptoms and signs: Pulse is deficient, deep and tight (1), with shortness of breath, abdominal contraction, dysuria, pallid facial complexion, abdominal distention, epistaxis and occasional reluctance to open the eyes (2). But the patient does not feel cold and feverish (3).

NOTES

1. Deficient, deep and tight pulse reflects Interior Deficiency, or Deficiency of both the Vital Energy and the Blood. (01-62)
2. Reluctance to open the eyes: In another version, "dimness in vision caused by vertigo."
3. But the patient does not feel cold and feverish: He is not suffering from Exterior syndrome (Initial Yang syndrome).

CLAUSE 6-6

Consumptive disease: The pulse is floating-huge, with burning sensation on palms of hands and feet. The disease becomes aggravated in spring and summer but subsides in autumn and winter. Seminal emission occurs due to Yin and Cold (1). Weak and emaciated legs make the patient unable to walk. (2)

NOTES

1. Cheng Lin: "Yin and Cold" should be understood as "Yin and Defi-

ciency." When Yin and Deficiency prevail, Vital Energy goes out of control and emission occurs. (05-498)

2. Explanation by Li Wen: Floating-huge pulse indicates outward dispersion of Vital Energy when Interior Deficiency prevails. The four extremities are Yang; thus when consumptive disease consumes the Yang, Deficiency in Yin nature will produce Interior Heat, which is reflected in the burning sensation on palms of hands and feet. Consumptive diseases generally belong to the category of Yin and Deficiency. In spring and summer, Yang Vital Energy prevails and tends to flow outward, causing the Interior to become more deficient and aggravating the case. In autumn and winter, the Vital Energy tends to conceal itself in the Interior, and the case will therefore be relatively less severe. The Kidney stores the Essence (including the congenital Essence and acquired Essence). When the patient is in a deficient state, the Kidney cannot control the emission of semen. As the Kidney regulates the bones, the legs are weak and emaciated when Deficiency prevails. (05-498)

CLAUSE 6-7

If the pulse of a male patient is floating-weak and hesitant, this indicates a case of sterility, as the seminal fluid is thin and cold. (1)

NOTES

1. Shen Mingzong: This clause deals with diagnosing sterility through judging the pulse. Fetus forms when both the male's sperm and female's blood are in a strong and normal state. When the sperm is strong and healthy, the pulse will also be strong and steady. Floating pulse indicates a case of Yin and deficient state; weak pulse indicates an insufficiency of congenital Yang; hesitant pulse exhibits exhaustion of the Vital Essence. Thus, this is a case with insufficiency of Yin, Yang and the Vital Essence. Thus the seminal fluid is thin and cold, resulting in sterility. (02-47)

CASES

Case 1 (65-162): Sterility Due to Kidney Deficiency

Mr. Kang, 28, first treatment on October 3, 1972. The patient and his wife, married five years, had no children. His wife was diagnosed as normal. Mr. Kang's diagnosis was male sterility due to azoospermia. The patient reported normal sex appeal. He was of thin build, had vertigo, soreness and lassitude over lumbar region and legs.

Diagnosis: This was a case of Deficiency of both Kidney Yin and Yang, needed to be tonified.

Treatment: A decoction was given to tonify and warm the Kidney, nourish

the Vital Essence and Blood. The patient told to restrain sexual activity.
Prescription:

Radix Aconiti Praeparata	9 grams
Cortex Cinnamomi (grind into powder, blend in the already-stewed decoction before service)	3 grams
Actinolitum	12 grams
Cornu Cervi Pantotrichum (blend in the already-stewed decoction before service)	1 gram
Placenta Hominis (blend in the already-stewed decoction before service)	3 grams
Rhizoma Rehmanniae Praeparata	12 grams
Radix Ophiopogonis	9 grams
Fructus Lycii	12 grams
Radix Morindae Officinalis	12 grams
Fructus Corni	9 grams
Semen Cuscutae	15 grams
Radix Achyranthis Bidentatae	9 grams

One dose of the decoction every day and Pills of *Guilingji* (a general tonic) were given. Two months later, he reported some improvement. The doctor prescribed the decoction with minor alterations. Treatment lasted several months until another sperm examination in May 1973 showed it had reached normal level. The patient looked energetic and vigorous. The medication was discontinued. Later the same year, his wife became pregnant.

CLAUSE 6-8

A patient suffering from frequent seminal emissions is also troubled by the following ailment: Abdominal contraction, cold over glans penis, vertigo and baldness. When pulse is extremely deficient and void-slow, this indicates diarrhea with undigested cereals, and loss of blood and sperm. Void, moving, or feeble and tense pulse indicates seminal emission for the male patient or dreaming of sexual intercourse for the female patient. Decoction of Ramulus Cinnamomi adding Os Draconis and Concha Ostreae can provide a cure.

Decoction of Ramulus Cinnamomi adding Os Draconis and Concha Ostreae*
(*Guizhi Jia Longgu Muli Tang*):

Ramulus Cinnamomi	3 *liang*
Radix Paeoniae	3 *liang*
Rhizoma Zingiberis Recens	3 *liang*
Radix Glycyrrhizae	2 *liang*
Fructus Ziziphi Jujubae	12 pcs.
Os Draconis	3 *liang*
Concha Ostreae	3 *liang*

Stew drugs in seven *sheng* of water until three *sheng* remain. Serve lukewarm in three doses.

**Xiao Pin Fang*, a collection of prescriptions by Chen Yanzhi, contains the annotation for this prescription: "When the patient is feverish with perspiration due to Deficiency and weakness, subtract Ramulus Cinnamomi and add three *fen* each of Radix Cynanchi Atrati and Radix Aconiti Praeparata."

Explanation of the Prescription: Decoction of Ramulus Cinnamomi is effective in dispersing the pathogenetic factors from the muscle to eliminate the Exterior syndrome, in tonifying the Interior Deficiency, and in harmonizing the Vital Energy with the Blood. Os Draconis and Concha Ostreae are added as an astringent to stop the emission. (01-63)

CASES

Case 1 (65-164):

A boy of 17 had nocturnal emission and spat blood whenever he contracted a cold.

Diagnosis: Syndrome caused by Fire stored in the Kidney. It tended to induce invasion of pathogenetic Wind to the Liver. When the Liver was in trouble, emission and spitting of blood occurred.

Treatment: Decoction of Ramulus Cinnamomi adding Os Draconis and Concha Ostreae was prescribed. In this prescription, Decoction of Ramulus Cinnamomi was designed to harmonize the Nutrient Essence and disperse the pathogenetic factors. Os Draconis and Concha Ostreae were added to tranquilize the Liver function and pacify the disturbed soul. Four doses of the decoction cured the ailment.

Case 2 (65-164): Dreaming of Sexual Intercourse, Case Recorded in Journal of *New Chinese Medicine*, 4:29, 1980

Li, 24, married woman, had an abortion six months ago with profuse loss of blood. She often had vertigo, tinnitus, anorexia and excessive leukorrhea. A month after, she dreamed of sexual intercourse, which lasted the whole night.

This occurred repeatedly. The next morning, she would have severe fatigue and trance. She consulted the doctor, accompanied by her husband.

Examination: Pallid complexion, emaciated build, low spirit, faint voice, vertigo, dim vision, tinnitus, palpitation, weak limbs, poor appetite, profuse leukorrhea of white, non-smelly and clear discharge, retarded menstruation with scanty and thin discharge and falling hair, tongue covered with thin, white coating, pale lips, deep-slender pulse.

Diagnosis: Symptoms suggested weakness and Deficiency due to loss of blood. Loss of blood (loss of Yin) caused Yang Deficiency. When both were deficient she lost control of mental activity and dreams of sexual intercourse occurred.

Treatment: Decoction of Ramulus Cinnamomi adding Os Draconis and Concha Ostreae combined with Decoction of *Guipi* was prescribed:

Ramulus Cinnamomi	9 grams
Radix Paeoniae Alba	12 grams
Fructus Ziziphi Jujubae	12 pcs.
Rhizoma Zingiberis Recens	10 grams
Os Draconis	30 grams
Concha Ostreae	30 grams
Radix Glycyrrhizae Praeparata	9 grams
Radix Astragali Hedysari	30 grams
Radix Codonopsis Pilosulae	30 grams
Rhizoma Atractylodis Macrocephalae	12 grams
Radix Polygalae	9 grams
Semen Ziziphi Spinosae	15 grams
Cinnabaris (wash down with the decoction)	6 grams

Eleven doses of the decoction were given. Dreams faded, appetite and complexion improved. Her lassitude, fatigue in extremities and leukorrhea remained.

Second treatment: Six doses of the original decoction were given with the following additions:

Semen Coicis	18 grams
Flos Celosiae Gristatae Alba	30 grams

Ailment was totally cured.

Case 3 (65-165): Enuresis (Involuntary Discharge of Urine)

A patient of eighteen had involuntary discharge of urine for several years and had been treated by different doctors.

Diagnosis: The patient was suffering Cold and Deficiency at Lower Portion of Body Cavity, with clear urination and cold feeling when urinating. There was a jumping feeling under the umbilicus. He was mentally distressed. Coldness of feet was reported. This was a case of Cold nature.

Treatment: Decoction of Ramulus Cinnamomi adding Os Draconis and Concha Ostreae combined with Pills of Eight Ingredients was given. A few days of treatment reduced the trouble. Six months later the syndrome was gone.

Case 4 (51-145):

Mr. Li, 29, masturbated frequently when young and had an active sex life when married. He had lumbago, general lassitude, which developed into insomnia, nocturnal emission in dream of sex. He had vertigo and tinnitus, shortness of breath, palpitation and easy perspiration. Tongue was pale-red with little coating. Pulse was moving and shaking when pressed slightly and became feeble and tense when pressed deeply. Drugs of Yin-tonification and warm quality had been taken, but did not help.

Diagnosis: This syndrome could be treated by Decoction of Ramulus Cinnamomi adding Os Draconis and Concha Ostreae.

Prescription:

Ramulus Cinnamomi	9 grams
Radix Paeoniae Alba	15 grams
Radix Glycyrrhizae Praeparata	9 grams
Os Draconis	15 grams
Concha Ostreae	15 grams
Rhizoma Zingiberis Recens	3 slices
Fructus Ziziphi Jujubae	10 pcs.
Poria	15 grams
Flos Albiziae	9 grams

Fifteen doses of decoction cured the ailment.

Case 5 (64-215): Case Recorded in Journal of *Jiangsu Chinese Medicine,* 3:13, 1981

Mr. Zhou, 37, first treatment in August 1976. The patient had falling hair seven or eight years ago and his forehead was bald. He had bitterness in mouth, red tongue with slightly purple edge covered by yellow, greasy coating. Pulse was slender-tight.

Treatment: Decoction of Ramulus Cinnamomi adding Os Draconis and Concha Ostreae was given:

Ramulus Cinnamomi
Os Draconis
Concha Ostreae

Radix Glycyrrhizae
Fructus Ligustri Lucidi
Herba Ecliptae
Fructus Schisandrae
Cortex Moutan Radicis
Radix Gentianae
Radix Paeoniae Rubra

After five doses of the decoction, hair began to grow. More doses were given. After nine doses, he had almost a full head of hair.

Powder of Rhizoma Aconiti (*Tianxiong*) (*Tianxiong San*):

Rhizoma Aconiti (*Tianxiong*)*	3 *liang*
Rhizoma Atractylodis Macrocephalae	8 *liang*
Ramulus Cinnamomi	6 *liang*
Os Draconis	3 *liang*

Pound the drugs into powder. Take one half *qianbi* with wine three times a day. If not effective, increase the dosage slightly.

*Rhizoma Aconiti (*Tianxiong*), Rhizoma Aconiti (*Wutou*) and Radix Aconiti Praeparata (*Fuzi*) all are drugs taken from the same plant Aconitum Carmichaeli Debx. Radix Aconiti Praeparata is processed from the lateral root, Rhizoma Aconiti (*Wutou*) is the parent root, Rhizoma Aconiti (*Tianxiong*) is the main root that does not bear lateral roots.

Explanation of the Prescription: When Rhizoma Aconiti (*Tianxiong*) and Ramulus Cinnamomi are taken in one decoction, they have the function of tonifying the deficient Yang at the Lower Portion of Body Cavity. Rhizoma Atractylodis Macrocephalae tonifies the Spleen. Os Draconis acts upon the Vital Essence as an astringent to stop the emission. (01-63)

CASES

Case 1 (65-166): Emission

The patient had involuntary emission occasionally. He was given pills made of Powder of Rhizoma Aconiti (*Tianxiong*), which cured the ailment.

Case 2 (65-166): Headache, Case Recorded in Journal of *Guangdong Medicine*,

Chinese Medicine Edition, 6:40, 1964

Mr. Liu, 42, driver, suffered from headache for more than a year. Recently his pain was aggravated with a feeling of emptiness in the head with difficulty in moving the head. He could not eat or sleep normally and was diagnosed as suffering from nervous headache. The prescribed treatment did not help.

Examination: Tongue was pale-red, covered with thin, white and moist coating. Pulse was deep-tight-slender and became strengthless when pressed deeply. Emission was also reported.

Diagnosis: Headache caused by Deficiency in Blood. Decoction of *Bazhen* with additions was prescribed. The decoction did not help.

Second treatment: Treated with Powder of Rhizoma Aconiti (*Tianxiong*) for Deficiency in the Kidney.

Prescription:

Radix Aconiti Praeparata	18 grams
Rhizoma Atractylodis Macrocephalae	24 grams
Ramulus Cinnamomi	18 grams
Os Draconis	18 grams

Blend thirty grams of rice wine into the already-stewed decoction before service.

Third treatment: Three doses of the decoction were served, which reduced the headache. Treatment continued. Headache was completely gone after twenty-three doses of the decoction were consumed.

CLAUSE 6-9

In normal male patients, if pulse is deficient, weak, slender and feeble, he is likely to sweat at night (1).

NOTES

1. The patient is deficient in Yin and Yang, Vital Energy and Blood. Thus the pulse is deficient, weak, slender and feeble. When both Yin and Yang Vital Energy are deficient, the Interior Vital Energy is unstable and likely to emanate in the form of sweat at night. (02-46)

CLAUSE 6-10

The pulse of a patient at the age of fifty or sixty is huge. He has a feeling of numbness in the region along the spine. Consumptive disease will cause borborygmus, and armpit and cervical tubercles. (1)

NOTES

1. You Yi: A patient at the age of fifty or sixty is weak in Vital Essence. When the pulse is huge, it indicates a disease caused by exogenous pathogenetic Wind. Numbness along the spine is caused by invasion of pathogenetic factors when Yang Vital Energy is insufficient. Borborygmus and armpit and cervical tubercles occur when the consumptive disease forces Yang Vital Energy to disperse outward. Thus the exuberant movement of the internal Cold causes the borborygmus. Consumptive disease also causes the ascending pathogenetic Heat to intermingle with the sputum, and forms armpit and cervical tubercles.

CLAUSE 6-11

The pulse of a patient suffering from a consumptive disease is deep-slender-slow. Such cases are called "exhaustion of the Vital Energy" (1). When the patient walks quickly, he begins to pant. Other symptoms include coldness in the extremities (2), abdominal distention, and loose stool caused by indigestion (3).

NOTES

1. Wu Qian: Exhaustion of the Vital Energy (*tuoqi*) occurs when Vital Energy is lacking in the chest, thus hampering breathing. The patient has to pant hard when walking quickly. (05-501)

2. Wu Qian: When there is Deficiency of Yang Vital Energy, Cold prevails, and exuberant Cold will affect the Exterior, causing coldness in the extremities. (05-501)

3. Wu Qian: When pathogenetic Cold is active in the Interior, abdominal distention, loose stool and indigestion will occur. (05-501)

Commentary: This clause gives the pulse and symptoms of Deficiency and exhaustion of both the Spleen and the Kidney Yang Vital Energy. Deep-slender-slow pulse reflects deficient Spleen and Kidney Yang Vital Energy. Ancient scholars suggest that the syndrome be treated with Decoction of *Lizhong** adding Radix Aconiti Praeparata, which serves as a warming agent for the Spleen and the Kidney Yang Vital Energy. (02-47)

*Decoction of *Lizhong*: See *Shanghan Lun*, Clause 386.

CLAUSE 6-12

The pulse is tight and huge. When pressed deeply, it is not as strong as a true tight pulse. Though huge, it is void within. Such pulse is called "void-tight" pulse (1). Tight pulse of reduced strength indicates prevalence of pathogenetic Cold. Void pulse reflects Interior Deficiency. When void-tight pulse occurs in female patients, this indicates premature delivery or mild, chronic bloody vaginal discharge. In male patients, it indicates loss of blood and sperm.

NOTES

1. Void-tight and void pulses are characterized by tight and huge pulses, but are weak, though void-tight pulse is somewhat stronger than void. These two pulses generally appear in severe cases with loss of blood. With loss of blood, Yin Vital Essence is greatly exhausted, and deficient Yang flows outward. This pathological state is reflected by void and void-tight pulse. (02-48)

CLAUSE 6-13

Consumptive disease: Decoction of Lesser *Jianzhong* can be given for the following symptoms and signs: Abdominal contraction, palpitation, epistaxis, abdominal pain, nocturnal emission, weakness and aching in the extremities, burning sensation on palms of hands and feet, parched mouth and throat.

Decoction of Lesser *Jianzhong**
(*Xiao Jianzhong Tang*)

Ramulus Cinnamomi	3 *liang*
Radix Glycyrrhizae Praeparata	2 *liang*
Fructus Ziziphi Jujubae	12 pcs.
Radix Paeoniae	6 *liang*
Rhizoma Zingiberis Recens	3 *liang*
Saccharum Granorum (malt extract)	1 *sheng*

Stew the drugs in seven *sheng* of water until three *sheng* remain. Filter the decoction, add Saccharum Granorum and stew again over slow fire until Saccharum Granorum melts. Serve one *sheng* of lukewarm decoction per dose three times a day.

*This prescription also appears in *Shanghan Lun*, Clause 100.

Remark: People who vomit frequently should not take the decoction, since it is sweet in taste.

Explanation of the Prescription: Jianzhong means literally "building up the Interior Spleen and Stomach Vital Energy." In this prescription, Decoction of Ramulus Cinnamomi tonifies the Deficiency and weakness and harmonizes the Nutrient Essence with the Vital Resistance. A strong dose of Radix Paeoniae is given to aid Ramulus Cinnamomi in treating the syndrome of upper Heat and lower Cold (upper Heat: epistaxis, burning sensation on palms of hands and feet, parched mouth and throat; lower Cold: abdominal contraction and pain, nocturnal emission). Saccharum Granorum, sweet in taste, is the principal ingredient, since sweet tasting drugs have the function of tonifying the Spleen. (01-66)

Appendix:

Decoction of Radix Astragali Hedysari *Jianzhong* (adding two *liang* Radix Ginseng), in Clause 6-14, is also recorded in *Qianjin* with the following commentary:

This prescription is efficacious in treating consumptive diseases in male and female patients having the following symptoms and signs: Owing to accumulation of chronic pathogenetic Cold and stagnation of Vital Energy, or because the patient has not completely recovered from a serious disease, he still suffers from heaviness in the extremities, weakness and aching in bones and muscles, difficulty in breathing, wheezing and fatigue when moving around, a sense of fullness in the chest and a feeling of adverse ascending air, stiffness and pain in the back and the waist, palpitations, parched lips and throat, dark facial and skin complexion, poor appetite, distention in the chest, costal regions and abdomen, difficulty in lifting the head, and preference for lying down. When disease lasts from one hundred days to even a year, the patient becomes thin and weak. When the Vital Energy of the Five Viscera is exhausted, recovery is difficult. Pulses on the Inch, Bar and Cubit of both wrists are deficient and weak, and Deficiency and Cold prevail. The patient feels lack of vitality, with constant abdominal contraction and numerous other diseases of a deficient nature.

CLAUSE 6-14

Consumptive disease with abdominal contraction and symptoms and signs of deficient case can be treated with Decoction of Radix Astragali Hedysari *Jianzhong*.

Decoction of Radix Astragali Hedysari *Jianzhong* (*Huangqi Jianzhong Tang*):

Decoction of Lesser *Jianzhong* adding
Radix Astragali Hedysari 1.5 *liang*

Additions and Subtractions:

1. When fullness in the chest and shortness of breath are observed, add Rhizoma Zingiberis Recens;
2. When abdominal distention is observed, subtract Fructus Ziziphus Jujubae and add 1.5 *liang* of Poria;
3. Add three *liang* of Rhizoma Pinelliae to tonify Vital Energy of deficient Lung.

Explanation of the Prescription: When Radix Astragali Hedysari is added to Decoction of Lesser *Jianzhong*, the decoction can more effectively tonify the Deficiency. In cases of fullness in the chest and shortness of breath, Rhizoma Zingiberis Recens is added to disperse the adverse ascending air. With abdominal distention, Fructus Ziziphi Jujubae, which is sticky in nature, is subtracted since it is not suitable for treating abdominal distention. Poria is then added to raise the light and clear element and reduce murkiness. When Lung is deficient and subsequently causes a cough, Rhizoma Pinelliae is added to eliminate sputum and stop the cough, so as to tonify the Deficiency of the Lung. (01-67)

CASES

Case 1 (64-227):

Zhang, 12-year-old boy, first treatment on August 2, 1978. The boy had abdominal pain for more than two years. Parasiticides and other drugs had been given, but they aggravated the condition.

Examination: The patient was emaciated with pale face, general fatigue and anorexia. There was afternoon fever with discomfort in abdomen and chronic pain around umbilicus. When the abdomen was warmed, the patient felt some comfort. He had soreness and lassitude in the muscles, which was reduced slightly when massaged.

Diagnosis: A consumptive disease. Use of parasiticides consumed the Interior Vital Energy, making the Body Resistance weaker. That caused soreness and lassitude in the muscles. A syndrome of Cold nature needed warmth and a syndrome of deficient nature was relieved when pressed. Pulse was moderate and tongue coating was pale and thin. The symptoms indicated a syndrome of deficient and consumptive type with abdominal trouble.

Treatment: Decoction of Radix Astragali Hedysari *Jianzhong* was prescribed:

Radix Astragali Hedysari	9 grams
Radix Paeoniae Alba	6 grams
Ramulus Cinnamomi	3 grams
Rhizoma Zingiberis Recens	2 grams
Radix Angelicae Sinensis	5 grams
Fructus Ziziphi Jujubae	3 grams
Radix Glycyrrhizae Praeparata	3 grams
Saccharum Granorum	9 grams

Second treatment: Seven doses of the decoction were served. Abdominal pain disappeared. There remained an uncomfortable feeling. Pulse was moderate, tongue covered with thin, white coating. The patient was instructed to continue treatment.

Third treatment: Five more doses alleviated the condition and appetite returned. The parents were instructed to give the boy no cold or uncooked food.

Case 2 (64-277): Case Recorded in Journal of *Shaanxi Chinese Medicine*, 5:34, 1980

Mr. Zou, 45, worker.

Diagnosis: The patient had chronic abdominal pain, no appetite and gastric upset, distention in chest and abdomen that was relieved by eating. There was fatigue, lasstiude and reluctance to speak. Skin was yellowish and withered. Extremities were cold, preferring warmth. Tongue was pale-white. Pulse was deficient-weak.

Treatment: Decoction of Radix Astragali Hedysari *Jianzhong* with alterations was prescribed:

Radix Paeoniae Alba	30 grams
Radix Glycyrrhizae	9 grams
Ramulus Cinnamomi	6 grams
Radix Astragali Hedysari	30 grams
Rhizoma Zingiberis Recens	3 slices

Fructus Ziziphi Jujubae	6 grams
Saccharum Granorum (wash down with the decoction)	45 grams

Case 3 (65-174):

A young girl suffered from fever accompanied by coughing, dyspnea and scanty urination. The syndrome developed into edema, which was cured by drugs expelling excessive fluid. The patient became very thin and weak.

Treatment: Decoction of Radix Astragali Hedysari *Jianzhong* was given one dose per day for thirty days. The patient had full recovery.

CLAUSE 6-15

Consumptive disease with symptoms and signs of lumbago, abdominal contraction and dysuria can be treated with Pills of Eight Ingredients of the Kidney Vital Energy.

For prescription, see "Appendix" to Chapter V.

CLAUSE 6-16

Consumptive disease with symptoms and signs of a deficient case, and all cases caused by exogenous pathogenetic Wind can be treated with Pills of Rhizoma Dioscoreae.

Pills of Rhizoma Dioscoreae
(*Shuyu Wan*):

Rhizoma Dioscoreae	30 *fen*
Radix Angelicae Sinensis	10 *fen*
Ramulus Cinnamomi	10 *fen*
Medicated leaven	10 *fen*
Radix Rehmanniae	10 *fen*
Semen Sojae Germinatum	10 *fen*
Radix Glycyrrhizae	28 *fen*
Radix Ginseng	7 *fen*
Rhizoma Ligustici Chuanxiong	6 *fen*
Radix Paeoniae	6 *fen*
Rhizoma Atractylodis Macrocephalae	6 *fen*
Radix Ophiopogonis	6 *fen*
Semen Armeniacae Amarum	6 *fen*
Radix Bupleuri	5 *fen*

Radix Platycodi	5 *fen*
Poria	5 *fen*
Colla Corii Asini	7 *fen*
Rhizoma Zingiberis	3 *fen*
Radix Ampelopsis	2 *fen*
Radix Ledebouriellae	6 *fen*
Fructus Ziziphi Jujubae (ground into paste)	100 pcs.

Pound the drugs into powder and mix with honey (Mel). Form into bullet-sized pills (the size of an egg yolk). Take one pill with wine before meals. This formula makes one hundred pills.

Explanation of the Prescription: Rhizoma Dioscoreae, the principal ingredient, tonifies the Spleen and Stomach, reinforced by Radix Ginseng, Rhizoma Atractylodis Macrocephalae, Poria, Radix Glycyrrhizae and Fructus Ziziphi Jujubae. The following ingredients nourish the Yin and tonify the Blood: Radix Rehmanniae, Radix Paeoniae, Radix Angelicae Sinensis, Rhizoma Ligustici Chuanxiong, Colla Corii Asini and Radix Ophiopogonis. The above drugs nourish the Yin and tonify the Vital Resistance to regulate the consumptive disease. The following ingredients are added to stimulate circulation of the Vital Energy and normalize its flow, preventing the tonic from being too sticky to function: Medicated leaven, Rhizoma Zingiberis, Radix Platycodi and Radix Ampelopsis. Ramulus Cinnamomi and Rhizoma Zingiberis regulate the normal flow of the Blood and the Vital Energy. Radix Bupleuri, Radix Ledebouriellae and Semen Sojae Germinatum are added to dissipate pathogenetic Wind. When the drug is prepared in pills, it has a prolonged efficacy. Thus the consumptive disease is gradually balanced and the pathogenetic Wind dispersed. (01-68)

CASES

Case 1 (46-106):

Mr. He, 40, suffered from consumptive disease for several years. He coughed and spat phlegm. Accompanying symptoms: Anorexia, emaciation, depression, hot feeling in palms of hands and feet, pale tongue free of coating, and slender-weak pulse. X-ray showed infiltrative pulmonary tuberculosis.

Treatment: it should be directed to replenish the Spleen, regulate Lung function, tonify Vital Energy and nourish the Blood. Pills of Rhizoma Dioscoreae were prescribed:

Radix Codonopsis Pilosulae	15 grams
Rhizoma Atractylodis Macrocephalae	10 grams
Poria	10 grams
Radix Rehmanniae	15 grams
Radix Angelicae Sinensis	10 grams
Radix Paeoniae Alba	10 grams
Radix Ophiopogonis	10 grams
Radix Bupleuri	10 grams
Semen Armeniacae Amarum	10 grams
Radix Platycodi	6 grams
Semen Sojae Germinatum	12 grams
Radix Glycyrrhizae Praeparata	6 grams
Fructus Ziziphi Jujubae	5 pcs.
Carapax Trionycis	15 grams
Radix Stemonae	12 grams
Bulbus Fritillariae Cirhosae	6 grams
Bulbus Lilii	10 grams
Rhizoma Anemarrhenae	6 grams
Cortex Mori Radicis	10 grams

The above drugs were stewed until the decoction was thick. Filtered the dregs and stewed again with additions of the following drugs:

Powder of Rhizoma Dioscoreae	30 grams
Powder of Placenta Hominis	30 grams
Colla Corii Asini	10 grams
Crystal sugar	30 grams
Honey	30 grams

The decoction was ready to serve when it turned to paste.

Served two spoonsful of extract per dose, three times a day. The treatment lasted a year. X-ray showed calcification of focus.

Case 2 (65-178): Case Recorded in Journal of *Harbin Chinese Medicine*, 2:52, 1965

Mr. Tang's daughter, 16, went to a feast in the neighboring village. She ate or drank more than she should and was exposed to cold wind. She began to cough, and had body pain, fever and diarrhea. The next February she was coughing, panting, having anorexia, diarrhea, abdominal pain, fever in the afternoon and pale face. She was weak and thin needing help when moving around. After consultation, she was given tonics such as Radix Ginseng, Radix Astragali

Hedysari, Radix Panacis Quinquefolii. Several doses of tonic were served, but she was worse. The patient had severe cough, insomnia and anorexia. Another doctor prescribed Pills of Rhizoma Dioscoreae in decoction form. Four doses relieved the patient. Another four doses were given. The syndrome was almost gone. The drug was then given in pill form; one pill in the morning, and one in the evening. Treatment continued for a month for full recovery.

Case 3 (55-163): Neurosis

Feng, 36, female teacher, suffered from palpitation, insomnia and vertigo for several years. Accompanying symptoms were tinnitus, fever, night sweat, and trance. She was sensitive and pessimistic, had anorexia, hypomnesia, diarrhea with intestinal booming sound and occasional constipation, general fatigue, delayed menstruation, profuse leukorrhea, and subject to colds. A doctor of Western medicine diagnosed neurosis.

In spring of 1963, the patient received treatment of Chinese medicine. Pills of Rhizoma Dioscoreae were prescribed. In a period of three months, she took 200 pills and recovered.

Case 4 (55-163): Meniere's Disease

Li, 40, female, suffered from consecutive cold after childbirth. She had headache and was treated. After recovering from headache, she had severe vertigo and could not get out of bed. Other symptoms: restlessness, nausea, tinnitus, deafness and anorexia. A doctor of Western medicine diagnosed Miniere's disease, while the TCM doctor said it was vertigo due to an excessive accumulation of phlegm. Both doctors treated the patient according to their respective diagnosis. Nothing seemed to help. The patient could only stay in bed most of the time. She had fatigue and lassitude, wanting to sleep. Sometimes she slept two full days and nights. The patient spat phlegm, had hypomnesia, trance and allophasis.

Pills of Rhizoma Dioscoreae were prescribed. Two months of treatment helped the patient. Treatment continued for two months, and returned the patient to normal.

CLAUSE 6-17

Consumptive disease with restlessness and insomnia can be treated with Decoction of Semen Ziziphi Spinosae.

Decoction of Semen Ziziphi Spinosae*
(*Suanzaoren Tang*):

Semen Ziziphi Spinosae 2 *sheng*

Radix Glycyrrhizae	1 *liang*
Rhizoma Anemarrhenae	2 *liang*
Poria	2 *liang*
Rhizoma Ligustici Chuanxiong	2 *liang*

Stew Semen Ziziphi Spinosae in eight *sheng* of water until six *sheng* remain. Add remaining drugs and stew again until three *sheng* remain. Serve the lukewarm decoction in three doses.

*According to *Prescriptions by Shenshi (Shenshi Fang)*, a collection of recipes from the Sui Dynasty (581-618), two *liang* of Rhizoma Zingiberis Recens are also added.

Explanation of the Prescription: Semen Ziziphi Spinosae has the function of nourishing the Liver, tranquilizing the Heart and eliminating restlessness. Radix Glycyrrhizae and Rhizoma Anemarrhenae are added to eliminate Heat. Poria acts as a general tranquilizer. Rhizoma Ligustici Chuanxiong is added to reinforce Rhizoma Anemarrhenae in eliminating Heat in the head, and acts as a hypnotic. (01-68)

You Yi: When a person is awake, the spirit (mental activity) is located in the eyes. When asleep the spirit is stored in the Liver. Patients suffering consumptive diseases also suffer Deficiency in the Liver Vital Energy. Thus the spirit cannot find a place to rest, resulting in insomnia. Semen Ziziphi Spinosae has the function of tonifying the Liver and acting as an astringent upon the wandering mental activity (spirit). Under such conditions, sputum, Dryness and Fire will find their way into the Interior, causing insomnia. Thus Rhizoma Anemarrhenae and Radix Glycyrrhizae are used to eliminate the Heat and moisten the Dryness, and Poria and Rhizoma Ligustici Chuanxiong are used to dissipate the sputum. This prescription mainly treats an imbalance of the Liver. When the Liver is restored to its normal function, the spirit will resume its proper place and there will be no more insomnia.

CASES

Case 1 (46-107): Neurosthenia

Ma, 45, female patient, suffered from neurosthenia. Symptoms: headache, vertigo, restlessness, insomnia, depression, fatigue, amnesia, blood pressure

130-145/80-90 mm.Hg., red tongue free from coating, tight-slender pulse.

Diagnosis: The syndrome was caused by pathogenetic Heat of deficient Liver. Pathological condition was affecting the Heart (mental activity) causing insomnia and restlessness, etc. Decoction of Semen Ziziphi Spinosae was prescribed:

Semen Ziziphi Spinosae Praeparata	12 grams
Rhizoma Ligustici Chuanxiong	3 grams
Rhizoma Anemarrhenae	10 grams
Poria	10 grams
Radix Glycyrrhizae	5 grams
Ramulus Uncariae cum Uncis	12 grams
Flos Chrysanthemi	10 grams
Fructus Tribuli	10 grams
Radix Rehmanniae	15 grams
Radix Paeoniae Alba	10 grams
Concha Ostreae	15 grams

Ten doses of the decoction were served. There was improvement. Pills of *Tianwang Buxin* were given for a longer period to complete treatment.

Case 2 (52-748): Schizophrenia and Insomnia

Zhang, 28, female worker, went insane due to severe fright. The patient talked nonsense, laughed and cried. She was sent to a mental hospital. Serious insomnia followed. Wintermin, miltown and perphenacine gave the patient only 2-3 hours of sleep every night.

Diagnosis: Pulse was slippery-speedy-slender, tongue red, covered with white and greasy coating. The syndrome was caused by accumulation of phlegm in a Yin-deficiency condition and mal-harmonization of Gall Bladder and Stomach. Combination of Decoction of Semen Ziziphi Spinosae and Decoction of *Wen Dan* was prescribed:

Semen Ziziphi Spinosae Praeparata	18 grams
Rhizoma Anemarrhenae	9 grams
Rhizoma Ligustici Chuanxiong	6 grams
Poria	15 grams
Os Draconis	30 grams
Radix Glycyrrhizae	10 grams
Pericarpium Citri Reticulatae	9 grams
Rhizoma Pinelliae	9 grams
Concha Ostreae	30 grams
Fructus Aurantii	9 grams
Caulis Bambusae	9 grams

Rhizoma Acori Graminei	9 grams
Radix Curcumae	9 grams

Ten doses were served. The patient slept four hours every night. Twelve doses were given in the second treatment, enabling the patient to sleep 6-7 hours at night. Symptoms subsided. Three doses were given to complete treatment.

Case 3 (51-153): Neurosthenia

Mr. Li, 24, had insomnia for years and was diagnosed as suffering from neurosthenia.

Symptoms: Headache, vertigo, daytime sleepiness, awakeful at night, restlessness, bitterness in mouth, red urine, red tongue covered with thin, yellow coating, tight-slender-weak pulse.

Diagnosis: The syndrome was caused by insufficient Yin Blood. Decoction of Semen Ziziphi Spinosae was prescribed to nourish the Yin Blood, clear deficient-Heat, and ease the disturbed spirit.

Prescription:

Semen Ziziphi Spinosae	15 grams
Poria	18 grams
Rhizoma Anemarrhenae	9 grams
Rhizoma Ligustici Chuanxiong	6 grams
Radix Rehmanniae	15 grams
Radix Paeoniae Alba	9 grams
Fructus Gardeniae	6 grams
Cinnabaris (wash down with the decoction)	1.5 grams
Folium Bambusae	4.5 grams

Six doses improved the condition. Nine more doses were given. The patient could then sleep normally. Pills of *Tianwang Buxin* were given, one morning and one at night to complete the treatment.

Case 4 (64-234): Night-walking

A man of 27, accompanied by his parents consulted the doctor in autumn of 1967. His mother told the doctor that for the past ten years, the son often got up at night to clean the house. He dressed, without a word, did not turn on the light, swept the floor, or cleaned the table. When his parents called, he did not answer. After 10-20 minutes, he took off his clothes, went to bed and fell asleep. The next morning when asked why he did this, he said he didn't know anything about it. His parents got used to the practice and let it go. In recent years, he got up almost every night and did a lot of house work. The next day, he could not recall what he did the previous night.

Examination: The patient said he had vertigo and sometimes became restless. The doctor found him indifferent, depressed, quiet with dull eyes. He had never had epilepsy or hysteria. Tip and edge of tongue were red with scant coating. Pulse was slender-tight and slightly speedy.

Diagnosis: The syndrome was caused by insufficiency of the Liver Yin and abnormal ascending of Kidney Vital Energy which impaired the normal condition of the Heart-spirit. Excessive phlegm resulting from impaired Yin disturbed the mental activity, ending in unconscious activities in sleep.

Treatment: Decoction of Semen Ziziphi Spinosae was prescribed:

Semen Ziziphi Spinosae Praeparata	30 grams
Semen Biotae	15 grams
Cortext Albiziae	12 grams
Caulis Polygoni Multiflori	12 grams
Rhizoma Ligustici Chuanxiong	10 grams
Rhizoma Anemarrhenae	12 grams
Poria cum Ligno Hospitae	12 grams
Os Draconis	12 grams
Concha Ostreae	12 grams
Cinnabaris (serve twice, wash down with decoction)	1.5 grams

Second treatment: After five doses, his parents reported improvement. Another five doses were given. The doctor asked his parents to keep close watch.

Third treatment: When the second five doses were consumed, the patient got relief from vertigo and restlessness. His mother reported that his night activities were reduced. Another five doses with minor alterations were given.

Fourth treatment: The patient improved, but not cured. One dose of the decoction was served daily for fifteen days.

Ten months later the mother reported a complete cure after the last 15-day treatment.

CLAUSE 6-18

The patient is extremely feeble and thin and suffers from the five strains (1), with abdominal distention and anorexia. This is caused by unregulated eating and drinking, melancholy, hunger and overexertion in sexual activity or physical labor. Channels and Collaterals, Nutrient Essence, Vital Resistance and Vital Energy are all impaired. In such cases blood stasis will result. The patient's skin is scaly, with rings around the eyes. The therapy aims to harmonize and ease the Interior and tonify the Deficiency. Pills of Radix et Rhizoma Rhei and Eupolyphaga seu Steleophaga is efficacious.

NOTES

1. The five strains: Five factors causing fatigue or overstrain. See note under Clause 1-13.

Pills of Radix et Rhizoma Rhei and Eupolyphaga seu Steleophaga (*Dahuang Zhechong Wan*):

Radix et Rhizoma Rhei (steamed)	10 *fen*
Radix Scutellariae	2 *liang*
Radix Glycyrrhizae	3 *liang*
Semen Persicae	1 *sheng*
Radix Paeoniae	4 *liang*
Radix Rehmanniae	10 *liang*
Lacca Sinica Exsiccatae	1 *liang*
Tabanus	1 *sheng*
Hirudo	100 pcs.
Holotrichia Diomphalia	1 *sheng*
Eupolyphaga seu Steleophaga	0.5 *sheng*

Pound the drugs into powder. Form pills the size of Semen Phaseoli with honey. Take five pills each time with wine three times a day.

Explanation of the Prescription: You Yi: Blood stasis in the Interior will promote further stasis. Thus stasis must be removed as soon as possible. In this prescription, moistening drugs are used to eliminate Dryness. Worms and insects are used to remove the stasis. Radix Rehmanniae, Radix Paeoniae and Radix Glycyrrhizae are used to tonify the Deficiency. In relieving the blood stasis, drugs which tonify the Blood are also used. (05-505)

CASES

Case 1 (51-155): Consumptive Disease Due to Blood Stasis, Case Recorded in *Dr. Ran Xuefeng's Case Studies*

A doctor's daughter of seventeen, suffered consumptive disease due to blood stasis.

Examination: Menstruation suspended for almost a year. Other symptoms:

fever, night sweat, coughing and dyspnea, insomnia, emaciation, scaly skin, distended abdomen, red, dry lips and tongue. Her father had not succeeded in treating the girl. He consulted Dr. Ran. The patient was restless, with tight-deficient-speedy pulse. Speedy pulse, fever and insomnia were three symptoms indicating consumptive disease. The girl had the three symptoms, but, blood stasis was the real cause.

Treatment: The following decoction was prescribed to go with Pills of Radix et Rhizoma Rhei and Eupolyphaga seu Steleophaga:

Radix Paeoniae Alba	18 grams
Radix Angelicae Sinensis	12 grams
Radix Rehmanniae	12 grams
Carapax Trionycis	15 grams
Radix Cynanchi Atrati	9 grams
Radix Asteris	9 grams
Radix Stemonae	9 grams
Radix Glycyrrhizae	3 grams

Ten Pills of Radix et Rhizoma and Eupolyphaga seu Steleophaga were given daily, in two servings with the decoction.

Second treatment: Ten days later, all symptoms had subsided. Another ten doses of the decoction with the following alterations were prescribed to go with the pills:

Subtract: Radix Asteris and Radix Stemonae.

Add: 2.5 grams of Flos Carthami, 2.5 grams of Powder of Succinum.

Third treatment: After ten decoction servings in ten days with the pills, the patient looked better. Decoction of Radix Glycyrrhizae Praeparata (see Appendix of this chapter) was given for a longer period of time. Three months later the girl had returned to good health with a lustrous complexion and healthy build.

Case 2 (64-238): Case Recorded in Journal of *Chinese Medicine*, 9:23, 1965

Mr. Chen, 47, first treatment on February 20, 1965. The patient had paroxysmal lower abdominal pain three days before he was hospitalized. The pain caused an uncomfortable feeling in the upper abdomen and back. He had severe nausea and vomiting, followed by yellow bitter fluid.

The patient was treated in department of Western medicine for a few days until February 25. Doctors of Chinese medicine were invited for consultation.

Examination: The patient was suffering and groaning. There was severe pain with tenderness on the left side of lower abdomen. Palpation showed a hard mass as big as an egg. There was no abdominal distention, no stool for five days, yellow urine, no fever and chill, no thirst. There was repeated retching. Lips and tongue were dark purple, tongue free of coating.

Pulse was tight-slender-hesitant.

Diagnosis: This was a syndrome of intestinal obstruction caused by formation of blood stasis.

Treatment: Pills of Radix et Rhizoma Rhei and Eupolyphaga seu Steleophaga were given to remove the stasis, produce new blood and harmonize the Interior, tonify the overall deficient condition. Two pills (each three grams) per dose, two times a day (morning and evening), were served.

Second treatment on February 26. In the morning the patient had black stool, which was hard at first, then became watery. Abdominal pain subsided significantly.

Third treatment on February 27. The patient could walk by himself in the room. Liquid food was given.

Fourth treatment continued to March 3, when abdominal pain subsided totally. Stool and urine returned to normal. Hard mass could not be palpated.

Appendix:

Prescription from *A Supplement to the Prescriptions Worth a Thousand Gold* (hereinafter: *Qianjin S.*):

Decoction of Radix Glycyrrhizae Praeparata*
(*Zhi Gancao Tang*)

Radix Glycyrrhizae Praeparata	4 *liang*
Ramulus Cinnamomi	3 *liang*
Rhizoma Zingiberis Recens	3 *liang*
Radix Ophiopogonis	0.5 *sheng*
Fructus Cannabis	0.5 *sheng*
Radix Ginseng	2 *liang*
Colla Corii Asini	2 *liang*
Fructus Ziziphi Jujubae	30 pcs.
Radix Rehmanniae	1 *jin*

*This prescription also appears in *Shanghan Lun*, Clause 177.

Stew all herbs except Colla Corii Asini in seven *sheng* of wine and eight *sheng* of water until three *sheng* remain. Filter the decoction and add Colla Corii Asini until it melts. Serve one *sheng* of lukewarm decoction per dose three times a day.

Efficacy of the Prescription: Decoction of Radix Glycyrrhizae

Praeparata is effective for all consumptive diseases with Deficiency and strain. Other symptoms may include perspiration, restlessness, and palpitations with slow-uneven pulse. The patient behaves normally. Within one hundred days, or eleven days in acute cases, the patient will not survive unless treated properly.

Prescription from *A Handbook of Prescriptions for Emergencies (Zhou Hou Bei Ji Fang)* by Ge Hong:

Otter Liver Powder is effective in curing consumptive diseases of a Cold nature, as well as an infectious disease called *Guizhu*.*

Otter Liver Powder
(*Ta Gan San*):

Bake one otter's liver and pound it into powder. Take one *fangcunbi* with water three times a day.

**Guizhu*: Infectious disease with symptoms of fever and chills, urinary disturbance and reluctance to speak. The patient does not know the cause of his discomfort. After a long period, he will die of inexplicable causes. People around him might be infected. (01-71)

CHAPTER VII

ON PULSE, SYMPTOM COMPLEX AND TREATMENT OF PULMONARY ASTHENIA, PULMONARY ABSCESS, COUGH AND INSPIRATORY DYSPNEA

CLAUSE 7-1

Question: When pathogenetic Heat is present in the Upper Portion of Body Cavity, the patient will suffer from coughing, followed by pulmonary asthenia. What is the cause of pulmonary asthenia?

Master: Exhaustion of the Body Fluid is the cause. Body Fluid may be exhausted by profuse perspiration, repeated vomiting, great thirst accompanied by frequent urination, incontinence of urination, constipation, or loose stool after administration of acute purgative.

Question: Pulse is speedy at the Inch (1). The patient coughs with sputum and saliva in his mouth. Why is this?

Master: This is a case of pulmonary asthenia. If the patient's mouth is parched and dry, if he experiences pain in his chest when coughing, and if pulse is slippery-speedy, it is a case of pulmonary abscess. Pulmonary asthenia always has symptoms of coughing with bloody pus and speedy-deficient pulse; whereas pulse of a patient suffering pulmonary abscess is always speedy-excessive.

NOTES

1. Pulse is speedy at the Inch: This indicates a case with pathogenetic Heat. When the patient coughs, it is "dry coughing" without sputum. This is because when the Lung is infected with pathogenetic Heat, normal secretion of Body Fluid is hampered and sputum accumulates. (01-73)

CLAUSE 7-2

Question: A patient coughs with inspiratory dyspnea. After feeling the pulse, a case of pulmonary abscess with bloody pus can be diagnosed. When the patient vomits bloody pus, death will follow. What is the pulse in such a situation? Could you kindly explain the syndrome?

Master: Pulse at the Inch is feeble (1) and speedy. Feeble pulse indicates pathogenetic Wind with spontaneous perspiration. Speedy pulse indicates pathogenetic Heat with aversion to cold. At the initial stage of the disease, pathogenetic Wind affects the Vital Resistance, though pathogenetic Wind will not accumulate at the Interior as it is expelled through expiration. When pathogenetic Heat enters the Nutrient Essence (2), it remains in the Interior and cannot be expelled through expiration. Pathogenetic Wind only harms the skin and the Exterior, whereas the Heat harms the Blood and the vessels. When pathogenetic Wind invades the Lung, the patient will exhibit the following symptoms and signs: coughing, parched feeling in mouth, wheezing with dyspnea, parched throat without thirst, repeated spitting of saliva and occasional shivering. When pathogenetic Heat is rampant in the Lung, the Blood stagnates and forms abscess and pus. The patient then vomits porridge-like sputum with bloody pus. The patient can be saved if treatment is given when the syndrome begins to manifest itself. But the patient will die if the abscess is completely formed. (3)

NOTES

1. Feeble pulse here means "floating-feeble," as floating pulse corresponds to pathogenetic Wind. (01-73)

2. Nutrient Essence: the Blood.

3. Recovery is possible even if the abscess is completely formed, though case is difficult to treat. This clause is a warning that the patient should obtain medical treatment before the syndrome becomes serious. (02-57)

CLAUSE 7-3

The patient with inspiratory dyspnea is likely to die if he is also suffering from facial dropsy, must shrug his shoulders to breathe, and exhibits floating-huge pulse (1). Case will be more serious if diarrhea is also present.

NOTES

1. Floating-huge pulse here is full of strength when felt lightly but feeble

and slender when pressed deeply. The deeper the fingers press, the smaller and emptier the pulse becomes. It may seem that the pulse is not beating at all. This is called "rootless pulse about to evanesce" (*wu gen yu tuo*). (01-74)

CLAUSE 7-4

The patient suffers from inspiratory dyspnea, wheezing and restlessness. This is a case of Lung-distention (1), which will lead to edema due to Wind-evil (2). Diaphoresis can be adopted to disperse the syndrome.

NOTES

1. Lung-distention (*Fei zhang*) is characterized by a sense of fullness in the chest in deficient nature, and coughing with wheezing. (01-75)

2. Edema due to Wind-evil (*Feng shui*): see Chapter XIV.

Commentary: Clauses 7-3 and 7-4 deal with syndromes of inspiratory dyspnea. Clause 7-3 describes a case of a deficient nature manifested in the "floating-huge pulse." Whereas case in Clause 7-4 is of an excessive nature. Lung-distention is caused by encroachment of pathogenetic Wind and Cold upon the Exterior, and stagnation of Water in the Interior. The Lung ceases its normal regulation of the Vital Energy, and pathogenetic factors accumulate there. When the flow of the Vital Energy is hampered, wheezing and dyspnea with restlessness occur. Since the Lung controls Water circulation, it directs the normal flow of Fluid from the Upper Portion of Body Cavity to the Urinary Bladder. When Water (Fluid) cannot find its way downward, it spills into the muscles and the Exterior, causing edema due to Wind-evil. Diaphoresis enables the stagnant Water to be dispersed together with the exogenous pathogenetic factors. The Lung may then resume its control over the Vital Energy, at the same time facilitating the normal flow of Water. (02-60)

CLAUSE 7-5

Patients suffering from pulmonary asthenia spit saliva repeatedly, though coughing and thirst are not present. They do suffer from enuresis and frequent urination though. When the Upper Portion of

Body Cavity (1) is extremely deficient, it loses control over the Lower Portion of Body Cavity (2). When pathogenetic Cold prevails in the Lung, the patient experiences vertigo (3) and copious salivation. Decoction of Radix Glycyrrhizae and Rhizoma Zingiberis can serve as a warming agent. After taking the decoction, if the patient begins to feel thirsty, he is suffering a case of great thirst with frequent urination. (4)

NOTES

1. The Lung.
2. The Urinary Bladder.
3. Vertigo may be caused by various factors. Stagnant Water is just one of the causes. (01-75)
4. This final sentence is not found in the *Pulse Classic*. The sentence appears in the Commentary of *Qianjin*. A note is appended which reads: "If the patient is thirsty, he is suffering a case of great thirst with frequent urination." (01-75)

Decoction of Radix Glycyrrhizae and Rhizoma Zingiberis*
(*Gancao Ganjiang Tang*):

Radix Glycyrrhizae Praeparata	4 *liang*
Rhizoma Zingiberis Praeparata	2 *liang*

Chop up the drugs. Stew in three *sheng* of water until 1.5 *sheng* remain. Filter the decoction and serve lukewarm in two doses.

*This prescription also appears in *Shanghan Lun*, Clause 29.

Explanation of the Prescription: This prescription treats pathogenetic Cold in the Lung. Radix Glycyrrhizae, of a sweet and warm nature, tonifies the Deficiency and reinforces the Vital Energy. Rhizoma Zingiberis, of a pungent and hot nature, warms the Lung and disperses the Cold. Thus this prescription can serve both to warm the Lung and to restore the Vital Energy. (01-76)

CLAUSE 7-6

The patient coughs with inspiratory dyspnea and a sound in his throat resembling the croaking of a frog. Decoction of Rhizoma

Belamcandae and Herba Ephedrae may be prescribed to cure the syndrome (1).

NOTES

1. Chao Yuanfang, in his *General Treatise on the Etiology and Symptomology of Diseases* (*Zhu Bing Yuan Hou Lun*), recorded the following symptoms and signs, which can be taken as a supplement to this clause. It reads: "Lung disease with inspiratory dyspnea is accompanied by the following symptoms and signs: Feeling of fullness caused by sputum in the chest and diaphragm, abnormal movement of Vital Energy, wheezing with uneven breathing which causes a sound in the throat resembling the croaking of a frog." In clinical observation, white and slippery tongue coating and floating-tense pulse are also visible in this syndrome. (02-61)

Decoction of Rhizoma Belamcandae and Herba Ephedrae (*Shegan Mahuang Tang*):

Rhizoma Belamcandae	13 pcs.*
Herba Ephedrae	4 *liang*
Rhizoma Zingiberis Recens	4 *liang*
Herba Asari	3 *liang*
Radix Asteris	3 *liang*
Flos Farfarae	3 *liang*
Fructus Schisandrae	0.5 *sheng*
Fructus Ziziphi Jujubae	7 pcs.
Rhizoma Pinelliae (large, washed)	8 pcs.**

Stew Herba Ephedrae in one *dou* two *sheng* of water. Skim off the foam and add the remaining drugs. Stew again until three *sheng* remain. Serve the lukewarm decoction in three doses.

*Or 3 *liang*, according to another edition.

**Or 0.5 *sheng*, according to another edition.

Explanation of the Prescription: You Yi: Coughing with inspiratory dyspnea indicates prevalence of pathogenetic factors in the Lung. With such pathogens, the normal down-flowing of the Vital Energy is hampered. Hence the feeling of gas ascending. The Body Fluid of a Cold nature stagnated in the Lung ascends to the throat, causing a sound resembling the croaking of a frog. Rhizoma

Belamcandae, Radix Asteris and Flos Farfarae reduce the abnormal ascent (of gas). Herba Ephedrae, Herba Asari and Rhizome Zingiberis Recens disperse the pathogenetic factors. Rhizoma Pinelliae eliminates the stagnant Water. Fructus Ziziphi Jujubae eases the Interior. Fructus Schisandrae acts as an astringent on the Lung. The latter two drugs are used with respect to the strong effect of the ingredients in the prescription, which are likely to harm Body Resistance.

CASES

Case 1 (48-127): Chronic Bronchitis

Chen, 53, female, suffered from chronic bronchitis almost eight years. Recently, when exposed to winter cold, she began to suffer. She made a croaking sound, while coughing, with salivation. The syndrome was aggravated at night, and the patient was unable to lie flat in bed. There was a chill, but no fever. Dropsy appeared below eyes. Fullness was experienced in chest and epigastrium. Tongue was covered with white-slippery coating. Pulse was floating-tense and slippery. The latest seizure had lasted ten days.

Diagnosis: Syndrome was caused when Cold Fluid-retention was accumulating at the Interior, hampering Lung function.

Treatment: Decoction of Rhizoma Belamcandae and Herba Ephedrae was prescribed. After three doses, coughing and asthma were reduced. Another three doses were given, and the syndrome brought under control.

Case 2 (48-128): Asthma, Case Recorded in Journal of *Chinese Medicine*, 1964, 12

Liu, 15-year-old boy, suffered from asthma since he was very young. The syndrome was aggravated in the last two years. When exposed to cold, he had an asthma attack. The patient had dyspnea, chest distress, coughing, spitting of phlegm, sweat on head and face, difficulty when lying down, anorexia, dropsy on face, and difficulty in opening mouth. Urination was normal. Pulse was slippery-speedy. Tongue was covered with white coating.

Diagnosis: Syndrome was caused by invasion of Cold fluid-retention over the Lung.

Treatment: Decoction of Rhizoma Belamcandae and Herba Ephedrae was prescribed:

Rhizoma Belamcandae	9 grams
Fructus Schisandrae	9 grams
Rhizoma Pinelliae	9 grams
Semen Armeniacae Amarum	9 grams
Bulbus Fritillariae	9 grams

Semen Raphani Praeparata	9 grams
Cortex Magnoliae Officinalis	9 grams
Haematitum	9 grams
Herba Ephedrae	3 grams
Herba Asari	1.5 grams
Poria	15 grams

Second treatment: Twelve doses of the decoction reduced the syndrome. Another two doses were given with alterations:

Subtract: Haematitum.

Add: Nine grams of Massa Fermentata Praeparata, nine grams of Cortex Mori Radicis Praeparata.

The syndrome was gone after the second treatment.

Case 3 (48-128): Whooping Cough, Case Recorded in Journal of *Chinese Medicine*, 1964, 12

A boy of four years had been coughing for almost a month. Whooping cough was diagnosed. When coughing, he had dyspnea and croaking. The syndrome was bad at night, making it hard for him to sleep. He had no appetite. His face was puffy, tongue covered with white-slippery coating.

Treatment: Decoction of Rhizoma Belamcandae and Herba Ephedrae was given:

Rhizoma Belamcandae	6 grams
Herba Ephedrae	1.5 grams
Fructus Schisandrae	6 grams
Rhizoma Pinelliae	6 grams
Semen Armeniacae Amarum	6 grams
Bulbus Fritillariae	6 grams
Gypsum Fibrosum	6 grams
Semen Raphani Praeparata	6 grams
Poria	9 grams
Rhizoma Zingiberis Recens	3 grams
Pericarpium Citri Reticulatae	3 grams
Natrii Sulfas Exsiccatus (wash down with the decoction)	3 grams
Cortex Mori Radicis Praeparata	4.5 grams

One dose alleviated the condition. Nine doses were taken and the syndrome subsided. After fifteen doses the syndrome was cured.

CLAUSE 7-7

The patient coughs with inspiratory dyspnea and spits saliva repeatedly. He cannot easily fall asleep but must sit upright to obtain relief. Pills of Fructus Gleditsiae Sinensis can be given as a remedy.

Pills of Fructus Gleditsiae Sinensis
(*Zaojia Wan*):

Fructus Gleditsiae Sinensis (fried in butter) 8 *liang*

Pound the drug into powder and form pills adding honey as big as seed of Chinese parasol. Blend three pills with paste of Fructus Ziziphi Jujubae and make a decoction. Give three doses in the day and one at night.

Explanation of the Prescription: This prescription treats cases of coughing with inspiratory dyspnea caused by accumulated sputum and saliva in the Lung. When the Lung ceases its normal function of purification and descendance, sputum and saliva form, causing coughing with inspiratory dyspnea. Sputum and saliva ascend with the ascending air and cause repeated spitting. When the patient lies in bed, inspiratory dyspnea is aggravated, the patient must remain upright for relief; otherwise there is a danger of suffocation. Therefore, Pills of Fructus Gleditsiae Sinensis, the most effective expectorant, are adopted to rapidly eliminate the sputum and saliva. Fructus Gleditsiae Sinensis, pungent and salty in nature, is a strong expectorant. In order to modify its effect, it is fried in butter and served with paste of Fructus Ziziphi Jujubae to protect the normal functioning of the Spleen and the Stomach. (02-62)

CASES

Case 1 (63-52): (Doctor: Cao Yingfu)

In 1910, Dr. Cao's mother suffered from coughing with dyspnea and spitting of yellow-greasy phlegm. Pills of Fructus Gleditsiae Sinensis were used. The patient had eaten rich and oily food and smoked a lot. This evolved into an accumulation of phlegm, causing coughing and dyspnea. Defication and urination were obstructed. Pills of Fructus Gleditsiae Sinensis were given to the patient, with paste made of Fructus Ziziphi Jujubae, four times within twenty-four hours. After the patient passed a stool and urinated, she could fall asleep. The following year there was a similar case not properly treated. The patient passed away.

Case 2 (63-54): (Dr. Cao Yingfu)

The doctor himself suffered from coughing and asthma with copious salivation and chest pain. He made Pills of Fructus Gleditsiae Sinensis and took four doses consecutively. His stool was loose and greasy two to three times a day. After recovering from the ailment, the doctor felt weak. He understood that Fructus Gleditsiae Sinensis was a severe expectorant, which was good at dispersing the phlegm but consumed one's energy. Paste of Fructus Ziziphi Jujubae should accompany the treatment to lessen its harm to the body.

Conclusion: Fructus Gleditsiae Sinensis is a good expectorant to be used only when there is a bad accumulation of phlegm, but care should be taken to protect the physique.

CLAUSE 7-8

Syndrome of coughing and floating pulse (1) can be treated with Decoction of Cortex Magnoliae Officinalis and Herba Ephedrae.

NOTES

1. The original text gives very little regarding the symptoms. According to *Qianjin*, the symptoms accompanying the same prescription are more detailed: Coughing with severe inspiratory dyspnea (gas from the Spleen and Stomach ascends abnormally) and sensation of fullness in the chest, discomfort and sound resembling croaking of frog in the throat with floating pulse can be treated with Decoction of Cortex Magnoliae Officinalis and Herba Ephedrae.

Decoction of Cortex Magnoliae Officinalis and Herba Ephedrae (*Houpo Mahuang Tang*):

Cortex Magnoliae Officinalis	5 *liang*
Herba Ephedrae	4 *liang*
Gypsum Fibrosum	an egg-sized pc.*
Semen Armeniacae Amarum	0.5 *sheng*
Rhizoma Pinelliae	0.5 *sheng*
Rhizoma Zingiberis	2 *liang*
Herba Asari	2 *liang*
Fructus Tritici	1 *liang*

Fructus Schisandrae	0.5 *sheng*

Stew Fructus Tritici in one *dou* two *sheng* of water until well-cooked. Filter the decoction and add remaining drugs. Stew until three *sheng* remain. Serve one *sheng* of lukewarm decoction per dose three times a day.

Explanation of the Prescription: See "Commentary" of Clause7-9

*Or three *liang* according to *Qianjin*.

CASES

Case 1 (46-122): Bronchial Asthma

A boy of thirteen suffered from bronchial asthma occasionally. The symptoms were chest distress, restlessness, coughing with spitting of yellow-greasy phlegm, dyspnea, wheezing sound, thirst, yellow coating on tongue, floating-speedy pulse.

Diagnosis: Syndrome was caused by pent-up fluid-retention evolving in pathogenetic Heat which obstructed the normal respiratory function.

Treatment: Decoction of Cortex Magnoliae Officinalis and Herba Ephedrae was given:

Cortex Magnoliae Officinalis	10 grams
Herba Ephedrae	3 grams
Semen Armeniacae Amarum	10 grams
Gypsum Fibrosum	10 grams
Rhizoma Pinelliae Praeparata	10 grams
Rhizoma Zingiberis	3 grams
Herba Asari	1.5 grams
Fructus Schisandrae	1.5 grams
Fructus Tritici	10 grams

Three doses of the decoction cured the condition.

Case 2 (52-600):

A boy of eighteen months, first treatment on December 10, 1981. At five months, the baby had a big appetite and indigestion. He developed diarrhea followed by several colds and pneumonia.

Examination: The week before the consultation, the baby had a cold, fever, abdominal distention and coughing, vomit of saliva, and anorexia. Coughing was aggravated at night. Pulse was floating-slippery. Tongue was covered with thin-white, slightly greasy coating.

Diagnosis: This syndrome was caused by constipation, indigestion and fluid-retention.

Treatment: Decoction of Cortex Magnoliae Officinalis and Herba Ephedrae was given:

Cortex Magnoliae Officinalis	3 grams
Herba Ephedrae	3 grams
Gypsum Fibrosum	1.8 grams
Semen Armeniacae Amarum	2 grams
Rhizoma Pinelliae	1 gram
Herba Asari	0.3 gram
Fructus Schisandrae	0.6 gram
Fructus Tritici	6 grams
Pericarpium Trichosanthis	6 grams
Fructus Hordei Praeparata	10 grams
Massa Fermentata Praeparata	10 grams
Fructus Crataegi Praeparata	10 grams

One dose of the decoction in five servings was given within twenty-four hours. After two doses, cough was reduced and abdominal distention subsided. Two more doses completed the treatment.

CLAUSE 7-9

When the pulse is deep, Decoction of Herba Euphorbiae Helioscopiae can be adopted.

Decoction of Herba Euphorbiae Helioscopiae
(*Zeqi Tang*):

Rhizoma Pinelliae	0.5 *sheng*
*Zishen** (Radix Asteris, according to another edition)	5 *liang*
Herba Euphorbiae Helioscopiae (stew in 5 *dou* of stream water until 1.5 *dou* remain)	3 *jin*
Rhizoma Zingiberis Recens	5 *liang*
Rhizoma Cynanchi Stauntonii	5 *liang*
Radix Glycyrrhizae	3 *liang*
Radix Scutellariae	3 *liang*
Radix Ginseng	3 *liang*

Ramulus Cinnamomi 3 *liang*

Add above drugs to the decoction of Herba Euphorbiae Helioscopiae and stew until five *sheng* remain. Serve five *ge* of the lukewarm decoction per dose. Finish the decoction till midnight.

**Zishen* may refer to Rhizoma Bistortae or Radix Salviae Miltiorrhizae.

Commentary: This clause refers only to the pulse without mentioning the symptoms and signs. The ingredients in the prescription suggest it is not appropriate for coughing. The principal ingredient, Herba Euphorbiae Helioscopiae, is an excellent water-expellent, not an expectorant. Thus this must be a prescription for treating edema with wheezing and coughing. (01-78)

You Yi: Clauses 7-8 and 7-9 discuss no symptoms and signs but give only floating and deep pulse as means of differentiating the therapy. Generally speaking, coughing is caused by pathogenetic factors in the Lung. When the pulse is floating, the pathological condition is located mainly in the Exterior. Thus the therapy seeks to disperse the pathogenetic factors from the Exterior (as in Clause 7-8). When the pulse is deep, pathological condition is located in the Interior. Thus the therapy seeks to disperse the pathogenetic factors from below (as in Clause 7-9). The therapy consists of expelling pathogenetic factors from wherever they are located.

CASES

Case 1(51-181): Case Recorded in Journal of *Chengdu College of Chinese Medicine*, 2:106, 1978

Mr. Cao, a stout farmer in his fifties, had, for the past three years, experienced coughing with copious salivation and spitting of greasy phlegm. Asthma made sleeping difficult. Asthma and cough occurred winter and summer, irrespective of the weather or pathological condition. There was pitted edema on face and extremities. The patient was thirsty with tastelessness and greasiness in mouth, constipation with intermittent loose bowel, scanty urine, deep-slippery pulse.

Diagnosis: Syndrome was caused by fluid-retention at the Interior producing pathogenetic Heat.

Treatment: Decoction of Herba Euphorbiae Helioscopiae was given. After one dose, syndrome subsided. Four doses helped the patient recover.

CLAUSE 7-10

For inspiratory dyspnea with strong ascending gas (1) and uncomfortable feeling in throat, Decoction of Radix Ophiopogonis can be given to reduce adverse ascending and stop the inspiratory dyspnea.

NOTES

1. Strong ascending gas: According to *Jinjian*, this should read "ascending pathogenetic Fire."

Decoction of Radix Ophiopogonis
(*Maimendong Tang*):

Radix Ophiopogonis	7 *sheng*
Rhizoma Pinelliae	1 *sheng*
Radix Ginseng	3 *liang*
Radix Glycyrrhizae	2 *liang*
Semen Oryzae Nonglutinosae	3 *ge*
Fructus Ziziphi Jujubae	12 pcs.

Stew the drugs in one *dou* two *sheng* of water until six *sheng* remain. Serve one *sheng* of lukewarm decoction per dose three times during the day and one at night.

Explanation of the Prescription: Ge Hong, in his *A Handbook of Prescriptions for Emergencies*, states that Decoction of Radix Ophiopogonis is effective for pulmonary asthenia with coughing and repeated spitting of saliva, parched throat and thirst. *Jinkui S* states that the clause deals with the treatment of pulmonary asthenia in deficient and Heat nature. The mechanism of the syndrome is the ascent of pathogenetic Fire in deficient nature. The Fire is caused by the exhaustion of the Body Fluid in the Lung and the Stomach when pathogenetic Heat prevails in the Upper Portion of Body Cavity. When the Body Fluid is exhausted, the Yin Vital Essence is weakened. When Yin is weakened, pathogenetic Fire will spread upward, causing the abnormal ascent of the Vital Energy in the Lung and Stomach, resulting coughing and wheezing. When there is little Body Fluid, it cannot ascend to moisten the throat, and causes an uncomfortable parched feeling. Other similar symptoms and signs include an inclination towards taking cool drinks to moisten the dryness, redness of the tongue with a thin coating, and a deficient and speedy pulse. This appears to be a syndrome of the Lung, but actually originates from a disorder of the Stomach. When the Stomach Yin Vital Essence is in a deficient state, the Lung is lacking Body Fluid (according to the producing sequence of the Five Elements, Spleen or Stomach produces Lung). So Decoction of Radix Ophiopogonis is given to nourish and clear the Lung and the Stomach, reducing the abnormal ascending of gas and relieving the inspiratory dyspnea. In this prescription, a strong dose of Radix Ophiopogonis is given as the principal ingredient to moisten the Lung, nourish the Stomach and drive away the deficient Heat. Rhizoma Pinelliae brings down the adverse ascending and dissolves the sputum (because Rhizoma Pinelliae is too dry in quality, it is given in small quantities). Radix Ginseng, Radix Glycyrrhizae, Fructus Ziziphi Jujubae and Semen Oryzae Nonglutinosae nourish and tonify the Stomach Vital Energy. Once the Vital Energy in the Stomach is restored, it will aid production of Body Fluid. When Body Fluid is sufficient, the deficient Fire will restrain itself, and coughing and inspiratory dyspnea will subside. If the case is one of strong pathogenetic Fire, Folium Bambusae and Gypsum Fibrosum may be added. (02-56)

CASES

Case 1 (48-432): Dry Cough

Lu, a boy of eighteen, busy with college entrance examination, began to cough due to overwork. He tried Chinese and Western medicine but nothing seemed to help.

Examination: Dry cough without phlegm, pain in chest, thirst, red tongue free of coating, slippery-slender-speedy pulse.

Treatment: Decoction of Radix Ophiopogonis was prescribed to relieve cough and smooth flow of Vital Energy:

Radix Ophiopogonis	15 grams
Rhizoma Pinelliae	6 grams
Radix Glycyrrhizae	3 grams
Folium Eriobotryae	9 grams
Radix Glehniae	15 grams
Radix Adenophorae	15 grams

Four doses of the decoction cured the ailment.

Case 2 (48-433): Retrograde Menstruation

Chen, 32, married female, had never menstruated. Every month, she had two to three times of epistaxis. Accompanying symptoms: Epigastric distress, retching with feeling of suffocation, scaly skin, slender-tight pulse, purple edge of tongue covered with thin coating.

Treatment: Decoction of Radix Ophiopogonis was prescribed:

Radix Ophiopogonis	15 grams
Radix Codonopsis Pilosulae	12 grams
Rhizoma Pinelliae	9 grams
Rhizoma Dioscoreae	12 grams
Radix Paeoniae Alba	9 grams
Radix Slaviae Miltiorrhizae	9 grams
Radix Glycyrrhizae	6 grams
Semen Persicae	6 grams
Radix Rubiae	15 grams
Herba Lycopi	9 grams
Fructus Ziziphi Jujubae	3 pcs.

The decoction worked effectively.

Case 3 (46-123):

A boy of fifteen suffered from bronchitis, with coughing and parched mouth and throat, constipation, red tongue, deficient-speedy pulse.

Diagnosis: Syndrome was caused by insufficient Stomach-Yin causing deficient Fire to ascend.

Treatment: The decoction to produce Body Fluid and nourish Lung and Stomach was prescribed:

Radix Ophiopogonis	12 grams
Radix Glehniae	15 grams
Radix Glycyrrhizae	6 grams
Fructus Ziziphi Jujubae	3 pcs.
Semen Oryzae Nonglutinosae	10 grams
Folium Mori	10 grams
Herba Dendrobii	12 grams
Folium Eriobotryae	10 grams
Crystal sugar	30 grams
Juice of pear	1 cup

Five doses of the decoction cured the ailment.

CLAUSE 7-11

The patient suffers from pulmonary abscess with serious wheezing which makes it difficult for him to lie quietly in bed. Decoction of Lung-purgation with Semen Lepidii seu Descurainiae and Fructus Ziziphi Jujubae may be prescribed.

Decoction of Lung-purgation with Semen Lepidii seu Descurainiae and Fructus Ziziphi Jujubae
(*Tingli Dazao Xie Fei Tang*)

Semen Lepidii seu Descurainiae

Stew until it turns yellow. Pound it and form a pill the size of a bullet. (According to the prescription in *Compendium of Materia Medica*, this sentence should read: "Pound it with honey and form a pill the size of a bullet.")

Fructus Ziziphi Jujubae 12 pcs.

Stew Fructus Ziziphi Jujubae in three *sheng* of water until two *sheng* remain. Remove Fructus Ziziphi Jujubae and add Semen Lepidii seu Descurainiae. Stew again till one *sheng* remains. Take the decoction in one dose.

Explanation of the Prescription: Zhao Liang: This is an important prescription for severe cases of pulmonary abscess. When abscess forms in the Lung, purgation must be carried out immediately, or else, it will be too difficult to remove. Moreover, when the abscess exists in the Lung for a long time, Lung Vital Energy is consumed, purgation will be too intense for the Lung to stand. Thus when the Blood begins to stagnate but before the abscess has taken shape, purgative should be given. In addition, when the patient suffers from a syndrome of wheezing which makes it difficult for him to lie quietly in bed, the case requires urgent attention. (05-510)

Semen Lepidii seu Descurainiae has a strong and immediate effect of purging the stagnant Water and reducing wheezing in an excessive case. Fructus Ziziphi Jujubae is added to tonify the Spleen and lessen the acute effect of Semen Lepidii seu Descurainiae. When the pathogenetic factors are driven out with strong drugs, Body Resistance is not weakened at the same time. (01-79)

CASES

Case 1 (48-156): Case Recorded in Journal of *Liaoning Medicine and Pharmacology*, Vol. 2, 1976

Decoction of Lung-purgation with Semen Lepidii seu Descurainiae and Fructus Ziziphi Jujubae had been used to treat pulmonary heart disease, pulmonary emphysema, bronchial asthma and chronic bronchitis. Good therapeutic effect was achieved when the syndromes were caused by excessive pathogenesis. It was especially effective when used in acute cases. For example:

Mr. Zhou, 72, suffered from asthma and cough for several years. Diagnosis was pulmonary emphysema.

Examination: The patient had attacks of severe asthma in the past three days. He was a plump build, with shortness of breath and palpitation. Asthma and cough were extremely bad at night. There was dyspnea and difficulty in urination and passing a stool. Pulse was floating-slippery-speedy. Tongue was red, covered with yellow coating.

Diagnosis: Syndrome was caused by failure of Lung function in normal flow of Vital Energy, complicated by accumulated phlegm and Humidity.

Treatment: Decoction of Lung-purgation with Semen Lepidii seu Descurainiae and Fructus Ziziphi Jujubae was given.

Three doses relieved the syndrome and full recovery was achieved.

Case 2 (48-156): Whooping Cough

A boy of five had a cough and fever, stuffy and sneezing nose. Later the boy had spastic cough and wheezing occurring many times consecutively. His face and ears flushed, accompanied by tears, sneezing and dropsy of face. Repeated attacks occurred at night. When coughing, phlegm, saliva, or food was spat out. The boy could not sleep well. This lasted almost a week.

Treatment: Decoction of Lung-purgation with Semen Lepidii seu Descurainiae and Fructus Ziziphi Jujubae was given:

Semen Lepidii seu Descurainiae	9 grams
Fructus Ziziphi Jujubae	10 pcs.
Fructus Chaenomelis	9 grams

Small servings of the decoction were given at short intervals. After three doses, the syndrome subsided.

Second treatment: Decoction of Malt Sugar (30 grams per dose) was served daily to help the patient recover, worked as anticipated.

Case 3 (48-157): Thoracic Hydrops, Cases Recorded in *Collection of Papers in the 1962 Annual Convention of Shandong Chinese Medicine Association*

Decoction of Lung-purgation with Semen Lepidii seu Descurainiae and Fructus Ziziphi Jujubae was used to treat tuberculous thoracic hydrops with satisfactory result.

Prescription (with alterations according to individual case):

Semen Lepidii seu Descurainiae
Fructus Ziziphi Jujubae
Radix Euphorbiae Kansui
Rhizoma Atractylodis Macrocephalae
Radix Paeoniae Alba
Cortex Mori Radicis
Radix Scutellariae

One group of patients were treated with the decoction only. An average of 8.3 doses cured the disease within 19.6 days on average. Thoracic hydrops were totally absorbed. Another group of patients were treated with the decoction and isoniazid. An average of 10.1 doses cured the disease within 14.8 days on average. Thoracic hydrops were totally cured.

Case 4 (52-735): Bronchial Asthma

Du, 68-year-old lady, first treatment on November 4, 1976. The patient reported that twenty years ago, after a cold, she began to cough with dyspnea. This was not treated and developed into bronchial asthma. The syndrome was always related to cold weather. The patient had to shrug her shoulders to help her breathe. She had profuse cold sweat, copious salivation, dark-red tongue covered with white-slippery coating. Pulse was deep-tight.

Diagnosis: Syndrome was caused by Fluid-retention of Cold to the Lung and obstruction of respiratory tract by greasy phlegm.

Treatment: Decoction of Lung-purgation with Semen Lepidii seu Descurainiae and Fructus Ziziphi Jujubae combined with Decoction of Lesser *Qinglong* (prescription see Clause 12-21) was given:

Semen Lepidii seu Descurainiae	9 grams
Fructus Ziziphi Jujubae	8 pcs.
Rhizoma Zingiberis	9 grams
Ramulus Cinnamomi	9 grams
Herba Ephedrae	9 grams
Radix Paeoniae Alba	10 grams
Radix Glycyrrhizae	9 grams
Herba Asari	4 grams
Rhizoma Pinelliae	9 grams

Fructus Schisandrae	10 grams

When three doses were consumed, coughing and asthma subsided with minor attacks at night. The patient could sleep 3-4 hours.

Second treatment: Six more doses of the decoction cured the disease. One year later, no recurrence was reported.

CLAUSE 7-12

A pulmonary abscess accompanied by the following symptoms and signs can be treated with Decoction of Radix Platycodi: Coughing with a sensation of fullness in the chest, shivering with cold, speedy pulse, a parched feeling in the throat without thirst, bad-smelling dense sputum, chronic spitting of purulent sputum as thick as porridge.

Decoction of Radix Platycodi*
(*Jiegeng Tang*):
Also effective in treating arthralgia due to stagnation of Blood.**

Radix Platycodi	1 *liang*
Radix Glycyrrhizae	2 *liang*

Stew the drugs in three *sheng* of water until one *sheng* remains. Serve the decoction warm in two doses. The patient will vomit purulent blood (a sign of recovery).

*This prescription also appears in *Shanghan Lun*, Clause 311.
***Qianjin* and *Waitai* do not give this annotation.

Explanation of the Prescription: Radix Platycodi is effective in treating the syndrome of pulmonary abscess, as it can eliminate both the abscess and the sputum. Radix Glycyrrhizae eliminates the pathogenetic Heat and functions as an antidote. Nevertheless, this prescription is not strong enough to treat the syndrome of pulmonary abscess, as clinical observation suggests. Prescriptions recorded in "Appendix" of this chapter can be used to cure more severe cases. (01-80)

The text gives one of its symptoms as "chronic spitting of purulent sputum as thick as porridge." From this, we can infer that the syndrome is becoming one of a deficient nature. Purgatives will no longer suit to the case. Thus Decoction of Radix Platycodi is used to eliminate the abscess and function as an antidote. (02-59)

CLAUSE 7-13

Lung-distention is a syndrome characterized by symptoms and signs of coughing with inspiratory dyspnea, wheezing, proptosis, and floating-huge pulse. Decoction of *Yuebei* adding Rhizoma Pinelliae can be adopted as a curative.

Decoction of *Yuebei* adding Rhizoma Pinelliae
(*Yuebei Jia Banxia Tang*):

Herba Ephedrae	6 *liang*
Gypsum Fibrosum	0.5 *jin*
Rhizoma Zingiberis Recens	3 *liang*
Fructus Ziziphi Jujubae	15 pcs.
Radix Glycyrrhizae	2 *liang*
Rhizoma Pinelliae	0.5 *sheng*

Stew Herba Ephedrae in six *sheng* of water. Skim off the foam and add the remaining drugs. Stew again until three *sheng* remain. Serve the decoction lukewarm in three doses.

Explanation of the Prescription: Wheezing with ocular proptosis indicates a severe case with pathogenetic Wind and Heat prevailing over the Lung. Decoction of *Yuebei* can be used to dredge through the stagnation of the Lung Vital Energy. Rhizoma Pinelliae is added to reverse the adverse ascending and eliminate the sputum. (01-81)

CASES

Case 1 (46-126): Bronchopneumonia

A female boy of one year old was suffering from bronchopneumonia. Two days earlier, the patient had a cold with fever, cough, stuffy and running nose. Temperature was 39℃. Other symptoms: Wheezing with spitting of saliva and phlegm, flaring nose, dry lips and oral cavity. Tongue was covered with white-slippery coating. Fingers were purple.

Diagnosis: Syndrome was caused by Fluid-retention in Heat nature invading to the Lung and the obstruction of respiratory tract.

Treatment: Intramuscular injection of penicillin was given, and Decoction of *Yuebei* adding Rhizoma Pinelliae was prescribed:

Herba Ephedrae	2 grams
Gypsum Fibrosum	10 grams
Rhizoma Pinelliae Praeparata	6 grams
Radix Glycyrrhizae	3 grams
Rhizoma Zingiberis	2 slices
Fructus Ziziphi Jujubae	1 pc.

One dose brought down the fever, and another dose eased the cough and asthma.

Case 2 (65-214): Lung-distention, Case Recorded in *Required Readings of Medical Professionals (Yi Zong Bi Du)*, Doctor: Li Zhongzi (1588-1655)

Mr. Sun's daughter suffered from chronic cough with asthma. Drugs to dissolve phlegm and eliminate Lung-fire had been given repeatedly but did not cure the condition. The doctor was sent for. She panted, was restless and irritated, eyes protruded, nose flared, pulse was floating and huge. This was a syndrome of Lung-distention.

Treatment: Decoction of *Yuebei* adding Rhizoma Pinelliae was prescribed.

One dose reduced the syndromes and another dose completed the treatment.

CLAUSE 7-14

Lung-distention with coughing, inspiratory dyspnea, restlessness and wheezing as well as floating pulse will indicate existence of stagnant Water in the epigastrium. Decoction of Lesser *Qinglong* adding Gypsum Fibrosum can be adopted.

Decoction of Lesser *Qinglong* adding Gypsum Fibrosum (*Xiao Qinglong Jia Shigao Tang*):

Qianjin gives the following additional symptoms: A referred pain from the costal regions to Quepen* (ST 12).

Herba Ephedrae	3 *liang*
Radix Paeoniae	3 *liang*
Ramulus Cinnamomi	3 *liang*
Herba Asari	3 *liang*
Radix Glycyrrhizae	3 *liang*
Rhizoma Zingiberis	3 *liang*
Fructus Schisandrae	0.5 *sheng*
Rhizoma Pinelliae	0.5 *sheng*
Gypsum Fibrosum	2 *liang*

Stew Herba Ephedrae in one *dou* of water. Skim off the foam and add remaining drugs. Stew again until three *sheng* remain. Serve one *sheng* of decoction to a strong person but reduce dosage for a weak patient. Give three doses a day. Four *ge* can be given to children.

Explanation of the Prescription: Decoction of Lesser *Qinglong*** simultaneously treats the Exterior syndrome (pathogenetic Cold) and the stagnant Water. Syndrome described in this clause is a complication of Decoction of Lesser *Qinglong* syndrome with restlessness of a Heat nature. Gypsum Fibrosum is added to eliminate the Heat. (01-81)

*An acupoint located in the supraclavicular fossa.
**See Clause 40 of *Shanghan Lun* as well as Clause 12-21 below.

CASES

Case 1 (46-127): Emphysema

Chen, lady of seventy-six, suffered from emphysema for many years. She coughed and spat saliva. When she moved around, she panted. Following a cold, she had chills and fever, with coughing, spitting of greasy phlegm and dyspnea. She was restless, had a parched mouth, but could drink only small amount.

Treatment: Decoction of Lesser *Qinglong* adding Gypsum Fibrosum was prescribed:

Herba Ephedrae	3 grams
Ramulus Cinnamomi	10 grams

Radix Paeoniae Alba	10 grams
Rhizoma Pinelliae Praeparata	10 grams
Rhizoma Zingiberis	3 grams
Herba Asari	2 grams
Fructus Schisandrae	3 grams
Radix Glycyrrhizae	3 grams
Gypsum Fibrosum	10 grams

After two doses, chill and fever subsided, clear phlegm discharged (used to be greasy).

Second treatment: The following prescription was given in three doses to complete the treatment:

Radix Ginseng
Pericarpium Citri Reticulatae
Rhizoma Pinelliae
Poria
Radix Glycyrrhizae
Rhizoma Atractylodis Macrocephalae
Rhizoma Zingiberis
Fructus Schisandrae
Herba Asari

Case 2 (65-216): Adenoviral Pneumonia, Case Recorded in *Clinical Experience of Dr. Pu Fuzhou*

A syndrome of Exterior Cold with Interior Fluid-retention, or adenoviral pneumonia in Western medicine, attacked Feng, a 6-year-old girl. She received three weeks of hospital treatment of Western medicine. Consultation held on March 14, 1961 and Dr. Pu was invited to examine the patient.

Examination: Fever, cough and panting, dyspnea, blue-pale face, diarrhea, pulmonary rales, pale tongue covered with gray-black coating, slippery-speedy pulse.

Diagnosis: Syndrome was caused by stagnation of Fluid-retention complicated by a cold, which should be treated by dispersing the stagnation of Vital Energy in the Lung.

Treatment: Decoction of Lesser *Qinglong* adding Gypsum Fibrosum was given:

Herba Ephedrae	1.5 grams
Rhizoma Zingiberis	0.9 gram
Herba Asari	0.6 gram
Fructus Schisandrae	10 pcs.
Rhizoma Pinelliae Praeparata	3 grams

Ramulus Cinnamomi	1.5 grams
Gypsum Fibrosum	6 grams
Radix Glycyrrhizae	1.5 grams
Semen Armeniacae Amarum	10 pcs.
Radix Paeoniae Alba	1.5 grams
Fructus Ziziphi Jujubae	2 pcs.

The drugs were stewed in 300 ml of water. Served the warm decoction in three servings.

Second treatment on March 16. Symptoms: Fever, flushed face, wheezing, appetite improving, diarrhea healing, color of tongue coating fading. Pulse was slippery and speedy. Treatment directed to harmonize the Stomach function and regulate the Lung function to disperse phlegm was adopted.

Prescription:

Rhizoma Pinelliae Praeparata	3 grams
Exocarpium Citri Grandis	2.4 grams
Radix Glycyrrhizae	1.5 grams
Radix Asteris	2.4 grams
Fructus Schisandrae	10 pcs.
Herba Asari	0.9 gram
Fructus Perillae Praeparata	3 grams
Radix Peucedani	1.5 grams
Rhizoma Zingiberis Recens	2 slices
Fructus Ziziphi Jujubae	2 pcs.

Third treatment on March 17. Fever subsided with good appetite, moderate pulse, better tongue condition. More doses of the decoction were served to achieve full recovery.

CLAUSE 7-15

Pulmonary abscess accompanied by the following symptoms and signs can be treated with Decoction of Lung-purgation with Semen Lepidii seu Descurainiae and Fructus Ziziphi Jujubae*: Fullness and distension in the chest, facial and body dropsy, stuffy and running nose, inability to distinguish flavors, coughing with inspiratory dyspnea, wheezing and difficulty in breathing.

*Prescription is found in Clause 7-11. Take one dose every three days. For serious cases, three or four doses can be given. Prior to this, give one dose of Decoction of Lesser *Qinglong*, see Clause 12-21.

Appendix:

Decoction of Radix Glycyrrhizae Praeparata (*Zhi Gancao Tang*) as recorded in *Waitai* is effective in treating pulmonary asthenia with copious saliva and sputum and nausea.

For prescription, see Chapter VI.

Decoction of Radix Glycyrrhizae (*Gancao Tang*) as recorded in *Qianjin* is effective in treating pulmonary asthenia with copious spitting of saliva, sputum and blood, and nausea.

Radix Glycyrrhizae	2 *liang*

Stew the drug in three *sheng* of water until one half remains. Serve the decoction lukewarm in three doses.

Explanation of the Prescription: This prescription first appeared in *A Handbook of Prescriptions for Emergencies*. Radix Glycyrrhizae has the function of eliminating the Heat, easing the cough, quenching the thirst and smoothing the normal flow of the Vital Energy. This prescription is suitable for the early stages of pulmonary asthenia.

Decoction of Rhizoma Zingiberis Recens and Radix Glycyrrhizae (*Shengjiang Gancao Tang*) as recorded in *Qianjin* is effective for pulmonary asthenia with repeated spitting of saliva and sputum, a parched feeling in throat, and thirst.*

Rhizoma Zingiberis Recens	5 *liang*
Radix Ginseng	3 *liang*
Radix Glycyrrhizae	4 *liang*
Fructus Ziziphi Jujubae	15 pcs.

*Parched feeling in throat and thirst: *Waitai* contains the following: Another edition states, "Parched feeling in throat *without* thirst." This may be a miscopying of the text, as symptoms of pulmonary asthenia generally do not include thirst. (01-83)

Decoction of Ramulus Cinnamomi subtracting Radix Paeoniae

adding Fructus Gleditsiae Sinensis (*Guizhi Qu Shaoyao Jia Zaojia Tang*) as recorded in *Qianjin* is effective in treating pulmonary asthenia with spitting of saliva and sputum.

Ramulus Cinnamomi	3 *liang*
Rhizoma Zingiberis Recens	3 *liang*
Radix Glycyrrhizae	2 *liang*
Fructus Ziziphi Jujubae	10 pcs.
Fructus Gleditsiae Sinensis (remove pericarp and seeds and fry)	1 pc.

Stew the drugs in seven *sheng* of water over a slow fire until three *sheng* remain. Serve the lukewarm decoction in three doses.

Commentary: This prescription eliminates the sputum and relieves wheezing; it is applicable to severe cases of an excessive nature. As pulmonary asthenia is generally of a deficient nature, this prescription is not suitable. It is doubtful that this is a correct version of the original text. (01-83)

Baisan Powder with Radix Platycodi (*Jiegeng Baisan*) as recorded in *Waitai* is effective for pulmonary abscess with symptoms and signs of coughing, fullness in the chest, shivering, speedy pulse, parched throat without thirst, repeated spitting of bad-smelling saliva and sputum, and chronic vomiting of abscess resembling porridge.

Radix Platycodi	3 *fen*
Bulbus Fritillariae Thunbergii	3 *fen*
Fructus Crotonis (remove skin and core, stew, pound into oiled powder)	1 *fen*

Pound the drugs into powder. Give one half *qianbi* for a strong person and less for a weak person. If the syndrome is located above the diaphragm, the patient will vomit abscess and blood. When the syndrome is below the diaphragm, the patient will have loose stool. In case the stool is excessive, drink one cup of cold water for relief.

Commentary: This prescription is from *Shanghan Lun* quoted by Wang Dao in his *Waitai*. (See Clause 141 of *Shanghan Lun*.) It is effective in acute cases of pulmonary abscess. In the course of application, careful attention should be paid to the patient's build, as this prescription is very strong.

Decoction of Rhizoma Phragmitis (*Weijing Tang*) as recorded in *Qianjin* is effective in treating pulmonary abscess with coughing, low fever, restlessness, sensation of fullness, and scaling skin on the chest.*

Rhizoma Phragmitis	2 *sheng*
Semen Coicis	0.5 *sheng*
Semen Persicae	50 pcs.
Semen Benincasae	0.5 *sheng*

Stew Rhizoma Phragmitis in one *dou* of water until five *sheng* remain. Filter the decoction and add remaining drugs. Stew again until two *sheng* remain. Serve one *sheng* as the first dose. When second dose is served, the patient should vomit abscess.

*Scaling skin on the chest: The skin in the chest region is coarse and scaling due to the formation of an abscess in the Interior. In such cases, the Blood and Vital Energy stagnate and cease providing nourishment to the skin. Scaling skin results. (02-60)

Explanation of the Prescription: This prescription is frequently used in the treatment of pulmonary abscess. Before the abscess forms, add the following ingredients to eliminate Heat, disperse the pathogenetic factors, and serve as an antidote: Herba Houttuyniae, Herba Taraxaci, Herba Violae, Flos Lonicerae, Fructus Forsythiae, etc. Once the abscess has formed, Radix Platycodi, Radix Glycyrrhizae, Bulbus Fritillariae Thunbergii and the like can be added to reinforce elimination of sputum and abscess.

This prescription can also be adopted for the following cases, with necessary additions and substraction: Lobar pneumonia, empyema, bronchiectasis, chronic bronchitis and pulmonary tuberculosis, etc. (02-60)

CASES

Case 1 (65-224): Pulmonary Abscess, Case Recorded in *Case Studies of Dr. Wu Jutong* (1758-1836)

My cousin, 40, addict of alcohol, liked to sit on hot *kang* (heatable brick bed) during winter. He suffered serious insomnia, and frequent perspiration. He was once given Folium Eriobotryae and Herba Ephedrae to improve Lung function, this consumed the Body Fluid. Pulmonary abscess was formed, with smelly discharge. The patient spat two *sheng* (liter) of purulent substance every day.

Treatment: Decoction of Rhizoma Phragmitis of *Qianjin* was prescribed:

Rhizoma Phragmitis
Radix Platycodi
Semen Persicae
Semen Coicis
Semen Benincasae
Radix Glycyrrhizae

The decoction was stewed in two bowls and served one and a half bowls in twenty-four hours. Spitting of purulent substance reduced. After other half dose of decoction was taken the spit was no longer smelly. Drugs regulating the Spleen and Stomach function were given to finish the treatment.

Case 2 (64-277):

Mr. Liang, 45, first treatment on October 25, 1962. The patient had a cold with coughing in April, but was unable to get treatment. He began having chest pain, spat purulent and bloody sputum almost four months when the syndrome was aggravated: the patient was spitting copious greasy and white smelly purulent sputum. He was hospitalized.

Examination: Temperature was 39 ℃. Respiration was 100/minute. He had parched feeling and pungent taste in mouth, slippery-speedy pulse, foul and greasy tongue coating.

Treatment: Decoction of Rhizoma Phragmitis was prescribed:

Rhizoma Phragmitis	30 grams
Semen Coicis	30 grams
Semen Benincasae	24 grams
Semen Persicae	9 grams
Flos Lonicerae	30 grams
Fructus Forsythiae	10 grams
Folium Isatidis	9 grams
Herba Houttuyniae	30 grams
Radix Platycodi	10 grams

Bulbus Fritillariae Thunbergii	9 grams
Fructus Trichosanthis	15 grams

Second treatment on October 30. Three doses of the decoction were served. The patient felt better. Another four doses were given.

Third treatment on November 4. Chest pain and cough subsided, spitting of sputum continued. The following drugs were added to the prescription:

Rhizoma Imperatae	20 grams
Cortex Moutan Radicis	6 grams

Fourth treatment: Four doses of amended decoction were served. All symptoms subsided. Pulse was speedy-slender, tongue red free from foul, greasy coating. There was still parched feeling in mouth. Decoction to Clear the Lung and Dissolve Phlegm (*Qing Zao Jiu Fei Tang*) with additions was prescribed:

Folium Mori	12 grams
Gypsum Fibrosum	10 grams
Semen Armeniacae Amarum	10 grams
Radix Glycyrrhizae	4 grams
Radix Ophiopogonis	12 grams
Radix Ginseng	9 grams
Colla Corii Asini	10 grams
Folium Eriobotryae Praeparata	9 grams
Fructus Trichosanthis	15 grams
Radix Glehniae	15 grams
Bulbus Fritillariae Thunbergii	9 grams

Fifth treatment: After five doses were consumed, all symptoms subsided. Pulse became moderate. Another six doses of decoction were given for the patient to take at home.

Case 3 (64-278): Case Recorded in Journal of *Zhejiang Chinese Medicine*, 10:19, 1957

Mr. Ma, 34-year-old farmer, first treatment on August 10, 1954. The patient had a cold, then pneumonia. Chronic coughing induced formation of purulent ulcer, causing chest pain, fever, restlessness, profuse perspiration, spitting of smelly and bloody sputum, emaciation and anorexia.

Treatment: Decoction of Rhizoma Phragmitis was prescribed as follows:

Rhizoma Phragmitis	10 grams
Semen Persicae	3 grams

Semen Coicis	4 grams
Semen Benincasae	3 grams
Talcum	4 grams
Gypsum Fibrosum	5 grams
Radix Scutellariae	2 grams
Bulbus Fritillariae Thunbergii	2 grams
Flos Lonicerae	4 grams
Caulis Bambusae in Taeniam	3 grams

Second treatment on August 14. After four doses, fever subsided. Spitting was still smelly. The following drugs were prescribed:

Rhizoma Phragmitis	10 grams
Semen Persicae	3 grams
Semen Coicis	4 grams
Talcum	4 grams
Semen Benincasae	3 grams
Flos Lonicerae	3 grams
Fructus Gardeniae	3 grams
Radix Scutellariae	2 grams
Semen Armeniacae Amarum	3 grams
Bulbus Fritillariae Thunbergii	2 grams

Third treatment on August 19. Five doses of the decoction were given. Spitting reduced and was no longer smelly. Perspiration and fever subsided. The following drugs were prescribed:

Radix Glehniae	3 grams
Radix Adenophorae	3 grams
Semen Coicis	8 grams
Semen Benincasae	3 grams
Talcum	4 grams
Rhizoma Phragmitis	8 grams
Radix Scutellariae	2 grams
Radix Ophiopogonis	3 grams
Radix Glycyrrhizae Praeparata	1 gram
Semen Armeniacae Amarum	3 grams
Radix Asteris	2 grams
Folium Eriobotryae	3 grams

Fourth treatment on August 25. After six doses of the decoction were consumed, the patient coughed less and had a good appetite. The following prescription to tonify the Deficiency and clear the remaining pathogenesis was given:

Radix Codonopsis Pilosulae	2 grams
Radix Ophiopogonis	3 grams
Radix Asteris	2 grams
Bulbus Lilii	3 grams
Semen Coicis	5 grams
Semen Benincasae	3 grams
Rhizoma Phragmitis	10 grams
Rhizoma Pinelliae	2 grams
Radix Glycyrrhizae	1 gram
Folium Eriobotryae	3 grams

CHAPTER VIII

ON PULSE, SYMPTOM COMPLEX AND TREATMENT OF *BENTUN* SYNDROME

CLAUSE 8-1

Master: *Bentun* (1), vomiting of pus, fright and Fire-evil are four diseases caused by fright. (2)

NOTES

1. *Bentun*, or *Bentunqi*: Syndrome characterized by a feeling of gas rushing up through the thorax to the throat from the lower abdomen. *Jinkui S*: *Bentunqi* is an attacking disease originating in the lower abdomen. At the onset, pain is felt in the lower abdomen suggesting the presence of compressed gas. The patient then feels the gas ascending to the Heart and the thorax and finally to the throat. The patient experiences great pain. Then the syndrome diminishes and finally subsides. You Yi writes in *The Gist of the Golden Chamber* (*Jinkui G*): The text says that *Bentun* is caused by fright; this is because the Kidney is hurt by fright. *Bentun* originates from a Kidney disorder. When the Vital Energy of the Kidney is disturbed, it ascends to the thorax and throat, like a pig running within the body. Liver disorders may also cause *Bentun*, as both the Kidney and the Liver are located in the Lower Portion of Body Cavity and their Vital Energy tends to rush upward.

2. This clause discusses the pathology and symptoms of *Bentun*. *Bentun*, vomiting of pus, fright and Fire-evil are related to the Heart Channel. Fright resembles convulsions and palpitations (see Chapter XVI). As to the mechanism of the syndrome with vomiting of pus caused by fright, further study is required. Fire-evil is a disease accompanied by fright caused by pathogenetic Fire. See Clause 119 of *Shanghan Lun*, which reads: "Initial Yang syndrome, febrile disease caused by Cold: The patient will become manic if warming needle is adopted." See also Clauses 65 and 117. (02-67)

CLAUSE 8-2

Bentun syndrome originates in the lower abdomen and rushes upward to the throat. An attack of the syndrome causes the patient unbearable suffering, which gradually reduces and subsides. The cause of the disease is fright and terror (1).

NOTES

1. *Bentun* syndrome is caused by fright and terror. The disease is related to the Heart, the Liver and the Kidney. The mechanism of ascent is related to *Chongmai*.* Fright injures the Heart, terror injures the Kidney. When the Yang Vital Energy of the Heart and the Kidney is deficient, pathogenetic Cold and Water will ascend through the channel of *Chongmai*. Or when the patient is frightened or experiences spiritual distress. Liver Vital Energy may accumulate and ascend through the *Chongmai*. Hence the causa morbi of *Bentun*.

**Chongmai* is one of the Eight Extra Channels. It originates in the pelvis (uterus) and runs upwards along the Interior of the vertebrae. It also begins from the sides of the genitalia and passes by both sides of umbilicus, ending in the chest. When this channel is diseased, such symptoms as dyspnea, abdominal pain, borborygmus, abnormal menstruation and infertility appear.

CLAUSE 8-3

Bentun syndrome with ascending gas rushing to the thorax, abdominal pain, and alternating episodes of chills and fevers can be treated with Decoction of *Bentun*.

Decoction of *Bentun*
(*Bentun Tang*):

Radix Glycyrrhizae	2 *liang*
Rhizoma Ligustici Chuanxiong	2 *liang*
Radix Angelicae Sinensis	2 *liang*
Rhizoma Pinelliae	4 *liang*
Radix Scutellariae	2 *liang*
Radix Puerariae	5 *liang*
Radix Paeoniae	2 *liang*
Rhizoma Zingiberis Recens	4 *liang*
Cortex Prunus Armeniacae	1 *sheng*

Stew the drugs in two *dou* of water until five *sheng* remain. Give one *sheng* of lukewarm decoction per dose, three in the day, and one at night.

Explanation of the Prescription: This prescription is only effective for *Bentun* syndrome caused by pathogenetic Fire which originates with an abnormal accumulation of Liver Vital Energy. If the case is of a Cold nature, therapy should follow that of Clauses 8-4 and 8-5. (02-68)

You Yi: This prescription treats *Bentun* syndrome originating with pathogenetic factors in the Liver. Alternating episodes of chills and fevers suggest a Lesser Yang syndrome. To disperse the abnormal accumulation in the Liver, Rhizoma Zingiberis Recens, Rhizoma Pinelliae and Radix Puerariae may be adopted. Radix Glycyrrhizae is added to relieve stress in the Liver Vital Energy. Rhizoma Ligustici Chuanxiong, Radix Angelicae Sinensis and Radix Paeoniae regulate the normal functioning of the Blood. Radix Scutellariae and Cortex Prunus Armeniacae are used to reverse the abnormal ascending. Ramulus Cinnamomi and Poria, the principal ingredients of *Bentun*, are not included as this is not a case originating in the Kidney.

CASES

Case 1 (64-288): Case Recorded in *Collection of Case Studies of Doctors in Hubei Province*

Master Zhang Zhongjing, author of the book, said *Bentun* was caused by fright. I agree. When I was younger, I treated a syndrome of *Bentun* successfully with Decoction of *Bentun*:

Mr. Shi, a young man, was gambling in a den when policemen came to catch the gamblers. Shi escaped by jumping the courtyard wall. A few days later, he began to have chills and fever, and gas rushing from lower abdomen. When attacked, the patient had so much pain he did not recognize people around him. Decoctions to regulate the Vital Energy and stop pain were given, but did not help. The patient consulted me. Three large doses of Decoction of *Bentun* were prescribed. The patient recovered.

Case 2 (64-289): Case Recorded in *Journal of Zhejiang College of Chinese Medicine*, 1:7, 1982

Li, 64-year-old lady, first treatment on October 24, 1965. One year prior to the consultation, her grandson was drowned. Her sadness made her restless and irritable and apt to lose her temper. She had dreams and insomnia. *Bentun* occurred: first, pain in the lower abdomen with a growing hard mass, bringing with it an ascending gas rushing to the throat, vertigo, dimness of vision, and feeling of suffocation. This lasted about half an hour and subsided gradually. It attacked two or three times a week. Tongue was covered with thin, yellow coating. Pulse was tight and slightly speedy.

Diagnosis: *Bentun* syndrome caused by emotional stimulation that induced the stagnation of Vital Energy in the Liver. Decoction of *Bentun* was adopted.

Prescription:

Cortex Prunus Armeniacae	15 grams
Radix Puerariae	12 grams
Rhizoma Pinelliae Praeparata	9 grams
Radix Scutellariae	9 grams
Rhizoma Zingiberis Recens	5 grams
Radix Paeoniae Alba	12 grams
Radix Angelicae Sinensis	6 grams
Rhizoma Ligustici Chuanxiong	5 grams
Os Draconis (stewed prior to other drugs)	15 grams
Concha Ostreae (stewed prior to other drugs)	30 grams
Haematitum	15 grams

The above decoction (with alterations every time) was served for a month. Thirty-nine doses were given before the syndrome was gone. Ten doses were finally served to complete the treatment.

Case 3 (46-136): Case recorded in *Tun Yuan Case Studies (Tun Yuan Yi An)*, (Dr. Xiao Zhuoru)

Bentun syndrome, caused by abnormal ascending of gas originating in the Kidney (in Cold nature), was a common disease. Decoction of Ramulus Cinnamomi adding Ramulus Cinnamomi was the cure. It was not common to see *Bentun* syndrome caused by ascending gas of the Liver-fire, here was one case:

An old lady said her daughter-in-law suffered from abdominal pain, with alternating chill and fever, parched throat and bitterness in mouth. The doctor thought this could be cured by Decoction of Lesser Bupleuri. The old lady insisted the doctor see the patient in person.

Examination: Abdominal pain accompanied by rushing of gas upward to the chest and throat. This occurred at intervals. Pulse was tight-speedy, tongue covered with white coating.

Diagnosis: *Bentun* syndrome caused by ascending of Liver-fire.

Treatment: Decoction of *Bentun* was given. One dose alleviated the condition, three doses completed the treatment.

Case 4 (52-566): Gastric Neurosis

Mr. Xu, 46-year-old worker. Since March 1965, he suffered from gastric upset with acid regurgitation and vomiting. When this happened, he felt gas rushing from lower abdomen to the chest, suffocating him, vomiting occurred as a consequence. The syndrome attacked every three to five days and had lasted for years. The patient consulted the doctor of Chinese medicine on February 15, 1979. Pulse was deep-slender, tongue covered with thin, white coating and coating at root of tongue thick and greasy. Decoction of *Bentun* was prescribed:

Rhizoma Ligustici Chuanxiong	9 grams
Radix Angelicae Sinensis	9 grams
Rhizoma Zingiberis Recens	15 grams
Rhizoma Pinelliae	9 grams
Radix Scutellariae	9 grams
Radix Glycyrrhizae	9 grams
Radix Puerariae	15 grams
Radix Paeoniae Alba	15 grams
Cortex Prunus Armeniacae	12 grams

Six doses were taken, one per day. There was no attack for fifteen days. There had been some vomiting.

Second treatment: The decoction was prescribed with additions:

Ramulus Cinnamomi	9 grams
Fructus Evodiae	9 grams
Poria	15 grams
Rhizoma Curculiginis	9 grams
Herba Epimedii	9 grams

Six doses were served. Vomiting subsided. The patient was in good spirits with good appetite. In February 1982, no recurrence was reported.

CLAUSE 8-4

After adopting a diaphoretic, warming needle is administered to induce another perspiration. If locus of puncture hole is left unprotected and comes into contact with cold, it will turn red and swell. An impulsive feeling will rise from the abdomen to the chest resulting in a *Bentun* syndrome. Treat with moxibustion and give Decoction of Ramulus Cinnamomi adding Ramulus Cinnamomi.

Decoction of Ramulus Cinnamomi adding Ramulus Cinnamomi (*Guizhi Jia Gui Tang*):

Ramulus Cinnamomi	5 *liang*

Radix Paeoniae	3 *liang*
Radix Glycyrrhizae Praeparata	2 *liang*
Rhizoma Zingiberis Recens	3 *liang*
Fructus Ziziphi Jujubae	12 pcs.

Stew the drugs over a slow fire in seven *sheng* of water until three *sheng* remain. Filter the decoction and give one *sheng* of lukewarm decoction as a serving.

Explanation of the Prescription: Ramulus Cinnamomi has the function of dispersing the Cold and reversing the adverse ascent of gas. Radix Paeoniae eases abdominal pain. Radix Glycyrrhizae and Fructus Ziziphi Jujubae harmonize the Stomach Vital Energy and ease the strained condition of the Interior. Rhizoma Zingiberis Recens nourishes the Stomach and reverses the adverse ascending. *Bentun* syndrome of a Cold nature can be eliminated by adopting this prescription, whether or not it is induced by use of the warming needle. (01-87)

Remark: This clause also appears in Clause 117 of *Shanghan Lun* with slight variations in the text.

CLAUSE 8-5

After adopting diaphoretic, a "jumping" feeling, resembling a baby pig running, is sensed below the umbilicus. Shortly afterwards, the feeling begins to move upward. This is called a *Bentun* syndrome. Prescribe Decoction of Poria, Ramulus Cinnamomi, Radix Glycyrrhizae and Fructus Ziziphi Jujubae to reduce the adversity.

Decoction of Poria, Ramulus Cinnamomi, Radix Glycyrrhizae and Fructus Ziziphi Jujubae
(*Fuling Guizhi Gancao Dazao Tang*):

Poria	0.5 *jin*
Radix Glycyrrhizae Praeparata	2 *liang*
Fructus Ziziphi Jujubae	15 pcs.

Ramulus Cinnamomi 4 *liang*

Stew Poria in one *dou* of *ganlan* water* until eight *sheng* remain. Add remaining drugs and stew until three *sheng* remain. Take three doses a day, one *sheng* per dose.

Remark: This clause also appears in Clause 65 of *Shanghan Lun*.

Explanation of the Prescription: This prescription deals with the onset of *Bentun* syndrome due to Water-retention. The mechanism of the disease is as follows: When a diaphoretic is adopted for a patient with Water-retention at the Lower Portion of Body Cavity, the Heart Yang Vital Energy becomes too deficient to control the Water circulation. Pathogenetic Water moves in the Interior. This can be seen from the jumping which takes place below the umbilicus and which is likely to ascend. The above decoction is adopted to stimulate the normal function of the Yang and facilitate Water circulation. Thus the ascending tendency is eliminated. (02-69)

**Ganlan* water (*ganlan shui*): Place two *dou* of water in a basin. With a spoon, drip the water repeatedly into the basin until it appears that 5,000-6,000 drops of dew are moving on the surface. This is *ganlan* water.

CHAPTER IX

ON PULSE, SYMPTOM COMPLEX AND TREATMENT OF CHEST OBSTRUCTION, HEART PAIN AND SHORTNESS OF BREATH

CLAUSE 9-1

Master: When feeling the pulse, excessiveness and deficiency should be diagnosed. Feebleness at Yang and tightness at Yin (1) indicate a Chest Obstruction syndrome (2) with pain. The extremely deficient state is the causa morbi. Feeble pulse at Yang indicates prevalence of a deficient state at the Upper Portion of Body Cavity. Chest Obstruction and Heart Pain (3) is manifested by a tight pulse at Yin.

NOTES

1. Feebleness at Yang and tightness at Yin: feeble pulse at the Inch (pulse under the first finger) and tight pulse at the Cubit (pulse under the ring-finger).

2. Chest Obstruction (*Xiong bi*): *Bi*, meaning "obstruction," is not only the name of the disease, but also indicates the mechanism and location of the syndrome. When normal physiological activities (such as the flow of the Vital Energy and the Blood) are obstructed, a feeling of pain will appear. Thus the principal symptom of the Chest Obstruction syndrome is pain. The mechanism of the syndrome is as follows: When Yang Vital Energy at the Upper Portion of Body Cavity is in a deficient state, the pathogenetic factors of a Yin nature will ascend to invade the former, causing the obstruction of Yang Vital Energy. Chest Obstruction generally bears the symptoms of a sensation of fullness and suffocation in the chest, with pain inside and outside the thorax. (02-70, 01-88)

Wu Qian: A mild case of the Chest Obstruction syndrome is called "fullness in the chest" and an acute case is called "Chest Pain." (05-523)

3. Heart Pain (*Xin tong*): Heart Pain includes pain in the thorax, the

Heart and the epigastrium. As the Heart is located in the chest, the syndromes of Heart Pain and Chest Obstruction always appear simultaneously, causing complications. Thus they are included in the same chapter. (01-88)

CLAUSE 9-2

A normal person who is not suffering from either a fever or a chill may feel a shortness of breath with hypopnea. This is an excessive case. (1)

NOTES

1. The syndrome is caused by an accumulation of phlegm and by indigestion which has obstructed normal physiological activities. It is different from the Chest Obstruction syndrome. (01-89)

CLAUSE 9-3

Chest Obstruction syndrome has the symptoms and signs of panting, coughing, spitting, shortness of breath and pain in the chest and back. The pulse is deep and slow in the Inch and slender-tense-speedy in the Bar (1). Decoction of Fructus Trichosanthis, Bulbus Allii Aacrostemi and Wine (2) can be adopted to eliminate the syndrome.

NOTES

1. In Cheng Lin's *Thorough Explanation of Synopsis of the Golden Chamber*, a note is added to the phrase "slender-tense-speedy in the Bar": "These few words must be wrong." *Jinkui E* provides the following explanation for the pulse mentioned in this clause: The pulse is deep and slow in the Inch and slender-tense-speedy in the Bar. The slow pulse and speedy pulse mentioned above do not refer to the jumping of the pulse but to the presentation of the pulse. Slow pulse here indicates an exhausted and weak state, whereas speedy pulse indicates the irritative and restless state of the pulsation.

2. Wine (*Baijiu*): This may refer to a) freshly brewed rice wine; or b) fermented glutinous rice. In clinical practice, the following may be used: Wine made of Chinese sorghum, *Shaoxing* rice wine, or rice vinegar, all which have the function of activating Yang Vital Energy and easing pain. (02-71)

Decoction of Fructus Trichosanthis, Bulbus Allii Aacrostemi and Wine
(*Gualou Xiebai Baijiu Tang*):

Fructus Trichosanthis (pound into pieces)	1 pc.
Bulbus Allii Aacrostemi	0.5 *jin*
Wine (*Baijiu*)	7 *sheng*

Stew the drugs in the wine until two *sheng* remain. Serve the decoction lukewarm in two doses.

Explanation of the Prescription: This prescription can dredge through the obstruction in the chest. Fructus Trichosanthis eliminates phlegm and reverse the adverse ascending of gas. Bulbus Allii Aacrostemi, of a warm quality, activates the Yang Vital Energy in the chest, disperses the accumulation and thus eases the pain. Wine (*Baijiu*) has the quality of ascending and carry the medicine upward. It can also strengthen the efficacy of Bulbus Allii Aacrostemi. (01-89)

CASES

Case 1 (65-238):

The patient suffered from pain in chest and back. Pulse was deep-hesitant and tense at Bar and Cubit positions. The patient had no cough or asthma. He was a tailor, who made fur coats. He worked very hard, often on cold nights. He had a feeling of suffocation in chest at night which developed into chest pain. Decoction of Fructus Trichosanthis, Bulbus Allii Aacrostemi and Wine was prescribed:

Fructus Trichosanthis	15 grams
Bulbus Allii Aacrostemi	9 grams
Wine	a small cup

Two doses cured the ailment.

Case 2 (65-239): Chest Obstruction (Angina Pectoris), Case Recorded in Journal of *Shanghai Chinese Medicine,* 2:21, 1964

Wei, 61, female, first treatment on October 26, 1962.

Examination: The patient had felt suffocation and severe pain in chest with dragging pain in the back for twenty days, with as many as ten attacks in a single day. When attacked, these symptoms appeared: shortness of breath, palpitation, nausea, acid regurgitation, perspiration. Examination by a hospital in Beijing showed it was a syndrome of angina pectoris. Pulse was deep-tense, tongue in normal condition.

Treatment: Decoction of Fructus Trichosanthis, Bulbus Allii Aacrostemi and Wine with additions was prescribed:

Fructus Trichosanthis	15 grams
Bulbus Allii Aacrostemi	9 grams
Ramulus Cinnamomi	7.5 grams
Fructus Aurantii Praeparata	9 grams
Herba Asari	3 grams
Rhizoma Cyperi Praeparata	9 grams
Rhizoma Curcumae Longae	6 grams
Exocarpium Citri Grandis	6 grams
Caulis Agastachis	9 grams
Rhizoma Acori Graminei	3 grams
Radix Salviae Miltiorrhizae	2 grams
Resina Olibani Praeparata	4.5 grams
Resina Commiphorae Myrrhae Praeparata	4.5 grams
Wine (blend into the already stewed decoction before service)	1/2 cup

Two doses were served. Two pills of *Su He Wan* (one pill per day) were also given.

Second treatment: Angina pectoris did not attack after taking the drugs. Another six doses of the decoction and pills were given. The following alterations were made in the decoction: Herba Asari reduced to 2.1 grams and Wine reduced.

The medicament worked. The patient was healthy again. In March 1963, no recurrence of angina pectoris was reported.

Case 3 (64-304): Exudative Pleurisy, Case Recorded in Journal of *Jilin Chinese Medicine*, 2:47, 1981

Mr. Zhou, 25-year-old farmer, first treatment on August 21, 1974. The patient was suffering from chill and fever, cough and a severe pain in the right chest. It was diagnosed by Western medicine as a syndrome of exudative pleurisy.

Decoction of Fructus Trichosanthis, Bulbus Allii Aacrostemi and Wine was prescribed:

Fructus Trichosanthis	50 grams
Bulbus Allii Aacrostemi	20 grams
Wine (blend into the already stewed decoction before service)	a small cup

The decoction was given once in the morning and once in the evening. Ten doses cured the syndrome. One month later the patient was examined and everything was normal.

Case 4 (48-439): 50 Cases of Intercostal Neuralgia, Cases Recorded in *Journal of Zhejiang Chinese Medicine*, Vol. 6, 1964

The journal reported on fifty cases of intercostal neuralgia cured by a combination of Decoction of Fructus Trichosanthis, Bulbus Allii Aacrostemi and Wine and Powder of *Si Ni* (prescription recorded in *Shanghan Lun*, Clause 318, listing the ingredients: Radix Glycyrrhizae Praeparata, Fructus Aurantii Immaturus, Radix Bupleuri and Radix Paeoniae). The basic prescription for all the fifty cases was:

Bulbus Allii Aacrostemi (prepared with wine)	9 grams
Pericarpium Trichosanthis Praeparata	9 grams
Radix Paeoniae Alba	9 grams
Radix Bupleuri	4.5 grams
Fructus Aurantii Immaturus Praeparata	4.5 grams
Radix Glycyrrhizae Praeparata	4.5 grams
Radix Curcumae	4.5 grams
Semen Persicae	6 grams
Rhizoma Cyperi Praeparata	6 grams

Additions and Subtractions:

When costal pain was severe, add:

Fructus Meliae Toosendan	9 grams
Radix Angelicae Pubescentis	9 grams
Radix Angelicae Dahuricae	6 grams
Folium Citri Reticulatae Viride	4.5 grams

When costal pain was too severe, add:

Resina Olibani	3 grams
Resina Commiphorae Myrrhae	3 grams

When there was stagnation of blood stasis, add:

Herba Artemisiae Anomalae	6 grams
Flos Carthami	3 grams

When there was coughing, add:

Semen Armeniacae Amarum	9 grams
Fructus Perillae Praeparata	9 grams

Among the 50 cases:

Three doses were given to complete the treatment in six cases;
Four doses were given to cure twenty-four cases;
Six doses were given to complete the treatment in sixteen cases;
Eight doses were served to complete the treatment in six cases.

On average, 4.8 doses were needed till the syndrome subsided. Of the fifty cases, five recurred within three months, but were treated again by the same decoction, which was effective.

CLAUSE 9-4

Chest Obstruction syndrome: The patient suffers an acute pain in the chest and a dragging pain in the back. The pain is so acute that he is unable to lie quietly in bed. Decoction of Fructus Trichosanthis, Bulbus Allii Aacrostemi and Rhizoma Pinelliae can be adopted to ease the pain.

Decoction of Fructus Trichosanthis, Bulbus Allii Aacrostemi and Rhizoma Pinelliae
(*Gualou Xièbai Banxia Tang*)

Fructus Trichosanthis (pound into pieces)	1 pc.
Bulbus Allii Aacrostemi	3 *liang*
Rhizoma Pinelliae	0.5 *jin*
Wine (*Baijiu*)	1 *dou*

Stew the drugs in the wine until four *sheng* remain. Serve one *sheng* of lukewarm decoction per dose three times a day.

Explanation of the Prescription: Rhizoma Pinelliae is added to eliminate the phlegm, as a large accumulation of phlegm stagnating in the chest is the cause of the syndrome.

Commentary: Prescriptions found in Clauses 9-3 and 9-4 are principal means of treating the Chest Obstruction syndrome. According to clinical reports, the above prescriptions are effective in curing angina pectoris caused by the obstruction of phlegm. If it is complicated with blood stasis, the following drugs, which can invigorate blood circulation and eliminate blood stasis, can be added (see Recipe No. 2 for Coronary Heart Disease): Radix Salviae Miltiorrhizae, Radix Paeoniae Rubra, Rhizoma Ligustici Chuanxiong, Flos Carthami and Lignum Dalbergiae Odoriferae.

Shixiao Powder, recorded in the *Formularies of the Bureau of the People's Welfare Pharmacies* (compiled by Chen Shiwen, et al., in 1151) can also be used to treat the disease.

Shixiao Powder:
(*Shixiao San*):

Faeces Trogopterorum
Pollen Typhae

Pound the drugs in equal quantities into powder. Give two *qian* per dose. Stew the powder in water with vinegar. Serve the hot decoction with the dregs. (02-72)

CASES

Case 1 (46-144): Pulmonary Heart Disease

Mr. Sheng, 60, retired, suffered from pulmonary heart disease.

Examination: He was coughing and spitting greasy phlegm, had chest pain and distention at back, palpitation and panting which made him difficult to lie flat. Stool and urine were normal. Tongue was red, covered with thin coating. Pulse was tight-slippery.

Diagnosis: Syndrome caused by distended Vital Energy in the Lung and stagnation of phlegm in the chest.

Treatment: To regulate the Vital Energy in the chest and disperse the stagnated phlegm.

Decoction of Fructus Trichosanthis, Bulbus Allii Aacrostemi and Rhizoma Pinelliae with additions was prescribed:

Fructus Trichosanthis	15 grams
Bulbus Allii Aacrostemi	10 grams
Rhizoma Pinelliae Praeparata	10 grams
Poria	10 grams
Semen Armeniacae Amarum	10 grams
Radix Glycyrrhizae	3 grams
Flos Inulae	10 grams
Cortex Magnoliae Officinalis	6 grams
Fructus Perillae	10 grams

Lumbricus	10 grams
Concha Margaritifera Usta	15 grams

The decoction relieved the ailment. Within two years, there had been two recurrences. When the syndrome attacked, the patient took the decoction accompanied by Pills of *Du Qi*,* which were effective.

*Pills of *Du Qi*: Rhizoma Rehmanniae Praeparata, Fructus Corni, Rhizoma Dioscoreae, Rhizoma Alismatis, Cortex Moutan Radicis, Poria, Fructus Schisandrae.

Case 2 (64-306): Case Recorded in Journal of *Jiangxi Chinese Medicine*, 1:34, 1981

Mr. Li, 60, suffered from chest pain and suffocation, which attacked once or twice a day. When there was mental distress or overwork, the attacks became more frequent and severe. He talked in his sleep (somniloquence). His extremities were cold. Pulse was deep-slow, tongue dark pale, covered with thin white coating. Pulsation was 60 times/minute. Blood pressure was 90-50 mm.Hg.

Diagnosis: Heart function hampered, complicated with stagnation of Blood and Vital Energy.

Treatment: To warm and regulate the Heart Yang and Vital Energy, and disperse blood stasis. Decoction of Fructus Trichosanthis, Bulbus Allii Aacrostemi and Rhizoma Pinelliae adding tonics and drugs removing stasis were given:

Pericarpium Trichosanthis	12 grams
Rhizoma Pinelliae	10 grams
Bulbus Allii Aacrostemi	10 grams
Ramulus Cinnamomi	6 grams
Radix Codonopsis Pilosulae	10 grams
Radix Aconiti Praeparata	6 grams
Radix Salviae Miltiorrhizae	15 grams
Radix Angelicae Sinensis	10 grams
Powder of Radix Notoginseng (blend in the already stewed decoction before service)	3 grams
Fructus Aurantii	10 grams
Rhizoma Cyperi	10 grams
Retinervus Citri Fructus	6 grams

The decoctions (with minor alterations) were served for two months. Chest pain reduced. Blood pressure raised to 103/65 mm.Hg. Pulsation was 65 times/minute. Appetite improved and the patient was able to work again. Decoction of Fructus Trichosanthis, Bulbus Allii Aacrostemi and Rhizoma

Pinelliae, with additions, was administered to stabilize the condition.

Case 3 (51-202):

Wang, 35, female. In autumn 1938, the patient had a feeling of distention and suffocation in chest, with pain referring to the back, dyspnea, panting and constipation. Pulse was deep-slippery, tongue covered with white-greasy coating.

Diagnosis: Syndrome caused by abnormal ascending of turbid Yin that accumulated and stayed in the Upper Portion of Body Cavity. Normal circulation was hampered.

Treatment: Decoction of Fructus Trichosanthis, Bulbus Allii Aacrostemi and Rhizoma Pinelliae was given to regulate the flow of the Yang Vital Energy and disperse turbidity to drain downward:

Fructus Trichosanthis	9 grams
Bulbus Allii Aacrostemi	6 grams
Rhizoma Pinelliae	6 grams
Fructus Aurantii Immaturus	4.5 grams
Semen Armeniacae Amarum	6 grams
Ramulus Cinnamomi	4.5 grams
Pericarpium Citri Reticulatae	3 grams

Four doses of the decoction were served. The syndrome was gone after several doses were taken.

CLAUSE 9-5

Chest Obstruction syndrome may be accompanied by either Vital-energy Stagnation (1) in the epigastrium or by stagnation of the Vital Energy in the chest with a sensation of fullness in the chest and gas ascending from the ribs rushing towards the Heart (2). Decoction of Fructus Aurantii Immaturus, Bulbus Allii Aacrostemi and Ramulus Cinnamomi can be adopted. Decoction of Radix Ginseng can be adopted as an alternative.

NOTES

1. Vital-energy Stagnation (*Pi*) is an ancient term for the syndrome which is commonly characteristic by a sensation of fullness and stagnation caused by stagnation of the Vital Energy in the chest, without pains or swelling mass. For details see Clause 131 of *Shanghan Lun*.

2. Wu Qian: Chest Obstruction with Vital-energy stagnation sensation of suffocation is a syndrome of a deficient nature. When Vital Energy is stagnating in the chest (but not in the epigastrium) with a sensation of fullness and gas as-

cending from the ribs rushing towards the Heart, this is a syndrome of an excessive nature. Syndrome of an excessive nature can be treated with Decoction of Fructus Aurantii Immaturus, Bulbus Allii Aacrostemi and Ramulus Cinnamomi. Note that Fructus Aurantii Immaturus and Cortex Magnoliae Officinalis are given in large quantities in the prescription. This is because this prescription is for an excessive syndrome and has the effect of dredging through the stagnation of the Vital Energy and reversing the adverse ascending of gas. Decoction of Radix Ginseng is used to treat the syndrome of a deficient nature by tonifying the Vital Energy and warming the Interior. (05-528)

Decoction of Fructus Aurantii Immaturus, Bulbus Allii Aacrostemi and Ramulus Cinnamomi
(*Zhishi Xiebai Guizhi Tang*)

Fructus Aurantii Immaturus	4 pcs.
Cortex Magnoliae Officinalis	4 *liang*
Bulbus Allii Aacrostemi	0.5 *jin*
Ramulus Cinnamomi	1 *liang*
Fructus Trichosanthis (broken open)	1 pc.

Stew Fructus Aurantii Immaturus and Cortex Magnoliae Officinalis in five *sheng* of water until two *sheng* remain. Filter the decoction and add remaining drugs. Stew again until it boils. Serve the lukewarm decoction in three doses.

Decoction of Radix Ginseng
(*Renshen Tang*):

Radix Ginseng	3 *liang*
Radix Glycyrrhizae	3 *liang*
Rhizoma Zingiberis	3 *liang*
Rhizoma Atractylodis Macrocephalae	3 *liang*

Stew the drugs in eight *sheng* of water until three *sheng* remain. Serve one *sheng* of lukewarm decoction per dose three times a day.

Explanation of the Prescriptions: Syndrome of an excessive nature can be treated with Decoction of Fructus Aurantii Immaturus, Bulbus Allii Aacrostemi and Ramulus Cinnamomi. Fructus

Aurantii Immaturus and Cortex Magnoliae Officinalis are used to disperse the stagnant Vital Energy in the Stomach and eliminate the sensation of fullness. Ramulus Cinnamomi disperses the stagnation and invigorates the flow of the Vital Energy to suppress the gas ascending from the ribs rushing to the Heart. Fructus Trichosanthis and Bulbus Allii Aacrostemi are effective in treating the Chest Obstruction syndrome.

Syndrome of a deficient nature should be treated by administering Decoction of Radix Ginseng. In treating this syndrome, the key is to tonify the Spleen and the Stomach. When the stagnant Cold and Yin substance in the Spleen and the Stomach are warmed with warming and tonifying drugs, the stagnation of a Cold and Yin nature will be dispersed simultaneously, and the Vital-energy Stagnation will diminish. Radix Ginseng strengthens Body Resistance, eases pain in the epigastrium and abdomen, and reduces the sensation of fullness. When taken with Rhizoma Zingiberis and Rhizoma Atractylodis Macrocephalae, Radix Ginseng can stimulate the Yang Vital Energy to overcome stagnation of Yin. Radix Glycyrrhizae tonifies the Body Resistance and harmonizes the drugs. (01-91)

CASES

Case 1 (64-310): Case Recorded in Journal of *Chinese Medicine and Pharmacology,* 4:31, 1982

Mr. Zhang, 32, first treatment on May 9, 1971. The patient suffered from ulcer with bloody stool, which made him weak. Accompanying symptoms: insomnia and dreamy sleep, spontaneous perspiration, shortness of breath, anorexia, severe pain in epigastrium, which moved to the back. He liked a warm environment. Tongue was red with bloody spot, covered with thin, yellow coating, that at root of tongue was greasy. Pulse was slender-hesitant.

Diagnosis: Syndrome caused by impaired condition of the Yang in the thorax with stagnation of Vital Energy and blood stasis.

Treatment: Decoction of Fructus Aurantii Immaturus, Bulbus Allii Aacrostemi and Ramulus Cinnamomi was given:

Fructus Aurantii Praeparata	12 grams
Fructus Trichosanthis	12 grams
Bulbus Allii Aacrostemi	12 grams
Rhizoma Pinelliae (prepared with ginger)	9 grams
Ramulus Cinnamomi	9 grams

Pollen Typhae (wrapped in cloth bag)	9 grams
Faeces Trogopterorum	9 grams
Radix Salviae Miltiorrhizae	15 grams
Rhizoma Zingiberis Recens	9 grams
Rhizoma Paridis	9 grams

Second treatment: Six doses of the decoction were served, effectively. Another fifteen doses were given. After this, there was full recovery.

Case 2 (62-176): Viral Pericarditis

Mr. Wang, 52, first treatment on December 2, 1981. The patient had a distended and stifled feeling in left thorax for three years. During Spring Festival of 1978, he had severe suffocation of left thorax and was hospitalized for three months. In 1981, the syndrome attacked often, so he consulted the doctor of Chinese medicine.

Examination: There was a distended and suffocated feeling in left thorax. Blood pressure was in normal range. Tongue was pale and fat, covered with greasy coating. Pulse was tight-hesitant.

Diagnosis: Syndrome of Chest Obsruction caused by stagnation of Vital Energy, blood stasis and impaired Heart Yang.

Treatment: Decoction of Fructus Aurantii Immaturus, Bulbus Allii Aacrostemi and Ramulus Cinnamomi was given to regulate the flow of Vital Energy, remove blood stasis and stimulate the stagnated Yang Vital Energy:

Pericarpium Trichosanthis	10 grams
Bulbus Allii Aacrostemi	10 grams
Fructus Aurantii Immaturus	10 grams
Ramulus Cinnamomi	10 grams
Cortex Magnoliae Officinalis	6 grams
Semen Persicae	12 grams
Flos Carthami	6 grams
Lignum Sappan	10 grams
Semen Biotae	20 grams
Herba Houttuyniae	30 grams

Second treatment on January 11, 1982. After six doses of the decoction, the patient felt relief. He resumed his travels, and the problem reoccurred (but not as severe as before). Tongue was pale and moist, covered with thin coating. Pulse was hesitant. The prescription based on the previous one was given:

Pericarpium Trichosanthis	60 grams
Bulbus Allii Aacrostemi	60 grams
Ramulus Cinnamomi	60 grams

Fructus Aurantii Immaturus	30 grams
Cortex Magnoliae Officinalis	30 grams
Semen Persicae	30 grams
Flos Carthami	30 grams
Herba Houttuyniae	30 grams
Semen Biotae	40 grams
Caulis Spatholobi	30 grams

Pounded the above drugs into powder and made pills of ten grams each with honey. One pill three times a day.

Third treatment on June 8. The patient took pills every day for a month. Following a relapse, the prescription, adding thirty grams of Radix Salviae Miltiorrhizae, was given. Two doses were consumed. No recurrence has been reported.

Case 3 (47-133):

Mr. Tian, 58, began to have chest pain three years ago. When he overworked or strained, pain attacked. At first, it was only once a month. It became more frequent. In the last two or three weeks, it attacked every 2-3 hours. The pain was severe, referring to the back and upper extremities. Shortness of breath and profuse perspiration occurred simultaneously. Nitroglycerin was given to relieve the pain, but soon it did not help.

Examination: Insomnia and dreamy sleep, bitterness in mouth, reluctance to drink water, plump build, flushed face, red tongue free of coating. Pulse was deep-tight-slender and weak at the Cubit position.

Diagnosis: Chest Obstruction syndrome complicated with ascending Liver Yang when Yin Deficiency prevailed.

Decoction of Fructus Aurantii Immaturus, Bulbus Allii Aacrostemi and Ramulus Cinnamomi with additions was prescribed:

Fructus Trichosanthis	30 grams
Bulbus Allii Aacrostemi	10 grams
Rhizoma Pinelliae	12 grams
Ramulus Cinnamomi	6 grams
Semen Ziziphi Spinosae Praeparata	30 grams
Radix Angelicae Sinensis	6 grams
Radix Rehmanniae	25 grams
Fructus Aurantii Immaturus	6 grams
Cortex Magnoliae Officinalis	10 grams
Radix Paeoniae Alba	12 grams
Poria cum Ligno Hospitae (prepared with Cinnabaris)	12 grams
Pericarpium Citri Reticulatae	10 grams
Rhizoma Zingiberis Recens	6 grams

One dose per day. Three doses brought relief. After twelve doses the syndrome was gone.

Case 4 (47-136):

A lady suffered from chest pain more than one year. When attacked, she could not eat, had coldness in extremities, distended feeling in chest. When palpated, chest was hard. Pulse was deep and slow-uneven. Decoction of Radix Ginseng was given. After taking the medication for one month, the syndrome was gone.

CLAUSE 9-6

Chest Obstruction syndrome with a feeling of suffocation in the chest and shortness of breath can be treated with either Decoction of Poria, Semen Armeniacae Amarum and Radix Glycyrrhizae, or Decoction of Pericarpium Citri Reticulatae, Fructus Aurantii Immaturus and Rhizoma Zingiberis Recens (1).

NOTES

1. In *Qianjin* and *Waitai*, the following does not appear: "... or Decoction of Pericarpium Citri Reticulatae, Fructus Aurantii Immaturus and Rhizoma Zingiberis Recens." (01-91)

Decoction of Poria, Semen Armeniacae Amarum and Radix Glycyrrhizae
(*Fuling Xingren Gancao Tang*):

Poria	3 *liang*
Semen Armeniacae Amarum	50 pcs.
Radix Glycyrrhizae	1 *liang*

Stew the drugs in one *dou* of water until five *sheng* remain. Serve one *sheng* of lukewarm decoction per dose three times a day. If the syndrome does not subside, additional doses should be given.

Decoction of Pericarpium Citri Reticulatae, Fructus Aurantii Immaturus and Rhizoma Zingiberis Recens
(*Ju Zhi Jiang Tang*):

Pericarpium Citri Reticulatae	1 *jin*

Fructus Aurantii Immaturus	3 *liang*
Rhizoma Zingiberis Recens	0.5 *jin*

Stew the drugs in five *sheng* of water until two *sheng* remain. Serve the lukewarm decoction in two doses.

Remark: *A Handbook of Prescriptions for Emergencies* and *Qianjin* both recorded the following regarding the efficacy of the prescription: (The prescription is) efficacious for Chest Obstruction syndrome with severe fullness in the chest, choking and suffocating feeling with itching, puckery and parched feeling in the throat, and copious salivation. (01-91)

Explanation of the Prescriptions: This clause discusses the treatment of a mild case of the Chest Obstruction syndrome. Chest Obstruction usually has the symptoms of chest pain and shortness of breath. But in this clause, only a feeling of suffocation in the chest and shortness of breath are listed. Thus the chest pain must be rather mild if it is included as one of its symptoms, while feeling of suffocation and shortness of breath are quite serious. This case may result from either of the two following pathological conditions:

a) Excessive pathogenetic Fluid-retention ascends to invade the Lung, causing a feeling of suffocation and shortness of breath. This syndrome may also be complicated with coughing and adverse ascending gas, copious salivation, and dysuria. Treat by adopting Decoction of Poria, Semen Armeniacae Amarum and Radix Glycyrrhizae, which serves to stimulate the flow of the Lung Vital Energy, and eliminate the Fluid-retention. Semen Armeniacae Amarum unblocks the obstruction of the Lung Vital Energy and Poria and Radix Glycyrrhizae disperse the phlegm. Once the Fluid-retention is eliminated, the Lung Vital Energy resumes its normal functioning, and the feeling of shortness of breath subsides.

b) If the syndrome is caused by stagnation of Vital Energy, symptoms may include a sense of suffocation and shortness of breath, with complications of adverse ascending gas, Vital-energy stagnation, and even vomiting. Treatment requires the dredging-through of the stagnant Vital Energy, reversal of the adverse ascending gas and dispersion of Fluid-retention. The prescription is

Decoction of Pericarpium Citri Reticulatae, Fructus Aurantii Immaturus and Rhizoma Zingiberis Recens. Pericarpium Citri Reticulatae is used to ventilate the normal flow of the Vital Energy. Fructus Aurantii Immaturus eliminates the phlegm and reverse the adverse ascending gas. Rhizoma Zingiberis Recens disperses Fluid-retention and harmonizes the Stomach Vital Energy, thus reversing the adverse ascending. When the obstruction in the chest is breached and the Vital Energy restored to its normal flow, the syndrome will disappear. (02-73)

CASES

Case 1 (46-146): Rheumatic Heart Disease

A boy of sixteen suffered from rheumatic heart disease, with the following symptoms: chest distress, coughing, spitting of phlegm and saliva, palpitation and dyspnea, pale face, dysuria, pitting edema on lower extremities, white slippery tongue coating, slow-uneven and interval pulse.

Diagnosis: Syndrome caused by hampered condition of the Heart Yang and accumulation of Fluid-retention at the Interior.

Treatment: To regulate the Vital Energy, disperse obstruction, reinforce the Yang to facilitate flow of Fluid. Combination of Decoction of Poria, Semen Armeniacae Amarum and Radix Glycyrrhizae and Decoction of Fructus Aurantii Immaturus, Bulbus Allii Aacrostemi and Ramulus Cinnamomi (see (see Clause 9-5) was prescribed:

Fructus Aurantii Immaturus	6 grams
Cortex Magnoliae Officinalis	10 grams
Fructus Trichosanthis	10 grams
Bulbus Allii Aacrostemi	10 grams
Ramulus Cinnamomi	10 grams
Poria	15 grams
Semen Armeniacae Amarum	10 grams
Radix Glycyrrhizae	3 grams
Rhizoma Pinelliae	10 grams

Second treatment: Five doses were served. The patient had relief. The following decoctions were combined to make another prescription:

Decoction of Pericarpium Citri Reticulatae, Fructus Aurantii Immaturus and Rhizoma Zingiberis Recens;

Decoction of Poria, Ramulus Cinnamomi, Rhizoma Atractylodis Macrocephalae and Radix Glycyrrhizae (Clause 12-15);

Decoction of Fructus Trichosanthis, Bulbus Allii Aacrostemi and Rhizoma Pinelliae (Clause 9-4)

Radix Stephaniae Tetrandrae was added to the combined decoction.

Five doses of the combined decoctions were effective. Edema on lower extremities disappeared.

Case 2 (64-312): Case Recorded in Journal of *Chinese Medicine*, 6:22, 1964

Mr. He, 34, suffered from chronic cough for five years. Treatments of Chinese and Western medicine had been used repeatedly, but the ailment still prevailed. The patient said there was an ascending gas from chest to throat with wheezing sound, shortness of breath, pain in epigastrium, costal regions, chest and back. The patient had anorexia, slow-slender pulse, white and thin tongue coating, and aversion to cold.

Treatment: Decoction of Pericarpium Citri Reticulatae, Fructus Aurantii Immaturus and Rhizoma Zingiberis Recens with additions was given:

Pericarpium Citri Reticulatae	12 grams
Fructus Aurantii Immaturus	9 grams
Rhizoma Zingiberis Recens	15 grams
Rhizoma Pinelliae (prepared with ginger)	12 grams
Poria	12 grams

Second treatment: After taking three doses of the decoction, pain over costal regions and back subsided. There was still pain in the epigastrium. The following decoction was prescribed:

Pericarpium Citri Reticulatae	12 grams
Fructus Aurantii Immaturus	9 grams
Rhizoma Zingiberis Recens	12 grams
Ramulus Cinnamomi	8 grams
Bulbus Allii Aacrostemi	9 grams
Fructus Trichosanthis	12 grams

Several doses were consumed. The ailment that had lasted five years was gone. More prescribed decoctions were given to stabilize the condition. Alterations were made:

Subtract: Bulbus Allii Aacrostemi, Rhizoma Zingiberis Recens and Ramulus Cinnamomi;

Add: Rhizoma Pinelliae, Poria and Radix Glycyrrhizae.

Case 3 (48-442):

Chen, 46, female patient, suffered from Chest Obstruction syndrome, with symptoms: distention and pain in epigastrium, nausea when syndrome was aggravated. Tongue was covered with greasy coating. Pulse was tight.

Diagnosis: Syndrome caused by obstruction of mingled phlegm and Vital

Energy which hampered normal physiological functions. Treatment to help promote circulation of Yang Vital Energy and dissolve phlegm was adopted. Combination of Decoction of Pericarpium Citri Reticulatae, Fructus Aurantii Immaturus and Rhizoma Zingiberis Recens and Decoction of Fructus Trichosanthis, Bulbus Allii Aacrostemi and Wine were prescribed:

Fructus Trichosanthis	12 grams
Bulbus Allii Aacrostemi	9 grams
Pericarpium Citri Reticulatae	12 grams
Fructus Aurantii Immaturus	9 grams
Rhizoma Zingiberis Recens	6 grams
Rhizoma Pinelliae	12 grams
Poria	12 grams

Four doses effectively eliminated Chest Obstruction and nausea.

CLAUSE 9-7

Chest Obstruction syndrome with sporadic mild and acute attacks can be treated with Powder of Semen Coicis and Radix Aconiti Praeparata. (1)

NOTES

1. According to *Jinkui S*, the clause should be interpreted: "To reduce acute attacks of Chest Obstruction, Powder of Semen Coicis and Radix Aconiti Praeparata can be adopted." The difference rises from varied interpretations of the original text.

Powder of Semen Coicis and Radix Aconiti Praeparata (*Yiyi Fuzi San*):

Semen Coicis	15 *liang*
Radix Aconiti Praeparata	10 large pcs.

Pound the drugs into powder. Serve one *fangcunbi* of powder per dose three times a day.

Explanation of the Prescription: This is an abbreviated clause which eliminates the symptoms and signs of the syndrome. Since this is a Chest Obstruction syndrome, the symptoms and signs can be inferred to include panting, coughing, spitting, and pains in the

the thorax and back. According to the ingredients listed in the prescription, the following symptoms and signs should also be present: Pale tongue with white and slippery coating; pulse deep-slow-tight or deep-slow-tense; contraction; and pains in the extremities. Radix Aconiti Praeparata is dosed as ten large pieces to strengthen its function of warming the Interior and dispersing Cold. Semen Coicis is used to eliminate Humidity, break through the obstruction, drain the Yin and murkiness downward and ease contraction of the extremities. (02-74)

Wei Litong: Semen Coicis reverses the adverse ascending and eases pain in the chest. Radix Aconiti Praeparata warms the Interior and disperses the pathogenetic factors. This recipe is a fine example of a cure of a syndrome with strong pathogenetic factors and weak Yang Vital Energy. Such cases are usually difficult to cure. (05-526)

CASES

Case 1 (46-147): Case Recorded in *Dr. Wu Jutong's Case Studies*

Mrs. Qian, 34, had a Chest Obstruction syndrome of Cold nature, with severe pain in lower abdomen, stomachache, coughing and spitting sputum. Pulse was tight-short-hesitant and tense. Powder of Semen Coicis and Radix Aconiti Praeparata with additions was prescribed:

Semen Coicis	8 *liang*
Radix Aconiti Praeparata	2 *liang*
Poria	8 *liang*
Rhizoma Atractylodis Praeparata	6 *liang*
Rhizoma Dioscoreae Hypoglaucae	4 *liang*
Pericarpium Zanthoxyli (carbonated)	3 *liang*
Fructus Foeniculi Praeparata	4 *liang*
Fructus Meliae Toosendan	3 *liang*
Caulis Akebiae	4 *liang*

Pounded the above drugs into powder, mixed with Massa Fermentata to make pills the size of Chinese parasol seeds. Three *qian* (nine grams) each dose were taken, washed down with decoction of ginger.

Case 2 (52-753):

Wu, 47, housewife, had chest pain with dragging pain in the back for more than five years. The disease attacked irregularly.

First treatment on April 26, 1981. The patient told the doctor that pain started in the back then referred to the chest. Overexertion and exposure to cold aggravated the syndrome. When attacked, the patient would have a family member pound her back to get relief. ECG was normal. Tongue was dark-pale with purple spots at tip, covered with white-greasy coating.

Diagnosis: Chest Obstruction syndrome caused by blood stasis, deficient Yang and prevalence of Cold-Humidity. Powder of Semen Coicis and Radix Aconiti Praeparata was prescribed with *Shen Su Yin*:

Semen Coicis	15 grams
Radix Aconiti Praeparata	9 grams
Radix Salviae Miltiorrhizae	20 grams
Lignum Sappan	10 grams
Resina Olibani Praeparata	9 grams
Resina Commiphorae Praeparata	9 grams
Semen Sinapis Albae	5 grams
Faeces Trogopterorum	10 grams
Rhizoma Corydalis	12 grams
Retinervus Luffae Fructus	10 grams
Radix Curcumae	10 grams
Rhizoma Acori Graminei	6 grams
Radix Bupleuri	12 grams
Retinervus Citri Fructus	10 grams

After three doses of decoction were consumed, pain subsided. Six doses more cured the ailment. To prevent relapse, pills made of the original prescription with additions and subtractions were given to be taken regularly:

Add: Radix Angelicae Sinensis, Radix Paeoniae Alba and Radix Codonopsis Pilosulae;

Subtract: Faeces Trogopterorum.

Case 3 (65-249): Intercostal Neuralgia, Case Recorded in Journal of *Henan College of Chinese Medicine*, 2:39, 1978

Mr. Cao, 50-year-old worker, suffered from intercostal neuralgia for more than ten years. The night of January 4, 1975, pain and distention of chest were seriously aggravated due to overexertion. The patient consulted the doctor on January 28. Anorexia, nausea, salivation, coldness of extremities were reported. Pulse was slender-tight, tongue pale, covered with white moist coating.

Diagnosis: Syndrome of Chest Obstruction of Cold-Humidity type, which should be warmed and fluid dispersed.

Treatment: Powder of Semen Coicis and Radix Aconiti Praeparata was given:

Radix Aconiti Praeparata	15 grams

Semen Coicis	30 grams

Second treatment on January 30. Two doses of the decoction were served. The same night, pain subsided and the patient could sleep 3-4 hours quietly. Combination of Powder of Semen Coicis and Radix Aconiti Praeparata, Decoction of *Lizhong** and Decoction of Fructus Trichosanthis, Bulbus Allii Aacrostemi and Rhizoma Pinelliae (Clause 9-4) was prescribed.

Third treatment: Pain was reduced, appetite good, but uneasy feeling in chest. Three doses of Decoction of *Lizhong* and Decoction of Lesser *Jianzhong* (Clause 6-13) were given effectively. Ten more doses were taken to complete the treatment.

* Decoction of *Lizhong*, see *Shanghan Lun*, Clause 386. Ingredients: Radix Ginseng, Rhizoma Zingiberis, Radix Glycyrrhizae, Rhizoma Atractylodis Macrocephalae.

CLAUSE 9-8

Symptoms and signs of Vital-energy Stagnation, adverse ascending feeling (1) and suspended pain of the Heart (2) can be eliminated by prescribing Decoction of Ramulus Cinnamomi, Rhizoma Zingiberis Recens and Fructus Aurantii Immaturus.

NOTES

1. Adverse ascending feeling: Ascending feeling caused by Fluid-retention or pathogenetic Cold stagnating in the epigastrium. (02-75)

2. Suspended pain of the Heart: Pain in the cardia including an upward dragging pain. (02-75)

You Yi: Suspended pain is caused by the adverse ascending of gas. (05-529)

Decoction of Ramulus Cinnamomi, Rhizoma Zingiberis Recens and Fructus Aurantii Immaturus
(*Guizhi Shengjiang Zhishi Tang*):

Ramulus Cinnamomi	3 *liang*
Rhizoma Zingiberis Recens	3 *liang*
Fructus Aurantii Immaturus	5 pcs.

Stew the drugs in six *sheng* of water until three *sheng* remain. Serve the decoction lukewarm in three doses.

Explanation of the Prescription: Syndrome described in this clause is caused by stagnation of Fluid-retention of a Cold nature in the epigastrium. According to the ingredients listed in the prescription, fullness in the chest and vomiting should also be present. Ramulus Cinnamomi and Rhizoma Zingiberis Recens invigorate the Yang Vital Energy and disperse the Cold. When Water-Fluid Stagnation is liquidated by warm drugs, adverse ascending will diminish. Fructus Aurantii Immaturus eliminates the Vital-energy Stagnation. (02-75)

CASES

Case 1 (46-148): Case Recorded in *Dr. Wu Jutong's Case Studies*

A man of eighty suffered from Fluid-retention syndrome. The ascending gas in the thorax caused distention in chest. Drugs to ventilate the Vital Energy and bring down the adversity had been given but did not help. This was because of age. There was deficient Yang, which not restored easily. Decoction of Ramulus Cinnamomi, Rhizoma Zingiberis Recens and Fructus Aurantii Immaturus with additions was given:

Ramulus Cinnamomi	6 *qian*
Rhizoma Zingiberis Recens	1 *liang*
Fructus Aurantii Immaturus	1 *liang*
Fructus Trichosanthis	3 *qian*
Bulbus Allii Aacrostemi	3 *qian*
Rhizoma Pinelliae	1 *liang*
Rhizoma Zingiberis	1 *liang*
Poria	1 *liang*
Lignum Aquilariae Resinatum (pound into powder, wash down with the decoction)	2 *qian*
Pericarpium Citri Reticulatae	5 *qian*
Lignum Dalbergiae Odoriferae	3 *qian*

The decoction relieved the condition as anticipated.

CLAUSE 9-9

Heart Pain with dragging pain leading towards the back and back pain with dragging pain leading to the cardia can be treated with Pills of Rhizoma Aconiti and Halloysitum Rubrum.

Pills of Rhizoma Aconiti and Halloysitum Rubrum*
(*Wutou Chishizhi Wan*):

Pericarpium Zanthoxyli	1 *liang*
Rhizoma Aconiti Praeparata	1 *fen*
Radix Aconiti Praeparata	0.5 *liang*
Rhizoma Zingiberis	1 *liang*
Halloysitum Rubrum	1 *liang*

Pound the drugs into powder and blend with honey. Make pills the size of Chinese parasol seeds. Take one pill before each meal, three times a day. If not efficacious, slightly increase the dosage.

*According to anther edition, dosages are as follows:

Pericarpium Zanthoxyli	2 *fen*
Rhizoma Aconiti Praeparata	1 *fen*
Radix Aconiti Praeparata	1 *fen*
Rhizoma Zingiberis	1 *fen*
Halloysitum Rubrum	2 *fen*

Explanation of the Prescription: Acute and continuous Heart Pain with dragging pain leading to the back and back pain with dragging pain leading to the cardia accompanied by coldness in the extremities and deep-tense pulse are caused by a solid accumulation of Yin and Cold. Rhizoma Aconiti Praeparata, Radix Aconiti Praeparata, Rhizoma Zingiberis and Pericarpium Zanthoxyli have the characteristics of great Heat and pungent taste, and serving as powerful agents to disperse the Cold and ease pain. Halloysitum Rubrum, warm and astringent, harmonizes the Interior and astringes the Yang Vital Energy. When the Cold is dispersed, pain will disappear at the same time.

CASES

Case 1 (56-82):

Mr. Jiang, 28, farmer, first treatment on April 8, 1954. The patient suffered from epigastric pain more than two years. The ailment was aggravated when he was exposed to cold weather. When attacked, there was cold sweat and anorexia. Tongue was pale, covered with white coating. Pulse was tense.

Diagnosis: Pain caused by accumulation of Cold and stagnation of Vital Energy. Pills of Rhizoma Aconiti and Halloysitum Rubrum was prescribed:

Rhizoma Aconiti	8 grams
Pericarpium Zanthoxyli	30 grams
Rhizoma Zingiberis	30 grams
Radix Aconiti Praeparata	15 grams
Halloysitum Rubrum	30 grams

Pounded the above drugs and made pea-sized pills with honey. Five pills taken after breakfast per day for a month worked effectively.

Case 2 (46-149):

Mr. Liu, 73, retired, suffered from coronary atherosclerotic cardiopathy and cardiac infarction and was hospitalized.

Examination: Chest pain with dragging pain leading to the back, cyanoderma face, perspiration, coldness of extremities, dark-purple tongue, deep-slender pulse.

Diagnosis: A pathological condition of exhaustion of Heart Yang and stagnation of Heart Blood. Pills of Rhizoma Aconiti and Halloysitum Rubrum were prescribed to restore the Yang, astringe the evanescent Vital Energy and remove stasis to stop pain.

Prescription (in decoction form):

Rhizoma Aconiti Praeparata	5 grams
Radix Aconiti Praeparata	10 grams
Pericarpium Zanthoxyli	3 grams
Rhizoma Zingiberis	5 grams
Halloysitum Rubrum	10 grams
Radix Ginseng	10 grams
Lignum Sappan	10 grams

Emergency treatment also adopted.

One dose of the decoction worked effectively to stop perspiration and bring warmth to extremities. Another dose stopped the pain. Pills of *Bozi Yang Xin** were given to complete the treatment.

*Pills of *Bozi Yang Xin* (Semen Biotae Nourishing the Heart): Semen Biotae, Fructus Lycii, Radix Ophiopogonis, Radix Angelicae Sinensis, Rhizoma Acori Graminei, Poria cum Ligno Hospitae, Radix Scrophulariae, Rhizoma Rehmanniae Praeparata, Radix Glycyrrhizae.

Case 3 (65-251): Cardiac Infarction

Mr. Zhi, 68-year-old worker, first treatment on November 6, 1969. The patient suffered from Fluid-retention syndrome which was aggravated in winter. He had no other disease. The morning of consultation, he had unbearable chest pain with shortness of breath, and cold sweat. ECG showed acute cardiac infarction and the patient was hospitalized.

Examination: Chest pain referring to back with dyspnea and suffocation, panting and groaning, pale face, cold extremities, cyanoderma lips and nails, cyan, slippery tongue coating, deep-slender-hesitant pulse.

Diagnosis: The patient's Spleen was in deficient condition, making possible an accumulation of phlegm. The Kidney was also deficient and exhausted, causing the turbid Yin ascending to disperse the Cold. Pills of Rhizoma Aconiti and Halloysitum Rubrum were prescribed:

Radix Aconiti Praeparata	9 grams
Rhizoma Aconiti Praeparata	6 grams
Rhizoma Zingiberis	9 grams
Radix Ginseng	6 grams
Poria	12 grams
Ramulus Cinnamomi	9 grams
Radix Glycyrrhizae Praeparata	6 grams
Halloysitum Rubrum (wrapped in cloth bag)	15 grams
Herba Asari	3 grams

Drugs were stewed to make two doses of the decoction, served in small quantity at short intervals, and finished within twenty-four hours.

Second treatment: The following afternoon, there was relief. Chest pain was reduced, no sweat on forehead, and extremities warm. Chest suffocation, shortness of breath, sporadic chest pain still existed. Pulse was deep-slender, tongue coating thinning. Lips and nails were slightly dark in color. New prescription was given with alterations:

Subtract: Ramulus Cinnamomi and Halloysitum Rubrum.

Add: Radix Salviae Miltiorrhizae 15 grams, Radix Ophiopogonis 9 grams.

Six doses were given, one dose two times a day.

Third treatment: Six doses cured the pain. Suffocation and shortness of breath reduced, pulse was slender-tight, tongue was light-red, covered with white coating. Combination of Decoction of Fructus Trichosanthis, Bulbus Allii Aacrostemi and Rhizoma Pinelliae (Clause 9-4) and *Sheng Mai San** was given for one month, which enabled the patient to walk around the room. He continued his treatment at home. Half a year later, the patient recovered fully.

**Sheng Mai San*: Radix Ginseng, Radix Ophiopogonis and Fructus Schisandrae.

Case 4 (65-252): Stomachache, Case Recorded in Journal of *Liaoning Chinese Medicine*, 4:39, 1978

Li, 13-year-old girl, first treatment on February 8, 1963. The patient suffered from frequent attacks of stomachache since she was eight. When exposed to cold and windy weather recently the stomachache attacked again. There was a twisting pain in the stomach with dragging pain to the chest and back. The patient also vomited fluid. There was aversion to cold, coldness in extremities, pale face, cyanoderma lips and nails. Tongue was covered with white, slippery coating. Pulse was small-tense.

Diagnosis: Stomachache caused by Cold and stagnation of Vital Energy. Pills of Rhizoma Aconiti and Halloysitum Rubrum were prescribed:

Rhizoma Aconiti Praeparata	6 grams
Rhizoma Zingiberis	6 grams
Pericarpium Zanthoxyli	6 grams
Halloysitum Rubrum	4.5 grams
Rhizoma Alpiniae Officinarum	6 grams
Radix Saussureae Lappae	3 grams

One dose of the decoction reduced pain and another dose relieved the patient.

Second treatment: She still had epigastric fullness and anorexia. Pulse was deep-tense. Tongue was covered with white-slippery coating. *Xiang Sha Ping Wei San** was prescribed with the following additions:

Add: Massa Fermentata, Fructus Hordei, Endothelium Corneum Gigeriae Galli, Radix Linderae, Radix Curcumae.

Three doses of the decoction worked effectively.

**Xiang Sha Ping Wei San*: Rhizoma Atractylodis, Cortex Magnoliae Officinalis, Pericarpium Citri Reticulatae, Radix Aucklandiae, Fructus Amomi, Radix Glycyrrhizae.

Pills for Treating Nine Types of Pain* (*Jiutong Wan*): Efficacious in relieving nine types of Heart Pain

Radix Aconiti Praeparata	3 *liang*
Herba Agrimoniae Praeparata	1 *liang*
Fructus Crotonis	1 *liang*
Radix Ginseng	1 *liang*
Rhizoma Zingiberis	1 *liang*
Fructus Evodiae	1 *liang*

Pound the drugs into powder. Blend with honey and make pills the size of Chinese parasol seeds. Give three pills with wine to a strong patient and two pills to a normal patient. This prescription is effective for sudden attack of disease due to exogenous pathogenetic factors, abdominal distention and pain, aphasia, wandering pain in the chest and the Heart due to long-term accumulation of pathogenetic Cold and ascending gas of a Cold nature. Also relieves pain caused by accidents such as falling off a horse or cart, bleeding, etc. General diet taboos should be practiced.

*According to *Qianjin*, the nine types of Heart Pain may be caused by: 1) Parasites; 2) Wandering Heart Pain; 3) Pathogenetic Wind; 4) Palpitations; 5) Indigestion; 6) Fluid-retention; 7) Pathogenetic Cold; 8) Pathogenetic Heat; 9) Paroxysmal pains.

Some annotators believe this prescription was appended by a later annotator. Cheng Lin states that this is not a prescription of Zhang Zhongjing.

Regarding the dosage and ingredients, *Qianjin* give the prescription as follows:

Radix Aconiti Praeparata	2 *liang*
Radix Euphorbiae Ebracteolatae	1 *liang*
Fructus Crotonis	1 *liang*
Radix Ginseng	1 *liang*
Rhizoma Zingiberis	2 *liang*
Fructus Evodiae	1 *liang*

CHAPTER X

ON PULSE, SYMPTOM COMPLEX AND TREATMENT OF ABDOMINAL DISTENTION, ABDOMINAL PAIN CAUSED BY COLD AND INDIGESTION

CLAUSE 10-1

Feeble and tight *Fuyang* pulse (1) generally indicates abdominal distention. If there is no abdominal distention, there will be constipation, pain on costal regions caused by the ascending of Deficiency and Cold. A warming agent (2) should be served. (3)

NOTES

1. *Fuyang* pulse: Located at the malleolus near the tarsal bones (arteria dorsalis pedis).

2. Warming agent: As this is a syndrome of a Cold and deficient nature with constipation, the warming agent mentioned here should be a laxative (or purgative) with warming ingredients. (01-95)

3. Mechanism of the disease: *Fuyang* pulse reflects the pathological conditions of the Stomach and indicates pathological changes in the Middle Portion of Body Cavity. Feeble pulse indicates deficient state of the Yang Vital Energy in the Middle Portion of Body Cavity. Tight pulse reflects a pathological condition in the Liver and indicates a case of a Cold nature and pain. When the Spleen and the Stomach are in a deficient and Cold state, the Vital Energy of the Greater Yin (Liver) Channel ascends abnormally, resulting in abdominal distention. If there is no abdominal distention, but rather constipation and pain in the costal regions, the mechanism of the disease remains the same. As the Spleen and the Stomach control transmission and digestion, so when they are in a deficient and Cold state, they will lose control of these functions resulting in constipation. The Liver has the functions of dispersion and discharge. When the Vital Energy of the Liver ascends abnormally, it loses the function of dispersion and discharge, resulting in either abdominal distention or constipation and pain in the costal regions. (02-78)

CLAUSE 10-2

Abdominal distention: When the abdomen is pressed, and the patient feels pain, it can be diagnosed as a case of an excessive nature (1). If there is no pain, it is a case of a deficient nature (2). For excessive cases, purgatives can be adopted. A yellowish coating on the tongue observed before administering purgative will diminish after purgative is given (3).

NOTES

1. Abdominal distention of an excessive nature is generally caused by indigestion in the Stomach or dried feces blocking the intestine. Thus the patient feels pain when the abdomen is pressed and the distention causes lasting suffering. (02-79)

2. Abdominal distention of a deficient nature is due to deficient and Cold state of the Spleen and the Stomach. Vital Energy lacks mobility and stagnates there causing abdominal distention. No pain is experienced and the distention reduces sporadically. (02-79)

3. Yellowish coating indicates accumulation of Heat and Excess. After adoption of purgative, Heat and Excess will be eliminated and the yellowish coating will diminish. If yellowish coating is still present after adoption of purgative, disease should be diagnosed again to determine its nature. In the following cases, though yellowish coating is observed, purgative cannot be given:

a) Acute febrile diseases caused by pathogenetic Humidity with yellowish tongue coating which has not yet become excessive with pathogenetic Dryness; or an excessive case which is becoming a deficient case, with the yellowish coating still present;

b) Dried feces accumulated in the intestine due to exhaustion of Body Fluid in a Greater Yang syndrome should be treated with ingredients serving both as a purgative and as an agent adding "water" to float the "boat."* If purgative with bitter ingredients is adopted, constipation will not be cured and yellowish tongue coating will not disappear. (02-79)

*A representative recipe is *Zengye Tang*, a decoction to increase the Fluid (to stimulate bowel movement), which includes Radix Scrophulariae, Radix Ophiopogonis and Radix Rehmanniae. *Zengye Tang* is found in *Detailed Analysis of Acute Febrile Diseases (Wen Bing Tiao Bian)* by Wu Tang (ca. 1758-1836).

CLAUSE 10-3

Abdominal distention which reduces sporadically and resumes afterwards indicates that the syndrome is of a Cold nature. Drugs with warming qualities should be prescribed. (1)

NOTES

1. You Yi: Abdominal distention with persistent suffering is a case of an excessive nature. Abdominal distention which reduces sporadically and resumes afterwards is a case of a Cold nature, since when the Yang Vital Energy is active temporarily in the abdomen, the distention will be reduced for a short while. When Yin prevails, distention resumes. This is a case of pathogenetic Cold germinating in the Interior; warm agent should therefore be prescribed.

CLAUSE 10-4

The patient's complexion is dark yellow (1). He is restless but does not feel thirsty. He suffers continuous diarrhea and a syndrome of accumulated excessive Cold in the chest. The case will be fatal (2).

NOTES

1. A dark yellow complexion without luster indicates Deficiency of the Spleen Vital Energy. (01-96)

2. This case is difficult to treat. The patient is suffering from a syndrome of excessive Cold in the chest, requiring a purgative with warm-quality drugs. But dark yellow complexion, restlessness and diarrhea indicate a syndrome of a deficient nature, which cannot be treated with purgatives. Thus the prognosis is unfavorable. (01-96)

CLAUSE 10-5

Pulse at the Inch (under the first finger) is tight. The patient has chills, contractions and pain throughout the costal regions (1).

NOTES

1. This is a case of an invasion of climatic pathogenetic Cold with a patient in a deficient state. The syndrome is half-Exterior, half-Interior. Annotators suggest prescribing Decoction of Radix Bupleuri and Ramulus Cinnamomi (subtract Radix Scutellariae and increase dosage of Radix Paeoniae). See Clause 146 of *Shanghan Lun* for Decoction of Radix Bupleuri and Ramulus Cinnamomi. Prescription includes:

Ramulus Cinnamomi
Radix Scutellariae
Radix Ginseng
Radix Glycyrrhizae
Rhizoma Pinelliae

Radix Paeoniae
Fructus Ziziphi Jujubae
Rhizoma Zingiberis Recens
Radix Bupleuri

CLAUSE 10-6

The patient susceptible to pathogenetic Cold (1) tends to yawn frequently with copious snivel. The patient who is feverish but with normal complexion sneezes frequently (2).

NOTES

1. The patient with weak build is easily affected by climatic Cold. (01-97)
2. The patient who has just caught a cold. (01-97)

CLAUSE 10-7

Interior Deficiency is the cause of diarrhea in patients who have been affected by pathogenetic Cold. He feels like sneezing but cannot sneeze. He also feels cold in the abdomen (according to another edition: He also feels *pain* in abdomen).

Commentary: Clauses 10-6 and 10-7 refer to the same etiopathology. Owing to differences in patients' physical constitution, pathological reactions are not the same. In patients suffering Exterior Deficiency, pathogenetic factors remain at the Exterior and bring about Exterior syndromes (such as the case discussed in Clause 10-6). In patients who suffer Interior Deficiency, pathogenetic factors will invade the Interior, causing illness there (such as the case discussed in Clause 10-7). (02-80)

Shen Mingzong: Symptoms and signs discussed in Clause 10-6 indicates a case caused by the invasion of pathogenetic Cold in the Lung. Clause 10-7 discusses a case caused by the invasion of pathogenetic Cold in the Spleen.

CLAUSE 10-8

When thin patients suffer abdominal pain around the navel, this is caused by the invasion of pathogenetic Wind and Cold (1). If Cereal Vital Energy ceases to move (2), a purgative is adopted, which will arouse the adverse ascending of gas. If gas does not ascend, Vital-energy Stagnation will occur in the epigastrium. (3)

NOTES

1. Thin and weak patients are apt to be susceptible to Wind and Cold, as their health is always in a deficient (weak) state. (01-97)

2. Cereal Vital Energy ceases to move: This suggests constipation. When the epigastrium is affected by Cold, Cereal Vital Energy (digestive activity) ceases, causing constipation. Bowels movement should be stimulated with drugs of a warm quality. Instead, purgative (generally with ingredients of a cold quality) is given to move the bowels. For patients with comparatively strong Body Resistance, physiological reaction will be the ascent of gas to resist drugs of a cold quality. In patients whose Body Resistance is weak, physiological reaction is not strong enough to resist the drug, and pathogenetic factors will descend to bring about a Vital-energy Stagnation. (01-97)

3. Abdominal pain around the navel may be of either an excessive or deficient nature. This clause discusses the treatment of abdominal pain caused by Cold. Clause 239 of *Shanghan Lun* discusses an excessive case caused by indigestion. The clause reads: "For five or six days in succession, the patient has no stool, pain around the navel and restlessness at regular times, all indicating formation of stercoroma, which hampers passage of normal stool for five to six days." (02-80)

CLAUSE 10-9

The patient suffers an abdominal distention. For ten days on end, he is feverish, with floating and speedy pulse and normal intake of food. Decoction of Cortex Magnoliae Officinalis with Seven Drugs can be adopted as a treatment. (1)

NOTES

1. This clause discusses complications of abdominal distention and Exterior syndrome. "The patient is suffering an abdominal distention. For ten days on end, he is feverish,..." means that the patient first has fever and then abdominal distention. Although the syndrome lasts for ten days, the pulse is floating and speedy, but not floating and tense (floating-tense corresponds to Initial Yang syndrome); abdominal distention is also observed, all indicating that the syndrome is not only at the Exterior but has invaded the Interior, with Interior syndrome becoming the main syndrome. Normal intake of food is evidence that the pathological condition is located in the intestine. Thus this is a case of Initial Yang syndrome complicated by Interior Excess of the Greater Yang syndrome. (02-83)

Decoction of Cortex Magnoliae Officinalis with Seven Drugs (*Houpo Qi Wu Tang*):

Cortex Magnoliae Officinalis	0.5 *jin*
Radix Glycyrrhizae	3 *liang*
Radix et Rhizoma Rhei	3 *liang*
Fructus Ziziphi Jujubae	10 pcs.
Fructus Aurantii Immaturus	5 pcs.
Ramulus Cinnamomi	2 *liang*
Rhizoma Zingiberis Recens	5 *liang*

Stew the drugs in one *dou* of water until four *sheng* remain. Give eight *ge* of the lukewarm decoction per dose, three times per day. For a patient who becomes nauseous, add five *ge* Rhizoma Pinelliae. Subtract Radix et Rhizoma Rhei for patients with diarrhea. For patients with prevailing syndrome of a Cold nature, increase dosage of Rhizoma Zingiberis Recens to 0.5 *jin*.

Explanation of the Prescription: This prescription treats both the Exterior and the Interior syndromes simultaneously. Ramulus Cinnamomi, Radix Glycyrrhizae, Rhizoma Zingiberis Recens and Fructus Ziziphi Jujubae harmonize the Nutrient Essence with the Vital Resistance and disperse the Exterior syndrome. Cortex Magnoliae Officinalis, Fructus Aurantii Immaturus and Radix et Rhizoma Rhei unblock the constipation and eliminate the sensation of fullness. (01-98)

CASES

Case 1 (02-83): Complete Intestinal Obstruction, Case Recorded in *Selected Readings of Case Studies of Veteran Doctors of Chinese Medicine* (Edited by Shenyang Science and Technology Commission)

A male baby of three months. The father said the baby cried with irritation. Abdominal distention was palpated. Since birth, the baby had been no stool. Every day, he vomited milk and then vomitus resembling stool in color. The baby could not take food and was sent to the hospital. Examination of Western medicine showed the baby suffered complete intestinal obstruction and an operation was planned. The parents doubted the three-month old baby could stand an operation and decided to try Chinese medicine.

First treatment on April 5, 1974. The patient was pale and in low spirit, with cold sweat, abdominal distention and resistance to palpation. Pulse was feeble, tongue coating gray-white.

Diagnosis: Syndrome caused by the impaired Spleen Yang and stagnation of indigestion.

Treatment: Help circulation of Vital Energy and warm the Interior Cold. Decoction of Cortex Magnoliae Officinalis with Seven Drugs was prescribed:

Cortex Magnoliae Officinalis	10 grams
Ramulus Cinnamomi	7.5 grams
Radix Glycyrrhizae	10 grams
Fructus Aurantii Immaturus	10 grams
Radix et Rhizoma Rhei	2.5 grams
Rhizoma Zingiberis Recens	5 grams

After one serving of decoction, the baby began to defecate stool with purulent substances. He had three stools within two to three hours, with lots of discharge. Abdominal distention reduced. After ten days of treatment, the baby was well.

Case 2 (46-159):

Mr. Pan, 43, had chill and fever, headache and pain over the body, epigastric fullness and nausea. These occurred after the patient was exposed to cold weather when sweating. He then overate. There was no stool three days. Tongue was covered with yellow-greasy coating, pulse floating-slippery.

Diagnosis: This was Interior Excess complicated by Exterior syndrome, to be treated by dispersing Interior and Exterior syndromes simultaneously. Decoction of Cortex Magnoliae Officinalis with Seven Drugs was prescribed:

Cortex Magnoliae Officinalis	10 grams
Fructus Aurantii Immaturus	6 grams
Radix et Rhizoma Rhei	10 grams
Ramulus Cinnamomi	10 grams
Radix Glycyrrhizae	3 grams
Rhizoma Zingiberis Recens	3 grams
Fructus Ziziphi Jujubae	3 pcs.
Radix Paeoniae Alba	10 grams

After two doses, there was a smooth stool. The patient was given forridge as a nourishing agent, which aided recovery.

Case 3 (55-106):

Cao, 34, female patient, suffering from acute hepatitis, was cured by drugs of cold quality, thus damaging the Yang in Spleen and Stomach. She had persistent abdominal distention aggravated in the afternoon. Improper intake of food could aggravate the case. Indigestion, repeated flatus, loose stool, coldness in extremities were reported. Pulse was slow-moderate. Tongue was pale covered with thin, white coating.

First treatment: Decoction of Cortex Magnoliae Officinalis with Seven Drugs was given.

Second treatment: Two doses of the decoction reduced abdominal distention. A few days later, distention resumed. Another two doses were served.

Third treatment: The same decoction was prescribed, with alterations subtracting Radix et Rhizoma Rhei, and increasing dosage of Ramulus Cinnamomi. The syndrome was gone after ten doses of decoction.

Case 4 (55-106):

Mr. Liang, 50, suffered from emphysematous asthma. When treated for asthma, abdominal distention was aggravated, causing chest distress and dyspnea; asthma became acute. This rotated repeatedly.

Decoction of Cortex Magnoliae Officinalis with Seven Drugs was given with increased dosage of Ramulus Cinnamomi (to warm the Interior). After taking the decoction, no loose stool was reported, and abdominal distention subsided. Emphysematous asthma was not cured, but abdominal distention never occurred again, making treatment of asthma easier.

CLAUSE 10-10

Pathogenetic Cold in the abdomen (1) will cause borborygmus, acute pain in the abdomen, adverse ascending of gas and a sensation of fullness in the chest and the costal regions, as well as vomiting and nausea. Decoction of Radix Aconiti Praeparata and Semen Oryzae Nonglutinosae can be prescribed to treat the case. (2)

NOTES

1. According to *Qianjin*, this should be "abdominal distention." (01-98)

2. This clause discusses the syndrome and treatment of abdominal distention caused by Cold and Deficiency in the Spleen and the Stomach with stagnation of Water-Humidity. The pathological condition is located in the abdomen and the principal symptom is borborygmus, due to inability of Spleen and Stomach to stimulate the normal flow of Water-Humidity. When the pathogenetic Cold ascends, adverse ascending and a sensation of fullness in the chest and the costal regions with vomiting and nausea result. (02-81)

Decoction of Radix Aconiti Praeparata and Semen Oryzae Nonglutinosae

(*Fuzi Gengmi Tang*):

Radix Aconiti Praeparata	1 pc.
Rhizoma Pinelliae	0.5 *sheng*
Radix Glycyrrhizae	1 *liang*
Fructus Ziziphi Jujubae	10 pcs.
Semen Oryzae Nonglutinosae	0.5 *sheng*

Stew the drugs in eight *sheng* of water until Semen Oryzae Nonglutinosae is thoroughly cooked. Filter the decoction. Give one *sheng* of lukewarm decoction per dose three times a day.

Explanation of the Prescription: When Cold prevails in the abdomen, Vital Energy cannot circulate normally, resulting in stagnation of Water-Humidity. Radix Aconiti Praeparata, hot in quality, is used to disperse the Cold and Humidity. Rhizoma Pinelliae eliminates fullness and reverses the adverse ascending. Radix Glycyrrhizae, Fructus Ziziphi Jujubae and Semen Oryzae Nonglutinosae harmonize the Stomach, relieve the pain, and reverse adverse ascending. (01-98)

CASES

Case 1 (65-265): Chronic Colitis

Mr. Li, 46, first treatment on November 8, 1977.

Examination: The patient reported abdominal pain with loose stool for more than six years. He was once hospitalized with a diagnosis of chronic colitis. When the abdomen was warmed or palpated, there was temporary relief. When exposed to cold, the pain was aggravated. Watery stool occurred two to three times a day. Every night the patient sensed cold gas in the abdomen with distention and gurgling sounds. Even on a hot summer night, the patient had to cover his abdomen tightly to keep warm. The cold feeling subsided in the morning. Accompanying syndrome: coronary insufficiency with chest distress, shortness of breath, sporadic chest pain, bradycardia. Pulse was deep-slender-weak, tongue red on tip, covered with thin-white moist coating.

Diagnosis: This syndrome was caused by Deficiency of Yang in Kidney and Spleen which failed to circulate the Fluid and Cereal. Stagnation of Fluid in Cold nature caused the trouble.

Decoction of Radix Aconiti Praeparata and Semen Oryzae Nonglutinosae was prescribed:

Radix Aconiti Praeparata	9 grams
Semen Oryzae Nonglutinosae (stewed later than other drugs)	30 grams
Rhizoma Zingiberis Recens	24 grams
Radix Paeoniae Alba	9 grams
Radix Glycyrrhizae Praeparata	6 grams
Fructus Foeniculi	6 grams
Fructus Litseae	9 grams
Cortex Magnoliae Officinalis	12 grams

Second treatment on November 15. Six doses of the decoction were served. Abdominal pain was reduced. Cold gas in abdomen became less frequent. The same decoction was prescribed, with alterations:

Add Rhizoma Atractylodis Macrocephalae, 9 grams; Poria, 12 grams.

Increase dosage of Radix Aconiti Praeparata to 12 grams.

Third treatment on December 8. Six doses of the above decoction were consumed. Stool was only once a day, but still watery. Cold gas in abdomen occurred occasionally. Chest distress and shortness of breath subsided. Pulse was deep-moderate, tongue coating thin and white. The patient continued taking the decoction till March 27, 1978. A total of 120 doses were served (Radix Aconiti Praeparata was used in every decoction). In some decoctions, the following alterations were made:

Add: Fructus Evodiae, Halloysitum Rubrum, Semen Coicis, Pericarpium Papiveris.

Subtract: Fructus Funiculi, Radix Paeoniae Alba, Semen Oryzae Nonglutinosae.

The syndrome was gone. In June 1978, Mr. Li was healthy and no recurrence was reported.

Case 2 (52-557):

Yang, 38, housewife, first treatment on March 15, 1981. The patient suffered from abdominal pain with borborygmus more than a month. A month before, when exposed to cold, she began to have abdominal pain which was always aggravated at night. Nausea, salivation, borborygmus, pain around umbilicus were accompanying symptoms. The patient had a pallid face. The abdomen was soft and relieved of pain when palpated. Stool was normal. No acid regurgitation or retching occurred. Tongue was pale, covered with white coating, pulse was deep-slender and moderate.

Diagnosis: Insufficiet Spleen Yang made it possible for the Cold gas to ascend.

Decoction of Radix Aconiti Praeparata and Semen Oryzae Nonglutinosae was prescribed:

Radix Aconiti Praeparata	10 grams
Semen Oryzae Nonglutinosae	9 grams
Rhizoma Pinelliae	9 grams
Radix Glycyrrhizae	6 grams
Fructus Ziziphi Jujubae	3 pcs.

Five doses of the decoction curved all the troubles.

Case 3 (64-338): Chronic Diarrhea, Case Recorded in Journal of *New Chinese Medicine*, 6:24, 1978

Yang, 39, female, suffered from chronic diarrhea. Yang Vital Energy was sinking, with stagnation of Vital Energy. Continuous diarrhea made the patient feel chest fullness and have anorexia. She was emaciated. Decoction of Radix Aconiti Praeparata and Semen Oryzae Nonglutinosae with alterations was given:

Radix Aconiti Praeparata	3 *qian*
Rhizoma Pinelliae	3 *qian*
Semen Oryzae Nonglutinosae	1 cup
Radix Glycyrrhizae	5 *qian*
Fructus Ziziphi Jujubae	10 pcs.
Halloysitum Rubrum	1 *liang*

One dose of the decoction stopped the diarrhea.

CLAUSE 10-11

Abdominal distention with constipation (1) can be eliminated by prescribing Decoction of Cortex Magnoliae Officinalis with Three Drugs.

NOTES

1. According to *The Pulse Classic*, this should read: "abdominal distention with fullness."

Decoction of Cortex Magnoliae Officinalis with Three Drugs (*Houpo San Wu Tang*):

Cortex Magnoliae Officinalis	8 *liang*
Radix et Rhizoma Rhei	4 *liang*
Fructus Aurantii Immaturus	5 pcs.

Stew Cortex Magnoliae Officinalis and Fructus Aurantii

Immaturus in one *dou* plus two *sheng* of water until five *sheng* remain. Add Radix et Rhizoma Rhei and stew it again until three *sheng* remain. Serve one *sheng* of lukewarm decoction. When stool loosens stop taking the decoction.

Explanation of the Prescription: You Yi: Abdominal distention with constipation is evidence of stagnation of the Vital Energy in the Six Bowels. Decoction of Cortex Magnoliae Officinalis with Three Drugs indicates the same ingredients as Decoction of Lesser *Chengqi* (see Clause 17-41 in this book and Clause 208 of *Shanghan Lun*). Decoction of Lesser *Chengqi* is prescribed to disperse the Interior Excess, so Radix et Rhizoma Rhei is heavily dosed as the principal ingredient. Decoction of Cortex Magnoliae Officinalis with Three Drugs is prescribed to stimulate the stagnant Vital Energy, thus Cortex Magnoliae Officinalis is taken as the principal drug and hence heavily dosed.

CASES

Case 1 (65-267): Case Recorded in *Dr. Ran Xuefeng's Case Studies*

Mr. Yu had mental strain in his work and had suffered from abdominal pain for several years. The pain attacked once every three to five months, or several times within a month. When attacked, the patient had abdominal discomfort, then distention and pain below diaphragm and above lower abdomen. He also vomited and could not eat. In his latest attack, he had a feeling of nausea but could not vomit, defecate, or urinate. The patient had cyanic face, with trismus, cold finger tips and nose tip. Pulse was tight and hesitant.

Decoction of Cortex Magnoliae Officinalis with Three Drugs was given:

Cortex Magnoliae Officinalis	2.4 grams
Fructus Aurantii Immaturus	5 grams
Radix et Rhizoma Rhei	12 grams
Rhizoma Coptidis	2.4 grams
Fructus Evodiae	3.6 grams

After one dose, pain subsided with borborygmus. Another dose was served, and loose stool resulted, relieving the symptoms. The pain was gone after another stool. Then drugs harmonizing the Stomach were given to complete the treatment.

Case 2 (48-272): Intestinal Obstruction, Cases Recorded in Journal of *Chinese Medicine*, Vol. 1, 1964

Two cases of intestinal obstruction were treated by Decoction of Cortex Magnoliae Officinalis with the additions of Natrii Sulfas Exsiccatus, Fructus Cannabis, Semen Trichosanthis, Semen Raphani, Pericarpium Citri Reticulatae. Also 60 ml peanut oil was taken to aid the decoction in loosing the bowels. After taking the decoction, abdominal pain became more acute for a moment, then repeated flatus occurred, followed by defecation of foul stool. All the symptoms were gone.

CLAUSE 10-12

When the doctor palpates the patient in the epigastrium, he feels distention and pain (1), indicating an excessive syndrome. A purgative such as Decoction of Greater Radix Bupleuri can be adopted. (2)

NOTES

1. Wu Qian: "with tidal fever" should be inserted here. Without such a symptom, Decoction of Greater Radix Bupleuri should not be given. This phrase must have been left out in the course of repeated copying. (05-537)

2. This clause discusses the symptoms and treatment of a syndrome with complications of Lesser Yang and Greater Yang syndromes. Distention and Vital-energy Stagnation in the epigastrium with tenderness suggests a case requiring a purgative. When the location of syndrome is in a higher position, this indicates a complication of the Lesser Yang and Greater Yang syndromes with Interior Excess as well as Exterior syndrome. Thus a purgative such as Decoction of Greater *Chengqi* (see Clause 2-13) should not be prescribed. Decoction of Greater Radix Bupleuri, which disperses both the Interior and the Exterior syndromes simultaneously, is the proper prescription for the case. In addition to the symptoms mentioned herein, the following apply to the symptoms and signs of Decoction of Greater Radix Bupleuri syndrome: Restlessness, chills and sporadic fever, fullness in the chest and the costal regions, a yellowish tongue coating and extremely tight pulse. (02-84)

Decoction of Greater Radix Bupleuri
(*Da Chaihu Tang*):

Radix Bupleuri	0.5 *jin*
Radix Scutellariae	3 *liang*
Radix Paeoniae	3 *liang*
Rhizoma Pinelliae	0.5 *sheng*
Fructus Aurantii Immaturus Praeparata	4 pcs.

Radix et Rhizoma Rhei	2 *liang*
Fructus Ziziphi Jujubae	12 pcs.
Rhizoma Zingiberis Recens	5 *liang*

Stew the drugs in one *dou* plus two *sheng* of water until six *sheng* remain. Filter the decoction and stew it again. Serve one *sheng* of lukewarm decoction per dose three times a day.

Explanation of the Prescription: This prescription also appears in Clause 103 of *Shanghan Lun*. In this prescription, Radix Bupleuri, Radix Scutellariae and Radix Paeoniae are used to eliminate the pathogenetic factors that have invaded the Lesser Yang Channel. Fructus Aurantii Immaturus and Radix et Rhizoma Rhei, cold in quality, disperse the Interior Excess of the Greater Yang Channel. Rhizoma Pinelliae, Rhizoma Zingiberis Recens and Fructus Ziziphi Jujubae harmonize the Interior and reverse the adverse ascending. (01-100)

Commentary: Decoction of Greater Radix Bupleuri with additions and subtraction is widely used in present-day clinical practice to treat various acute abdomen, such as acute cholecystitis, cholelithiasis, acute pancreatitis, acute and chronic appendicitis, syndrome following remission of acute ulcerative perforation and celiac infection, etc. (02-84)

CLAUSE 10-13

When abdominal distention is not reduced or only partially reduced, Decoction of Greater *Chengqi* should be prescribed as a drastic measure. (1)

NOTES

1. The clause also appears in Clause 255 of *Shanghan Lun* with the following note: When purgative has been adopted, abdominal distention is not reduced or only partially reduced. Greater Yang syndrome should be observed before Decoction of Greater *Chengqi* is adopted.

Decoction of Greater *Chengqi* (*Da Chengqi Tang*), prescription see Clause 2-13.

CLAUSE 10-14

Decoction of Greater *Jianzhong* can be adopted for syndromes having the following symptoms and signs: Acute pain in the chest and the epigastrium caused by Cold, nausea and vomiting that prevents the patient from eating, pathogenetic Cold in the abdomen that forms protruding mass in the shape of a head or foot which appears in different abdominal locations with tenderness that is extremely painful.

Decoction of Greater *Jianzhong*
(*Da Jianzhong Tang*):

Pericarpium Zanthoxyli Praeparata	2 *ge*
Rhizoma Zingiberis	4 *liang*
Radix Ginseng	2 *liang*

Stew the drugs in four *sheng* of water until two *sheng* remain. Filter the decoction, add one *sheng* of *Jiaoyi* (malt sugar) and stew again over a slow fire until one and a half *sheng* remain. Serve the decoction in two doses. After serving the decoction, wait as long as it takes to prepare a meal and then serve two *sheng* of porridge. Another dose of the decoction can be taken later. The patient should follow liquid diet for the entire day. Cover the patient and keep him warm.

Explanation of the Prescription: You Yi: Acute pain in the chest and the epigastrium caused by Cold, and nausea and vomiting that prevents the patient from eating indicate rampant excessive Yin and Cold and a debility in the Spleen and the Stomach Vital Energy. A protruding mass in the shape of a head or foot which appears in different abdominal locations with tenderness that is extremely painful indicates the forming of a mass of a Yin and Cold nature. Parasites in the abdomen may also take this opportunity to move about. Decoction of Greater *Jianzhong* is adopted to build up Interior (Spleen and Stomach) Yang Vital Energy so as to reverse the ascending Yin and Cold. Pericarpium Zanthoxyli and Rhizoma Zingiberis are used to warm the Stomach and disperse the parasites (ascarides). Radix Ginseng and *Jiaoyi* (malt sugar) tonify the Vital Energy and tranquilize the Interior.

CASES

Case 1 (48-72):

Mr. Zeng, 40, suffered from stomachache for several years. Epigastric region was cold. The patient had acid regurgitation and preferred hot drink or soup. When food was eaten, pain was reduced. Tongue was pale, covered with white coating; pulse was tight.

Diagnosis: Stomachache caused by prevalence of Cold and Deficiency, which was treated by Decoction of Greater *Jianzhong*:

Pericarpium Zanthoxyli	6 grams
Rhizoma Zingiberis	9 grams
Radix Codonopsis Pilosulae	12 grams
Radix Paeoniae Alba	12 grams
Ramulus Cinnamomi	9 grams
Radix Glycyrrhizae Praeparata	6 grams
Rhizoma Pinelliae	9 grams
Rhizoma Atractylodis Macrocephalae	9 grams
Saccharum Granorum (blend into the already-stewed decoction before service)	30 grams

Several doses dispersed the ailment.

Case 2: Biliary Ascariasis, Cases Recorded in Journal of *Zhejiang Chinese Medicine*, Vol. 2, 1964

The journal recorded forty-five cases of biliary ascariasis successfully treated with Decoction of Greater *Jianzhong*.

Prescription:

Pericarpium Zanthoxyli	9 grams
Rhizoma Zingiberis	9 grams
Fructus Mume	9 grams
Cortex Meliae	9 grams
Semen Arecae	9 grams
Radix Codonopsis Pilosulae	9 grams
Saccharum Granorum	60 grams
Rhizoma Coptidis	5 grams
Radix Coptidis	5 grams
Radix Glycyrrhizae	5 grams

The cases were categorized into three types, treated respectively by adding the following drugs:

1. Cases with Heat— add drugs of purgative, such as Radix et Rhizoma Rhei, Cortex Magnoliae Officinalis, Fructus Aurantii Immaturus.

2. Cases with Cold— add drugs of warm and dispersive quality, such as Fructus Evodiae, Herba Asari.

3. Cases with Cold and Stagnation or stasis— add such drugs as Rhizoma Alpiniae Officinarum, Rhizoma Cyperi, Lignum Santali.

Therapeutic effect: Among the 45 cases, 39 cases were fully cured, 4 cases were cured slowly, and 2 cases were not successfully treated.

Case 3 (65-271): Case Recorded in Journal of *Guangdong Chinese Medicine*, 2:46, 1959

Zhong, 67, female, first treatment on September 22, 1954. The patient was in good health until two days earlier when she had acute pain in chest and abdomen. Other symptoms were copious salivation, anorexia, white tongue coating, tight-slow pulse.

Diagnosis: Syndrome caused by ascending of Yin-Cold when the upper and middle portions were having Yang Deficiency. Decoction of Greater *Jianzhong* was prescribed:

Pericarpium Citri Zanthoxyli	18 grams
Rhizoma Zingiberis	30 grams
Radix Codonopsis Pilosulae	30 grams
Saccharum Granorum (blend into the already-stewed decoction before service)	30 grams

Second treatment: After taking the decoction, chest and abdominal pain was reduced by fifty percent. There was still salivation, but nausea stopped and the patient began to eat. Pulse condition was improved (not as tight-slow as before). Rhizoma Pinelliae was added to alleviate salivation. Prescription appeared as follows:

Pericarpium Zanthoxyli	24 grams
Rhizoma Zingiberis	36 grams
Radix Codonopsis Pilosulae	36 grams
Rhizoma Pinelliae Praeparata	18 grams
Saccharum Granorum (blend into the already-stewed decoction before service)	30 grams

Two doses of the decoction cured the ailment.

CLAUSE 10-15

Invasion of pathogenetic Cold will cause the following symptoms and signs to appear: Pain on one of the flanks, fever (1), and tense-tight pulse. Purgative with warm ingredients should be adopted to eliminate the constipation. Decoction of Radix et Rhizoma Rhei and Radix Aconiti Praeparata will provide the cure (2).

NOTES

1. According to *The Pulse Classic*, "fever" should not be included as one of the symptoms. (01-101)

2. Tense-tight pulse generally indicates prevalence of cold and pain, a syndrome with an accumulation of excessive Cold. The "fever" mentioned here does not refer to the fever of an Exterior syndrome, nor to that of the Interior Excess of a Greater Yang syndrome, but to a fever of an Exterior syndrome, nor to that of the Interior Excess of a Greater Yang syndrome, but to a fever caused by stagnation of the Yang Vital Energy due to the excessive Yin and Cold and imbalance of the Nutrient Essence with the Vital Resistance. In clinical observation, fever with excessive Yin and Cold may or may not appear as one of the main symptoms, though constipation will be present. Other symptoms and signs may include chill, cold in the extremities, and sticky tongue coating. (02-86)

Decoction of Radix et Rhizoma Rhei and Radix Aconiti Praeparata (*Dahuang Fuzi Tang*):

Radix et Rhizoma Rhei	3 *liang*
Radix Aconiti Praeparata	3 pcs.
Herba Asari	2 *liang*

Stew the drugs in five *sheng* of water until two *sheng* remain. Serve the decoction in three doses. For strong patients, stew the decoction until two and a half *sheng* remain and serve in three doses. After serving one dose, a second can be given in a time when a person has walked four to five *li* (two kilometers or more).

Explanation of the Prescription: The main syndrome in this case is constipation, and prognosis largely depends on whether loose stool is observed. As the stagnation of excessive Cold has made the Yang Vital Energy deficient, the appearance of loose stool means the case is curable. If Decoction of Radix et Rhizoma Rhei and Radix Aconiti Praeparata does not produce a stool but rather nausea and vomiting, a feeling of cold in the extremities and a slender pulse, the case is deteriorating. *Wenpi Tang*, a recipe from *Experiential Prescriptions for Universal Relief* (*Pu Ji Ben Shi Fang*) by Xu Shuwei, is applicable to the syndrome.

Decoction to Warm the Spleen (*Wenpi Tang*) includes the following ingredients: Cortex Magnoliae Officinalis, Radix Glycyrrhizae, Rhizoma Zingiberis, Cortex Cinnamomi, Radix Aconiti Praeparata, Radix et Rhizoma Rhei. (02-86)

CASES

Case 1 (64-352):

A gentleman had drunk heavily. Spleen and Kidney Yang was deficient and exhausted. One day he had acute abdominal pain, and tenderness and profuse perspiration. There was no stool for three days. Tongue was covered with greasy coating, pulse was deep-excessive.

Diagnosis: Accumulation of Humidity, phlegm and indigestion would be helped by purgative. But the Yang Deficiency did not allow the administration of purgative with drugs in cold quality, purgative with warm drugs was the right cure. Decoction of Radix et Rhizoma Rhei and Radix Aconiti Praeparata was prescribed:

Radix Aconiti Praeparata	5 *fen*
Cortex Cinnamomi	4 *fen*
Rhizoma Zingiberis	5 *fen*
Radix et Rhizoma Rhei	4 *qian*
Fructus Aurantii Immaturus	1.5 *qian*
Cortex Magnoliae Officinalis	1 *qian*

Case 2 (64-352): Case Recorded in Journal of *Zhejiang Chinese Medicine*, 4:171, 1983

Mr. Shen, 58, had gastrectomy surgery the previous year. After the operation, his stomach was weak. At noon one day after eating, pain and distention occurred, followed by vomiting the same evening. There was no stool for three days. Examination showed an acute case of intestinal obstruction. The patient had pale face, cold extremities, pale and swollen tongue covered with greasy coating. Pulse was deep-tense-tight.

Diagnosis: Obstruction caused by stagnation of indigestion and Cold.

Decoction of Radix et Rhizoma Rhei and Radix Aconiti Praeparata was prescribed:

Radix et Rhizoma Rhei	12 grams
Radix Aconiti Praeparata	10 grams

Rhizoma Zingiberis	10 grams
Rhizoma Pinelliae (prepared with ginger)	10 grams

After taking the decoction, there was a loose stool. Syndrome was gone.

Case 3 (02-86):

Mr. Zhong suffered from abdominal pain for several years. Drugs of warm quality such as Decoction of *Lizhong* (Radix Ginseng, Rhizoma Zingiberis, Radix Glycyrrhizae Praeparata and Rhizoma Atractylodis Macrocephalae) and Decoction of *Sini* (Radix Glycyrrhizae Praeparata, Rhizoma Zingiberis and Radix Aconiti Praeparata) were given. They worked temporarily, but the syndrome attacked irregularly. Intake of cold food induced attacks. When there was an attack, the patient had washed pepper down with decoction of fresh ginger, which gave him temporary relief.

Examination: Pulse was deep and tight-tense. Tongue was white, moist free from coating. Palpation of abdomen gave the patient pain, dragging to the lumbar and costal regions. Urination was normal. Stool, every other day, was not smooth, and was scanty.

Diagnosis: Syndrome of stagnation of Cold and indigestion, which should be warmed and dispersed. Drugs like Decoctions of *Lizhong* and *Sini* could warm the Cold but not remove the accumulation. Decoction of Radix et Rhizoma Rhei and Radix Aconiti Praeparata was prescribed:

Radix et Rhizoma Rhei	4 *qian*
Radix Aconiti Praeparata	3 *qian*
Herba Asari	1.5 *qian*

Two doses of the decoction worked effectively.

Case 4 (02-86):

Mr. Yuan, 45, had chest and abdominal distention, pain, and dyspnea. It was hard for him to lie flat. He also had a fever. There was no stool for five days. His deep pulse indicated the syndrome was in the Interior. Tight-tense pulse indicated the syndrome was in Cold nature.

Diagnosis: Syndrome caused by stagnation of Yin and Cold at the Interior, Yang (Heat) being resisted to the Exterior. Drugs should be adopted to warm the Interior Cold, and a purgative should be given to disperse the stagnation. Decoction of Radix et Rhizoma Rhei and Radix Aconiti Praeparata was prescribed.

Radix et Rhizoma Rhei	2 *qian*
Radix Aconiti Praeparata	2 *qian*
Herba Asari	1 *qian*

One dose of the decoction actuated a loose stool and subsidence of distention and pain. Fever also went down.

CLAUSE 10-16

Coldness in the extremities caused by pathogenetic Cold can be treated with *Chiwan* Pills. (1)

NOTES

1. From the ingredients used in the prescription, it can be inferred that the following symptoms and signs belong in this clause: abdominal pain, nausea, and adverse ascending of gas, symptoms caused by Fluid-retention. (01-101)

Chiwan Pills
(*Chi Wan*):

Poria	4 *liang*
Rhizoma Aconiti Praeparata	2 *liang*
Rhizoma Pinelliae*	4 *liang*
Herba Asari	1 *liang*

Pound the drugs into powder. Add Cinnabaris, which will make the powder red. Mix the powder with honey and form pills the size of Fructus Cannabis. Take three pills before meals, twice in the day and once at night. If not effective, increase dosage till cure is effected.

*According to another edition, Rhizoma Pinelliae is replaced by Cortex Cinnamomi.

Remark: Prescription for *Chiwan* Pills in *Qianjin* differs as follows:

Chiwan Pills
(*Chi Wan*):

Poria	4 *liang*
Cortex Cinnamomi*	4 *liang*
Herba Asari	1 *liang*
Rhizoma Aconiti	2 *liang*

Radix Aconiti Praeparata	2 *liang*
Fructus Ziziphi Jujubae	1 pc.

(01-102)

*According to another edition, Cortex Cinnamomi is replaced by Rhizoma Pinelliae.

Explanation of the Prescription: Rhizoma Aconiti and Herba Asari, warm in quality, disperse the pathogenetic Cold. Rhizoma Pinelliae and Poria reverse adverse ascending and eliminate Fluid-retention. Cinnabaris, heavy and tranquilizing, reverses the adverse ascending. This is a prescription applicable to syndromes caused by an intermingling of pathogenetic Cold with Fluid-retention. (01-102)

CASES

Case 1 (52-539):

Mr. Xu, 47-year-old farmer, first treatment on October 18, 1974. The patient suffered from abdominal pain due to stagnation of Cold for several years. When he was exposed to cold weather, there could be an attack. Twenty days prior to consultation, he contracted a cold, which caused abdominal pain with ascending and descending cold gas and distended testes. Tongue was covered with white-slippery coating, pulse was tight-slender and hesitant. Pills of *Chiwan* and Decoction of Greater *Jianzhong* (Clause 10-14) were combined to make a new prescription:

Poria	15 grams
Rhizoma Pinelliae	9 grams
Radix Aconiti	10 grams
Herba Asari	3 grams
Radix Linderae	15 grams
Pericarpium Zanthoxyli	9 grams
Rhizoma Zingiberis	10 grams
Semen Litchi	10 grams
Semen Citri Reticulatae	9 grams
Fructus Meliae Toosendan	9 grams

Three doses of the decoction worked effectively.

Case 2 (52-540):

Mr. Zhang, 27, first treatment on August 14, 1981. Testis on the right had convulsive pain for four months. Last April, his wife visited him in Beijing and when his wife left, he had a very strong sexual urge every night. His penis was erect all night. He began to feel pain and distention in his right testis, with pain in the lower abdomen. When weather changed, the syndrome was aggravated. Tongue was tender-red, covered with thin, white coating, and pulse was tight-tense. Yin-Deficiency was one pathological condition. Pills of *Chiwan* added to big dose of Radix Paeoniae Alba were prescribed:

Radix Aconiti	10 grams
Radix Aconiti Kusnezoffii	10 grams
Ramulus Cinnamomi	10 grams
Radix Paeoniae Alba	25 grams
Radix Glycyrrhizae	6 grams
Rhizoma Zingiberis Recens	6 grams
Fructus Ziziphi Jujubae	6 pcs.

Sixteen doses of the decoction cured the ailment.

CLAUSE 10-17

Abdominal pain with tight-tense pulse. Tight pulse indicates stagnation of Vital Resistance, creating aversion to cold. Tense pulse reflects anorexia. When pathogenetic Cold conflicts with Body Resistance, abdominal pain in the navel region results, accompanied by cold sweat, coldness in extremities and deep-tense pulse (1). Decoction of Greater Rhizoma Aconiti will provide a cure. (2)

NOTES

1. According to *The Pulse Classic, Qianjin* and *Waitai*, "deep-tense pulse" should read, "deep-tight pulse."

2. This clause discusses the mechanism, symptoms and treatment of abdominal pain caused by Cold. Both tight and tense pulses reflect Interior excessive Cold, which results from a Deficiency of the Yang Vital Energy. When the Yang Vital Energy fails to circulate in the Exterior, aversion to cold results. Deficiency of the Yang Vital Energy in the Interior brings about anorexia. When the Yang Vital Energy fails to circulate in the Interior, the Cold stagnates there, causing abdominal pain in the navel region, aggravating abdominal pain. Cold sweat and coldness in the extremities occur and the pulse turns from tight-tense to deep-tense. Thus Decoction of Greater Rhizoma Aconiti is adopted to disperse the Cold and ease the pain. (02-87)

Decoction of Greater Rhizoma Aconiti
(*Da Wutou Jian*):

Rhizoma Aconiti Praeparata	5 big pcs.

Stew the drug in three *sheng* of water until one *sheng* remains. Filter the decoction and add two *sheng* of honey. Then stew the decoction until all the water evaporates. Two *sheng* of the decoction will remain. Serve seven *ge* to a strong patient and five *ge* to a weak. If not effective, serve a second dose the next day. No more than one dose should be served per day.

Explanation of the Prescription: Rhizoma Aconiti, of an extremely hot quality, is often used in clinical practice to cure syndromes of a severe Cold nature such as acute abdominal pain with Cold in the extremities. It can disperse Cold, ease pain and stimulate the physiological functioning of Yang Vital Energy. But Rhizoma Aconiti is poisonous, it is decocted together with honey which reduces the poison and prolongs its efficacy. That the text says, "No more than one dose should be served per day," is evidence of the strong efficiency of the drug. Be cautious about its administration.

Decoction of Pericarpium Zanthoxyli for Emergencies, a recipe found in *Waitai*, has a function similar to Decoction of Greater Rhizoma Aconiti but is milder. Prescription is as follows:

Decoction of Pericarpium Zanthoxyli for Emergencies
(*Jie Ji Shujiao Tang*):

Pericarpium Zanthoxyli
Radix Aconiti Praeparata
Rhizoma Zingiberis
Rhizoma Pinelliae
Semen Oryzae Nonglutinosae
Radix Glycyrrhizae
Fructus Ziziphi Jujubae

(02-87)

CASES

Case 1 (51-231): Case Recorded in Journal of *New Medicine and Pharmacology*, 12:16, 1978

Mr. Shen, in his fifties, first treatment on June 1973. The patient suffered from paroxysmal abdominal pain for many years. When there was a serious attack, the patient was hospitalized with diagnosis of gastrointestinal neurosis. The patient told the doctor that whenever he was exposed to cold or worked too hard, there was an aggravation of the syndrome. When the syndrome attacked, there was no fixed locus, the pain moved around the umbilicus. Profuse perspiration occurred when the pain was severe. Locus invited warmth and massage. Tongue was pale, covered with thin-greasy-slippery coating.

Diagnosis: This syndrome was caused by accumulation of Interior Cold and malfunction of the Yang Vital Energy circulation. Warm drugs could disperse stagnation and relieve pain.

Decoction of *Lizhong* (Radix Ginseng, Rhizoma Zingiberis, Radix Glycyrrhizae Präeparata and Rhizoma Atractylodis Macrocephalae) was given. The decoction was not strong enough. Decocter Greater Rhizoma Aconiti was then served. In the first decoction, dosage of Rhizoma Aconiti was 4.5 grams. Honey should be used to stew the decoction, but it was not convenient to stew the drug with honey in the preparation room. Radix Glycyrrhizae and Semen Sojae Nigrum were used to replace honey. Two doses were served, which reduced the pain and perspiration effectively.

In the next treatment, dosage of Rhizoma Aconiti increased to nine grams.

Third treatment: Four doses were consumed, abdominal pain was gone. Tongue coating was diminishing and pulse became moderate. Decoction of Greater Rhizoma Aconiti, composed of drugs of hot quality, was the right cure for syndrome of cold nature. The patient was allowed to go home after receiving treatment in the hospital for a month.

CLAUSE 10-18

Abdominal pain caused by Cold with pain in the abdomen and the costal regions, and dragging pains can be reduced with Decoction of Radix Angelicae Sinensis, Rhizoma Zingiberis Recens and Mutton.

Decoction of Radix Angelicae Sinensis,
Rhizoma Zingiberis Recens and Mutton
(*Danggui Shengjiang Yangrou Tang*):

Radix Angelicae Sinensis	3 *liang*
Rhizoma Zingiberis Recens	5 *liang*
Mutton	1 *jin*

Stew the drugs and the mutton in eight *sheng* of water until three *sheng* remain. Serve seven *ge* of the lukewarm decoction per dose three times a day.

In cases caused by severe Cold, increase the dosage of Rhizoma Zingiberis Recens to one *jin* and stew the drugs in thirteen *sheng* of water until three *sheng* and two *ge* remain. In case of acute pain with nausea, add two *liang* of Pericarpium Citri Reticulatae and one *liang* of Rhizoma Atractylodis Macrocephalae to the original prescription.

Explanation of the Prescription: This clause discusses abdominal pain caused by Cold due to Deficiency in the Blood. When the Blood is deficient, the Vital Energy is also deficient. When the abdomen and costal regions lose their normal function of warming the Vital Energy and nourishing the Blood, pain in the abdomen and the costal regions occurs. The pain is generally mild and reduces somewhat when pressed or warmed locally. The pulse should be tight-hesitant, or feeble-tense. Decoction of Radix Angelicae Sinensis, Rhizoma Zingiberis Recens and Mutton is adopted to tonify the Deficiency, nourish the Blood and disperse the Cold. (02-88)

CASES

Case 1 (64-359): Case Recorded in *Ben Cao Yan Yi (Amplified Materia Medica)* written in 1116 by Kou Zongshi

Master Zhang Zhongjing's prescription, Decoction of Radix Angelicae Sinensis, Rhizoma Zingiberis Recens and Mutton, is effective in treating abdominal pain caused by Cold. One example:

A woman gave birth on a cold day, letting pathogenetic Cold invade the body through the reproductive tract. There was acute pain and distention of abdomen below umbilicus with tenderness. One doctor said this was caused by formation of blood stasis. Kou Zongshi told him: "No, the syndrome should be treated by Master Zhang's Decoction of Radix Angelicae Sinensis, Rhizoma Zingiberis Recens and Mutton." Two doses of the decoction were given, which worked as anticipated.

Case 2 (64-359): Case Recorded in Journal of *New Medicine and Pharmacology*, 12:16, 1978

A female patient of twenty-three suffered abdominal pain for a long time.

Examination: The patient was weak and thin. The pain moved around the umbilicus. When attack was acute, the patient perspired heavily. The pain attacked irregularly. She had no appetite, was depressed, pulse was deep-slender and tight, tongue pale, covered with thin, white coating. There was temporary relief when the abdomen was palpated or warmed. The patient drank hot water or soup to relax. Coldness on extremities was reported.

Diagnosis: Syndrome with Interior abdominal pain and Deficiency of Body Resistance (failure in warming the extremities) which should be treated simultaneously. Decoction of Rhizoma Aconiti and Ramulus Cinnamomi was given first:

Radix Aconiti Praeparata (stewed prior to other drugs)	9 grams
Ramulus Cinnamomi	9 grams
Radix Paeoniae Alba	9 grams
Fructus Ziziphi Jujubae	10 pcs.
Rhizoma Zingiberis Recens	3 slices
Radix Glycyrrhizae Praeparata	6 grams

Five doses were served. Abdominal pain subsided.

Second treatment: Another seven doses were given. The patient looked energetic, had better appetite. Pulse was slender, tongue was tender-red. Extremities became warm. Symptoms of Cold nature retreated. Later, Deficiency of Blood was treated mildly. Decoction of Radix Angelicae Sinensis, Rhizoma Zingiberis Recens and Mutton was given in ten doses. The doctor told the patient this decoction should be taken regularly for a long period of time to give gradual stimulus to blood.

Two months later the patient reported that she felt healthy.

Case 3 (52-522): Case Recorded in *Dr. Xie Yinglu's Case Studies*

Mr. Zhou's wife suffered from acute pain in lower abdomen after childbirth in a winter month. Drugs to remove stasis had been administered repeatedly, but syndrome became worse. When attacked, the pain was so acute that the slightest touch was unbearable. She had nausea and vomiting and urge to urinate and defecate. The pain dragged to lumbar and costal regions. Three doctors were consulted. Two suggested giving purgative to relieve pain, Doctor Xie did not agree. He said: A patient in such a weak condition could not stand a purgative. The syndrome was caused by invasion of pathogenetic Cold when she was in puerperium. As the patient had Deficiency both in Exterior and Interior with floating-huge pulse, drugs to disperse the Exterior syndrome could not be used, as the patient was too weak. Tonics could not be used as she was suffering from abdominal pain with tenderness. Decoction of Radix Angelicae Sinensis, Rhizoma Zingiberis Recens and Mutton was the cure. Since there was nausea and vomiting, Pericarpium Citri Reticulatae and Caulis Allii Fistulosi was added.

Prescription:

Radix Astragali Hedysari
Radix Ginseng
Radix Angelicae Sinensis
Rhizoma Zingiberis Recens
Mutton (stew the mutton separately and add the syrup to the decoction)
Pericarpium Citri Reticulatae
Caulis Allii Fistulosi

One dose of the decoction induced perspiration and the subsidence of pain.

CLAUSE 10-19

Abdominal pain caused by Cold with coldness and numbness in the extremities and pain throughout the body: Neither acupuncture, moxibustion or other drugs can cure the syndrome. Decoction of Rhizoma Aconiti and Ramulus Cinnamomi can be adopted as a curative.

Decoction of Rhizoma Aconiti and Ramulus Cinnamomi
(*Wutou Guizhi Tang*)

Rhizoma Aconiti	5 pcs.

Stew Rhizoma Aconiti in two *jin* of honey until half of the decoction remains. Filter the decoction. Mix five *ge* of the decoction with five *ge* of Decoction of Ramulus Cinnamomi* to make one *sheng* of decoction. For the first dose, serve two *ge* of the decoction. If not effective, increase dosage to three *ge*. If still not effective, increase to five *ge*. When the medicament takes effect, the patient behaves as if drunk. If the patient vomits, efficacy of the decoction is proven.**

*Decoction of Ramulus Cinnamomi
(*Guizhi Tang*)

Ramulus Cinnamomi	3 *liang*
Radix Paeoniae	3 *liang*
Radix Glycyrrhizae Praeparata	2 *liang*
Rhizoma Zingiberis Recens	3 *liang*
Fructus Ziziphi Jujubae	12 pcs.

Stew the drugs in seven *sheng* of water over a slow fire until three *sheng* remain. Filter the decoction.

**When the patient behaves as if drunk: it indicates Exterior syndrome is subsiding. If patient vomits, it is evidence that the Interior Coldness has disappeared. (01-104)

Explanation of the Prescription: This prescription is designed to treat syndrome with Interior and Exterior Coldness. Abdominal pain, the principal symptom, is caused by the stagnation of pathogenetic Cold in the Interior. When Yang Vital Energy is extremely deficient, it cannot reach the extremities, causing coldness and even numbness in the extremities. Pain throughout body is due to the disharmony between the Nutrient Essence and the Vital Resistance caused by the invasion of pathogenetic Cold. This is a case of pathogenetic Cold prevailing in both the Exterior and the Interior. Rhizoma Aconiti is used to disperse the Cold and ease the pain. Decoction of Ramulus Cinnamomi is adopted to harmonize the Nutrient Essence with the Vital Resistance. After taking the decoction, the patient may vomit or behave as if he were drunk. This is a physiological reaction which occurs after taking the decoction, though it is not always the same in all cases. (02-88)

CASES

Case 1 (02-88):

Yuan, female, a strong young farmer, mother of three children, had never suffered menstrual disorders. One day, she had an acute pain in her lower abdomen with contracture. Drugs to regulate the menses were given, but did not work. This lasted two weeks when the doctor was sent for.

Examination: Pulse was deep-tense. There was headache, pain all over the body, cold extremities, perspiration, moist tongue, salivation, chill, but no thirst and fever. When abdominal pain around umbilicus became acute, there was cold sweat. The patient sensed cold gas from vagina. When the abdomen was warmed, there was a relief.

Diagnosis: Since the patient had regular menstruation, blood stasis or stagnation of Vital Energy could be ruled out. The syndrome did not seem to be caused by indigestion or improper intake of food. It was a syndrome caused by prevalence of Cold at both Interior and Exterior (tense pulse and cold extremities were the respective symptoms and signs). Decoction of Rhizoma Aconiti and Ramulus Cinnamomi was the right cure.

Prescription:

Rhizoma Aconiti Praeparata	4 *qian*
Ramulus Cinnamomi	6 *qian*

Radix Paeoniae	4 *qian*
Radix Glycyrrhizae	2 *qian*
Fructus Ziziphi Jujubae	6 pcs.
Rhizoma Zingiberis Recens	3 slices

The decoction was served with honey. Two doses were given. Pain and coldness subsided.

Second treatment: Decoction to warm the Interior and smooth the flow of Channels and Collaterals was prescribed as follows:

Radix Angelicae Sinensis	5 *qian*
Ramulus Cinnamomi	2 *qian*
Herba Asari	1 *qian*
Radix Paeoniae	3 *qian*
Caulis Akebiae	3 *qian*
Radix Glycyrrhizae	2 *qian*
Fructus Evodiae	2 *qian*
Rhizoma Zingiberis Recens	3 slices

Case 2 (64-361): Case Recorded in *Clinical Experience of Dr. Zhao Xiwu*

Mr. Han, in his fifties, suffered from abdominal pain caused by Cold for two and a half years. Almost every day he had acute abdominal pain and distention, coldness of extremities, stiff legs, and cold sweat all over the body. Tongue was covered with thin, white coating, pulse was tight-slender. One dose of Decoction of Rhizoma Aconiti and Ramulus Cinnamomi worked. Twenty or thirty doses were taken. There was improvement but the syndrome was not totally gone.

Second treatment: Decoction of Radix Angelicae Sinensis, Rhizoma Zingiberis Recens and Mutton was given. Several dozen of doses cured the ailment.

Case 3 (64-362): Case Recorded in Journal of *New Medicine and Pharmacology*, 12:17, 1978

Mr. Yang, 32, first treatment on March 10, 1965. The syndrome started when the patient forded cold water on a winter day. He was also sexually active that day. There appeared an acute pain in his testes. Accompanying symptoms: Hard and swollen scrotum, acute pain with dragging pain to the lower abdomen, which was cold when palpated, cold sweat on scrotum, coldness on extremities. Pulse was deep-tight, face was cyan-black with depressed feeling. Tongue was moist and white. The patient preferred staying in warm environment.

Diagnosis: Syndrome caused by stagnation and accumulation of Yin and

Cold, which should be dispersed by warm drugs. Decoction of Rhizoma Aconiti and Ramulus Cinnamomi was given:

Radix Aconiti Praeparata (stew prior to other drugs)	30 grams
Radix Paeoniae Alba	30 grams
Ramulus Cinnamomi	30 grams
Radix Glycyrrhizae Praeparata	30 grams
Rhizoma Zingiberis Recens	30 grams
Radix Astragali Hedysari	60 grams
Fructus Ziziphi Jujubae	12 pcs.

Twelve doses were served. Simultaneausly, another stew was served, which contained:

Radix Angelicae Sinensis	120 grams
Rhizoma Zingiberis Recens	250 grams
Mutton	1,000 grams

Both the decoction and the stew eased the pain and brought warmth. The patient was able to go back to his work.

CLAUSE 10-20

The pulse is speedy-tense and becomes speedy-tight. When the pulse is pressed, it feels as tight as a bowstring. Even if it is pressed deeply, it remains equally tight. Treat such a case by prescribing a purgative with warm-quality drugs to disperse the Cold. Tense-huge and slow pulse indicates the existence of a hardened mass in the epigastrium. If the pulse is huge-tense, it indicates a case of Yin within Yang (1). A purgative can be adopted. (2)

NOTES

1. Wu Qian: Huge pulse indicates Excess of Yang. Tense pulse indicates Excess of Yin. This is a case of Yin within Yang. Purgative can be adopted to release the Excess. (05-535)

2. According to *Jinjian*, original text should read as follows: Tense-huge and slow pulse indicates the existence of a hardened mass in the epigastrium. A purgative with warm-quality drugs should be adopted to disperse the Cold. Huge-tense pulse indicates a case of Yin within Yang. Purgative can be adopted. (05-535)

Appendix: Prescriptions from *Waitai:*

Prescription A: Decoction of Rhizoma Aconiti, effective in treating acute abdominal pain caused by Cold, invasion of pathogenetic Wind in the Five Viscera, contraction which renders the patient immobile, constriction of genitals (flaccid constriction of penis) and coldness in the extremities.

Prescription see above.*

Prescription B: Decoction of Radix Bupleuri and Ramulus Cinnamomi, effective in curing syndrome of sudden attacks of pain in the epigastrium and abdomen. (According to the original text in *Waitai*, this should read: "effective in curing syndrome of abdominal pain caused by Cold.")

*Decoction of Rhizoma Aconiti in *Waitai* is the same as Decoction of Rhizoma Aconiti and Ramulus Cinnamomi found in Clause 10-19, the dosages are not the same:

Decoction of Rhizoma Aconiti
(*Waitai Wutou Tang*):

Rhizoma Aconiti	15 pcs.
Cortex Cinnamomi	6 *liang*
Radix Paeoniae	4 *liang*
Radix Glycyrrhizae	2 *liang*
Rhizoma Zingiberis Recens	1 *jin*
Fructus Ziziphi Jujubae	10 pcs.

Decoction of Radix Bupleuri and Ramulus Cinnamomi
(*Waitai Chaihu Guizhi Tang*):

This prescription also appears in Clause 146 of *Shanghan Lun*.

Radix Bupleuri	4 *liang*
Radix Scutellariae	1.5 *liang*
Radix Ginseng	1.5 *liang*
Radix Paeoniae	1.5 *liang*
Ramulus Cinnamomi	1.5 *liang*
Rhizoma Zingiberis Recens	1.5 *liang*
Radix Glycyrrhizae	1 *liang*
Rhizoma Pinelliae	2.5 *ge*
Fructus Ziziphi Jujubae	6 pcs.

Prescription C: Decoction of *Zouma*, effective in curing syndrome with attack of pestilent factors, Heart pain, abdominal distention and constipation.

Decoction of *Zouma*
(*Zouma Tang*):

Semen Armeniacae Amarum	2 pcs.
Fructus Crotonis Praeparata	2 pcs.

CLAUSE 10-21

Question: How does one diagnose a syndrome of indigestion?

Master: Pulse at the Inch (under the first finger) is floating-huge. When it is pressed deeply, it becomes hesitant. Pulse in the Cubit (under the ring-finger) is also feeble-hesitant. (1) This is evidence of indigestion. Decoction of Greater *Chengqi* can be adopted as a purgative. (2)

NOTES

1. According to *Jinjian*, "feeble-hesitant" is "huge-hesitant."

2. This clause discusses the pulse accompanying indigestion. You Yi: Pulse in the Inch is floating-huge, indicating strong Cereal Vital Energy. Excessive intake of cereal (causing indigestion) will not benefit the Spleen but harm it. When the pulse is deeply pressed, it becomes hesitant. This demonstrates that when the Spleen is damaged, the Blood and the Vital Energy cannot circulate smoothly, which is indicated by hesitant pulse. Pulse in the Cubit is also feeble-hesitant, demonstrating that the Interior Vital Energy cannot circulate normally. Thus the Vital Essence produced by cereal and water cannot flow downward to provide a nourishment. Since this is a case of indigestion, Decoction of Greater *Chengqi* is the proper medicine to purge the Excess (indigestion).

CLAUSE 10-22

Speedy-slippery pulse indicates an excessive case and indigestion. The purgative, Decoction of Greater *Chengqi*, can be considered as a cure. (1)

NOTES

1. Generally speaking, indigestion is evidenced by a slippery pulse. But according to Clause 10-21, a hesitant pulse also indicates a case of indigestion. What is the difference? When indigestion begins, the obstruction is not very seri-

ous, thus the pulse is generally slippery.

But if indigestion has lasted a comparatively long time, seriously obstructing the flow of Vital Energy in the intestine, the pulse will become hesitant. In such cases, purgative should be adopted immediately to disperse the indigestion, as the latter may consume too much Body Resistance. Clause 10-22 described the initial stage of indigestion, though a purgative is also necessary. Whether Decoction of Greater *Chengqi* (given as a drastic measure) is necessary depends on the overall syndrome. That is why the text says, "Decoction of Greater *Chengqi* can be considered as a cure."

CLAUSE 10-23

Diarrhea with anorexia (1) signifies a case of indigestion. A purgative should be prescribed. Decoction of Greater *Chengqi* will provide a cure.

NOTES

1. Wu Qian: When the patient first has diarrhea and anorexia, this is caused by indigestion, and he refuses all food. If the diarrhea has lasted for a long time, the patient cannot absorb food as his Spleen has been seriously damaged. The case in this clause is one of a fresh onset of diarrhea with anorexia. Thus a purgative can be adopted to disperse the indigestion. (05-540)

CLAUSE 10-24

When the indigestion remains in the upper gastric cavity (1), an emetic should be prescribed to help the patient eliminate the indigestion by vomiting. Powder of Pedicellus Melo should be adopted.

NOTES

1. The upper digestive tract.

Powder of Pedicellus Melo
(*Guadi San*):

Pedicellus Melo	1 *fen*
Semen Phaseoli	1 *fen*

Pound the drugs into powder. Stew Semen Sojae Praeparatum in seven *ge* of water. Take one *qianbi* of the powder with the warm decoction. If there is no emesis, increase the dosage gradually until a good emesis is observed.

Taboo: The patient who has lost blood or who is physically weak should not take this medicine.

Explanation of the Prescription: This emetic is applicable to all cases of a Yang and excessive nature with pathogenetic factors in the chest and near the throat with nausea and vomiting. Its application is not restricted to cases of indigestion. In an emergency, one cup of heavily salted water can also be used as an emetic. (02-90)

CLAUSE 10-25

Tense pulse resembling a twisting rope (1) indicates indigestion.

NOTES

1. This is a tense-slippery pulse. Unlike tense-tight pulse present in Exterior syndromes, pulse varies between tense and slippery, resembling a twisting rope. (01-108)

CLAUSE 10-26

Tense pulse (1) indicates either an Exterior syndrome with headache caused by pathogenetic Wind and Cold, or abdominal indigestion. (2)

NOTES

1. According to another edition, this should read, "tense pulse in the Inch (under the first finger)."

2. This clause discusses the meaning of a tense pulse. Generally speaking, a tense pulse is present in an Exterior syndrome with headache and aversion to cold caused by pathogenetic Wind and Cold. But tense pulse may also appear in cases of indigestion, wherein tense pulse will resemble a twisting rope. Other symptoms may include abdominal pain and distention. (01-108)

CHAPTER XI

ON PULSE, SYMPTOM COMPLEX AND TREATMENT OF ACCUMULATION OF PATHOGENETIC WIND AND COLD IN THE FIVE VISCERA

CLAUSE 11-1

When the Lung is affected by pathogenetic Wind, the patient will feel parched in throat and wheeze. He will also feel vertigo, heaviness of movement and swelling throughout the body. (1)

NOTES

1. The Lung dominates the Vital Energy and is related to the skin and hair. When the Lung is affected by pathogenetic Wind, the Vital Energy is affected as well, which will in turn affect the normal flow of the Body Fluid. Thus the patient feels parched in throat. When pathogenetic Wind injures the Lung, abnormal ascent of gas will result in wheezing. When the Vital Energy is injured, the patient experiences heaviness of movement. Swelling will occur when the Vital Energy fails to circulate the Water. (05-541)

CLAUSE 11-2

When the Lung is affected by pathogenetic Cold, the symptom of spitting sticky sputum will appear. (1)

NOTES

1. Wu Qian: When the Lung is affected by Cold, Yang Vital Energy in the chest is reduced to a debilitated state and fails to circulate the Body Fluid, causing an accumulation of Body Fluid. Spitting sticky sputum results. (05-541)

CLAUSE 11-3

Pulse of a Dead Lung (1) is deficient when pressed lightly and as weak and rootless as the leaves of a Chinese onion (2) when pressed deeply. This indicates a fatal case.

NOTES

1. Pulse of a Dead Lung (or other Viscera) is an expression of the decay of visceral energy (*zhen zang mai*). This pulse generally indicates an unfavorable prognosis. (01-110)

2. "As weak and rootless as the leaves of a Chinese onion" describes a kind of pulse with a sensation of inner emptiness and rootlessness. (01-110)

CLAUSE 11-4

When the Liver is affected by pathogenetic Wind, the patient feels pain on both flanks and walks with his back bent. His head shakes and eyelids jump. He begins to show a preference for sweet food. (1)

NOTES

1. Xu Bin: Head occupies the highest position in the body. Only pathogenetic Wind can attain such a high position. Wind is characteristic of movement, thus the head shakes and the eyelids jump. The Liver Channel passes by the diaphragm and causes pain in the flanks. The Liver dominates the tendons; when it is attacked by pathogenetic Wind, the tendons will constrict, causing the patient to bend his back. When the pathogenetic factor in the Liver is excessive, the Spleen and the Stomach will be conquered. As sweet food tonifies the Spleen and the Stomach, the patient changes his eating habit and begins to show a preference for sweet food. This physiological reaction is an act of self-rescue. (05-542)

CLAUSE 11-5

When the Liver is affected by pathogenetic Cold, the patient cannot raise his arms and feels parched at the root of the tongue (1). He sighs frequently and chest pain hampers his normal movements. After eating, he will vomit and perspire. (2) (*The Pulse Classic* and *Qianjin* give the following symptoms and signs: "... with occasional night sweating and coughing. After eating, the patient vomits the liquid portion of the food.")

NOTES

1. According to *Jinjian*, the original text should not include the following words: "The patient cannot raise his arms and feels parched at the root of the tongue" and "perspire." (05-542)

2. The Liver is characterized by being easy and smooth in movement. The

Vital Energy circulates in both sides of the chest. Thus when the Liver is affected by pathogenetic Cold, the Vital Energy stagnates, causing repeated sighing. When the Vital Energy stagnates, pain will result and normal movement will be hampered. Vomiting after eating is also due to the abnormal ascending of pathogenetic Cold. (05-542)

CLAUSE 11-6

Pulse of the Dead Liver is weak when pressed lightly. When pressed deeply, pulse is "as stale as a rope" (pulse does not rebound) or moves like a snake. Such pulsation is an indication of a fatal case. (1)

NOTES

1. Zhou Yangjun: When pressed deeply, the pulse is "as stale as a rope," this is a tight-tense pulse. Normal pulse has both "coming" and "going," which is the oscillation between Yin and Yang. But here the pulse is like a rope, meaning that it does not come back. This indicates the evanescence of the Stomach Vital Energy, which generally indicates a fatal case. When the pulse resembles a snake, it is an indication that it is struggling. This signifies the dispersion of the Body Resistance, which is also a signification of a fatal case. (05-543)

CLAUSE 11-7

Syndrome of Liver-affection (1): The patient enjoys having a strong pressure applied to his chest by another person. Before the onset of the syndrome, he prefers to drink hot beverages (2). Decoction of Flos Inulae (3) can be adopted.

NOTES

1. Liver-affection (*gan zhuo*): The Liver is affected by pathogenetic factors, resulting in the Vital Energy and the Blood stagnating in the Liver. (01-112)

2. Wu Qian: Liver-affection occurs when the Vital Energy is stagnated with Vital-energy Stagnation in the chest which produces a feeling of discomfort. Heavy pressure on the chest helps the flow of Vital Energy. Before the onset of the syndrome, the patient prefers hot beverages, evidence that the syndrome is caused by pathogenetic Cold. (05-543)

3. Wu Qian: Decoction of Flos Inulae is inappropriate for the syndrome. It is an error due to miscopying.

Decoction of Flos Inulae
(*Xuanfuhua Tang*):

Flos Inulae	3 *liang*
Allium Fistulosum	14 pcs.
*Xinjiang**	a little bit

Stew the drugs in three *sheng* of water until one *sheng* remains. Serve the decoction in one dose.

*Some annotators believe *Xinjiang* is a silk fabric freshly dyed with a red dyestuff (such as Flos Carthami or Radix Rubiae). Tao Hongjing (452-536) believes this indicates freshly gathered Radix Rubiae.

Explanation of the Prescription: Cao Jiada: In this syndrome, the Liver encroaches upon the Lung. When the Liver is affected, Vital Energy in the chest is blocked and is relieved somewhat when pressed. When the Yang Vital Energy cannot flow normally, the patient tends to have hot beverages as a self-rescue. Allium Fistulosum harmonizes the Liver and invigorates the Yang Vital Energy. Flos Inulae tonifies the Lung Vital Energy. *Xinjiang* dredges through the Collaterals to facilitate the normal functioning of physiological activities.

— *Detailed Exploration of the Golden Chamber*

CASES

Case 1 (65-295): Case Recorded in Journal of *Guangdong Chinese Medicine*, 7:36, 1962.

Mr. Zheng suffered from chest distress, restlessness and irritation for three months. Pulse on both Cubit positions was tight-huge. No fever, headache or palpitation was diagnosed. This was a Liver-affection syndrome, to be treated by Decoction of Flos Inulae. Prescription was as follows:

Flos Inulae	9 grams
Xinjiang	6 grams
Caulis Allii Fistulosi	7 pcs.

One dose of the decoction cured the ailment.

Case 2 (65-295): Case Recorded in *Case Studies from Famous Doctors Edited by*

Liu

A patient suffered from chronic cough and could not turn his body left. Syndrome was originated in the Liver, which caused ascending gas in the Lung (coughing). Mental depression was the cause. The syndrome should not be dispersed too quickly. Treatment was directed to the pathological condition in the Liver, not the Lung. Decoction of Flos Inulae was given:

Flos Inulae
Cortex Moutan Radicis
Semen Persicae
Radix Curcumae
Xinjiang
Radix Glycyrrhizae
Radix Achyranthis Bidentatae
Radix Paeoniae Alba

Case 3 (52-726):

Li, 50, female worker, first treatment on November 26, 1981. The patient suffered from myocardial ischemia for a long time with pain in chest, palpitation and shortness of breath. Overexertion and excessive anger aggravated the syndrome: there was a distention and pain in chest, a feeling of gas ascending, with repeated hiccups. Severe palpitation and suffocation occurred whenever she moved around, also insomnia and dreamy sleep. Pulse was slippery-tight-slender. Tongue was covered with white coating.

Decoction of Flos Inulae was given to regulate the flow of Vital Energy and bring down the adverse ascending:

Flos Inulae (wrapped in cloth sack)	10 grams
Ochra Haematitum	30 grams
Flos Carthami	3 grams
Caulis Polygoni Multiflori	30 grams
Radix Curcumae	12 grams
Cortex Albiziae	30 grams
Caulis Allii Fistulosi	1 pc.
Os Draconis	30 grams
Concha Ostreae	30 grams

Second treatment: Four doses of the decoction were served. Hiccups, chest pain and insomnia subsided. The patient looked refreshed. The same decoction adding thirty grams of Radix Pseudostellariae was given in four doses to achieve full recovery.

Case 4 (02-92): Case Recorded in Journal of *Chinese Medicine*, 6:29, 1964

Mr. Lu, 50, suffered from chronic stomachache for already eighteen years. Chronic gastritis was the diagnosis of a hospital of Western medicine. The patient was thin and was losing his appetite. He had chest pain and pain in costal regions. He preferred hot beverages. Massage and pressure on the chest gave him temporary relief.

Decoction of Flos Inulae was prescribed as follows:

Flos Inulae (wrapped in cloth sack)	30 grams
Radix Rubiae	6 grams
Caulis Allii Fistulosi	14 pcs.

Second treatment: After taking the decoction, chest pain was reduced. The patient still preferred hot beverages. There had been loose stools. Scrotum was cold and wet. The above decoction was given with additions as follows:

Flos Inulae (wrapped in cloth sack)	18 grams
Radix Rubiae	4.5 grams
Rhizoma Zingiberis	12 grams
Poria	12 grams
Fructus Aurantii Immaturus Praeparata	6 grams
Caulis Allii Fistulosi	7 pcs.

Two doses were given. Later, decoctions were prescribed with Decoction of Flos Inulae as the principal elements with alterations according to pathological changes. Eleven treatments were given before final recovery.

CLAUSE 11-8

When the Heart is affected by pathogenetic Wind, the patient has a fever and cannot get out of bed. He feels hungry, but immediately vomits whatever food he eats (1).

NOTES

1. Wu Qian: Fever is the principal symptom of diseases caused by Wind. It is difficult to understand why the patient is hungry but immediately vomits what he eats. There must be an error in the text. (05-543)

CLAUSE 11-9

When the Heart is affected by pathogenetic Cold, the patient suffers uneasiness in the Heart (in the chest), as if he has eaten too much garlic. In acute cases, there will be pain in the Heart (chest) dragging towards the back or pain in the back dragging towards the Heart (chest); this is similar to a *Guzhu* syndrome (1). If the pulse is floating, a spontaneous vomiting will bring about a recovery (2).

NOTES

1. According to different annotations, *Guzhu* syndrome indicates one of the following syndromes:

a) A disease similar to pulmonary tuberculosis or tuberculous peritonitis;

b) Abdominal distention caused by parasites such as schistosomiasis;

c) Syndrome with pains in the epigastrium and abdomen, restlessness, general fatigue and heaviness of movement.

2. Xu Bin: Floating pulse indicates that the pathogenetic factors have not accumulated solidly in the chest. Spontaneous vomiting will clear out pathogenetic factors and most likely lead to recovery. (05-544)

CLAUSE 11-10

When the Heart is affected and damaged, the following symptoms and signs will appear: When the patient is tired, his head and face will turn red. Other symptoms and signs include tenesmus, fever, restlessness, pain in the Heart, jumping movements in the region of navel and tight pulse (1) (2).

NOTES

1. Tight pulse: According to Wu Qian, "tight pulse" should read "deep pulse." Deep pulse indicates a pathological condition in the Kidney. (05-544)

2. You Yi: When the patient is tired, his head and face turn red because with Deficiency of Heart Vital Energy. Yang Vital Energy tends to flow upward, resulting in Deficiency of the Lower Portion and tenesmus. When the Heart lacks nourishment and becomes deficient, fever, restlessness and pain will occur. Jumping movements in the region of the navel is the movement of the Kidney Vital Energy.

CLAUSE 11-11

Pulse of a Dead Heart is excessive when pressed lightly, resembling the feeling of beans. When pressed deeply, the pulse becomes restless and swift. Such pulse suggests a fatal case.

CLAUSE 11-12

The patient cries out in restlessness as if he were haunted. This is due to a Deficiency of the Blood and the Vital Energy, and is classed as a Heart disease. When the Vital Energy in the Heart is deficient, the patient senses fright, closes his eyes and tends to sleep. He will have dreams of a long journey and experiences spiritual irritability and depression. Evanescence of the Yin Vital Essence will lead to a case of insanity with emotional depression. Evanescence of the Yang Vital Energy will result in mania. (1)

NOTES

1. According to Wu Qian, the last sentence reads, "Evanescence of the Yin Vital Essence will lead to a case of mania (*kuang*, agitated madness disorder). Evanescence of the Yang Vital Energy will result in insanity with emotional depression (*dian*, retarded madness disorder)." This must be a copying mistake. As the *Canon of Medicine* says, "When Yin is excessive, insanity with emotional depression results (Yin is excessive, resulting in evanescence of Yang). When Yang is excessive, mania occurs (Yang is excessive, resulting in evanescence of Yin)." (05-544)

CLAUSE 11-13

When the Spleen is affected by pathogenetic Wind, the patient will have a fever and behave as if he were drunk. (1) He feels discomfort and heaviness in the abdomen, and his skin and eyes (2) are jumping. He also experiences shortness of breath.

NOTES

1. Li Wen: Behave as if he were drunk: This means the patient's face is red and he experiences weakness in the extremities. (05-545)
2. Skin and eyes: According to *Qianjin*, this is "skin and muscle." According to Li Wen, it reads "eyelids."

CLAUSE 11-14

Pulse of a Dead Spleen is huge and strong when pressed lightly. When pressed deeply, it feels like an inverted empty cup, with swirling and restless pulsation. This indicates a fatal case.

CLAUSE 11-15*

Fuyang pulse (1) is floating and hesitant. Floating pulse indicates strong Stomach Vital Energy, whereas hesitant pulse indicates frequent urination. Conflict of floating and hesitant pulses (2) causes constipation and Spleen Restriction (3). Pills of Fructus Cannabis will provide a cure.

NOTES

1. *Fuyang* pulse: *Fuyang* pulse is located at the malleolus near the tarsal bones (arteria dorsalis pedis).

2. Conflict of floating and hesitant pulses: When syndromes of floating and hesitant pulses appear at the same time. Floating pulse indicates a strong Stomach Vital Energy and hesitant pulse indicates Deficiency of the Spleen Vital Energy, which fails to transmit Vital Essence to the Stomach in a normal way. Body Fluid only flows downward, bringing on frequent urination. When Stomach Vital Energy is too strong, the Spleen ceases to secrete Body Fluid, resulting in constipation. (01-114)

3. Spleen Restriction (*Pi Yue*): When Stomach Vital Energy is strong and that of the Spleen is weak, the function of the Spleen is restricted by the Stomach. As the Spleen dominates Humidity and is conducive to Humidity factors, when the Stomach's excessive Heat exhausts the Body Fluid, the Spleen's function of secreting Body Fluid is restricted by the Stomach, resulting in constipation. (See Clause 179 of *Shanghan Lun*.)

*This clause also appears in *Shanghan Lun* (Clause 247).

Pills of Fructus Cannabis
(*Maziren Wan*)

Fructus Cannabis	2 *sheng*
Radix Paeoniae	0.5 *jin*
Fructus Aurantii Immaturus	1 *jin*
Radix et Rhizoma Rhei	1 *jin*
Cortex Magnoliae Officinalis	1 *jin*
Semen Armeniacae Amarum	1 *sheng*

Pound the drugs into powder, and form pills the size of Chinese parasol seeds with honey. Take ten pills three times a day. Gradually increase dosage until normal defecation is observed.

Explanation of the Prescription: This prescription serves as a laxative with mild action. It is effective in treating habitual constipation and suitable to old and weak patients. (02-93)

Xu Bin: The recipe is made up in pill form rather than as a decoction. This is to obtain results through mild action, and avoid damage to the Body Resistance. When Spleen Restriction occurs, it can be inferred that Body Resistance is already weak and the Body Fluid exhausted. Thus no drastic cures or purgatives should be adopted. (05-546)

CLAUSE 11-16

Kidney-affection syndrome with the following symptoms and signs can be treated with Decoction of Radix Glycyrrhizae, Rhizoma Zingiberis, Poria and Rhizoma Atractylodis Macrocephalae: Heaviness in movement, and cold in the lumbar region as if the patient were sitting in water. Syndrome is similar to that caused by pathogenetic Water (1), but the patient is not thirsty. Other symptoms may include normal urination and intake of food, which indicates that the trouble is at the Lower Portion of Body Cavity. Pathology of the syndrome is as follows: when the patient performs work, he perspires which makes his clothes wet and cold. If this condition persists for a long period of time, the patient will be affected by the syndrome with cold, by a painful sensation in the region below the waist, and by a feeling of heaviness in the abdomen as if he were carrying a thousand coins around his waist. (2)

NOTES

1. Wu Qian: Syndromes caused by pathogenetic Water may refer to edema. But since the patient has normal urination, this is not a case of Water-retention but rather a syndrome caused by Humidity. (05-547)

2. In this syndrome the Kidney is affected by pathogenetic Cold and Humidity. Since the Kidney is located in the lumbar region, the syndrome is called Kidney-affection. The syndrome generally arises along with perspiration due to physical labor. When the lumbar region is affected by Cold and Humidity, the Yang Vital Energy cannot circulate normally, which causes cold, pain, and a sensation of heaviness in that region. Although the pathological condition is located in the Lower Portion of Body Cavity, the Viscera and Bowels are not yet affected, and the patient has no great thirst, has normal urination and normal

intake of food. The proper therapy is to warm the Cold and Humidity factors resting in the Channel, there is no need to warm the Kidney. (02-93)

Decoction of Radix Glycyrrhizae, Rhizoma Zingiberis, Poria and Rhizoma Atractylodis Macrocephalae
(*Gan Jiang Ling Zhu Tang*)

Radix Glycyrrhizae	2 *liang*
Rhizoma Atractylodis Macrocephalae	2 *liang*
Rhizoma Zingiberis	4 *liang*
Poria	4 *liang*

Stew the drugs in five *sheng* of water until three *sheng* remain. Serve the lukewarm decoction in three doses. This will cause the waist to warm up.

Explanation of the Prescription: As this is a case caused by pathogenetic Cold and Humidity in the lumbar region but not in the Kidney itself, drugs are used to disperse the Cold and Humidity. Rhizoma Zingiberis warms the Interior and disperses Cold. Poria, Rhizoma Atractylodis Macrocephalae and Radix Glycyrrhizae (it should be Radix Glycyrrhizae Praeparata) tonify the Spleen Vital Energy and eliminate the Humidity. New developments in the administration of the prescription have widened the efficacy of the decoction. Chronic gastroenteritis, intestinal disturbances, edema in the lower extremities due to pregnancy, incontinence of urination in the aged, enuresis, and chronic case of cold in lumbar region with morbid leukorrhea in women, can all be treated with the decoction. (02-93)

CASES

Case 1 (02-94): Case Recorded in Journal of *Guangdong Chinese Medicine*, 7:31, 1962

Du, 50, female, first treatment on October 20, 1958. The patient suffered from lumbago and a feeling of heaviness and numbness in lumbar region. Pain and contraction of hip muscles made it difficult for her to walk and move her body. General lassitude had lasted about five months. Pulse was deep-slow. This was a Kidney-affection syndrome, caused by pathogenetic Cold and Humidity to the lumbar region when the Kidney was in deficient condition. Decoction of Radix Glycyrrhizae, Rhizoma Zingiberis, Poria and Rhizoma Atractylodis

Macrocephalae was recommended to cure the syndrome:

Rhizoma Atractylodis Macrocephalae	30 grams
Poria	30 grams
Rhizoma Zingiberis	30 grams
Radix Glycyrrhizae Praeparata	15 grams

Two doses were served. The patient made three visits to doctor, each time were given eight doses of the docoction. In later treatments, Ramulus Cinnamomi and Cortex Eucommiae were added to strengthen the efficacy.

Case 2 (46-193):

Mr. Feng, 54, suffered from lumbar pain and cold feeling. He felt as if he were sitting in cold water. Appetite was poor, stool loose and watery. Tongue coating was white-slippery and pulse was soft-moderate. It was a syndrome caused by invasion of pathogenic Cold and Humidity in the lumbar muscles. As lumbar region houses the Kidney, thus Kidney-affection, it should be treated with Decoction of Radix Glycyrrhizae, Rhizoma Zingiberis, Poria and Rhizoma Atractylodis Macrocephalae:

Rhizoma Zingiberis	6 grams
Radix Glycyrrhizae	3 grams
Poria	10 grams
Rhizoma Atractylodis Macrocephalae	12 grams

Second treatment: Five doses of the decoction were given, which were effective, with moxibustion and physiotherapy. Another five doses of decoction adding twelve grams of Radix Codonopsis Pilosulae were served, which successfully cured the lumbago.

Case 3 (56-105):

Mr. Zhang, 42-year-old driver, first treatment on April 20, 1978. The patient suffered from chronic diarrhea more than ten years. Test report showed no bloody, or pus, in the stool or other irregularity.

Examination: The patient sensed a cold feeling in the lumbar region. Pulse was deep-slippery and strengthless. Tongue coating was thin-white. Decoction of Radix Glycyrrhizae, Rhizoma Zingiberis, Poria and Rhizoma Atractylodis Macrocephalae with additions was prescribed:

Poria	12 grams
Radix Glycyrrhizae Praeparata	6 grams
Rhizoma Atractylodis Macrocephalae	6 grams
Rhizoma Zingiberis	12 grams

Polyporus Umbellatus	9 grams
Rhizoma Alismatis	9 grams

Second treatment: Three doses of the decoction were served. Stool was less frequent with discharge in recognizable shape, feeling of warmth in the lumbar region. Another three doses of the decoction were given.

Third treatment: Stool was once a day, with shaped feces. Decoction of *Lizhong* was prescribed:

Radix Codonopsis Pilosulae	9 grams
Rhizoma Atractylodis Macrocephalae	9 grams
Rhizoma Zingiberis	9 grams
Radix Glycyrrhizae	9 grams

Fourth treatment: After taking Decoction of *Lizhong*, stool became more frequent and loose again. The original prescription was given. Three doses were served.

Fifth treatment: Three doses of the decoction was effective. More doses were given. The patient was instructed to stop medication for several months. No recurrence reported.

Analysis: Doctor Quan Yijing (author of the book No. 56): Cold feeling in lumbar region showed obvious invasion of pathogenetic Cold and Humidity. Kidney is a Viscus that controls Water circulation and mechanism of urination and stool. When Kidney was affected by prevalence of Cold and Humidity, it failed to function properly, loose stool resulted. In general practice, diarrhea was treated by adjusting the pathological condition of the Middle Portion of Body Cavity. (Decoction of *Lizhong* was the drug treating ailment in the Middle Portion, the Stomach and Spleen systems). Therefore, it did not work (as stated in the third treatment). So Decoction of Radix Glycyrrhizae, Rhizoma Zingiberis, Poria and Rhizoma Atractylodis Macrocephalae was used. Polyporus Umbellatus and Rhizoma Alismatis were added to strengthen its function of facilitating fluid circulation. When excessive Water expelled in urination, stool returned to normal.

CLAUSE 11-17

Pulse of a Dead Kidney is mighty and hard when pressed lightly. When pressed deeply, it feels like a swirling ball with an irregular movement. If this pulsation is more apparent in the Cubit (under the ring-finger), the case will be fatal.

CLAUSE 11-18

Question: Deficiency and exhaustion of the Three Portions of Body Cavity (1): When the Upper Portion of Body Cavity is deficient and exhausted, the patient will belch frequently. Why is this?

Master: The Upper Portion is nourished by the Middle Portion. When the Stomach (located in the Middle Portion) Vital Energy is out of harmony, cereal cannot be digested. Indigestion causes the belching. When the Lower Portion is deficient and exhausted, enuresis and fecal incontinence will occur due to a disorder of the Vital Energy, which can no longer control stool and urination. No therapy needs to be adopted. The disorder will subside after a period of time (2).

NOTES

1. Deficiency and exhaustion of the Three Portions of Body Cavity refers to the exhaustion of the functional activities of the Vital Energy. (01-117)

2. No therapy for the syndrome of the Lower Portion is necessary. After a length of time, when the functioning of the Vital Energy at the Upper Portion becomes normal again, the syndrome will be cured. (01-116)

CLAUSE 11-19

Master: When the Upper Portion of Body Cavity is affected by pathogenetic Heat, coughing (1) will develop into a syndrome of pulmonary asthenia. When the Heat rests in the Middle Portion, constipation results. When the Heat invades the Lower Portion, hematuria, urinary disturbance and constipation result. Pathogenetic Cold in the large intestine makes the stool watery, whereas Heat in the large intestine will bring stool with thick mucus. Pathogenetic Cold in the small intestine leads to tenesmus and bloody stool. Heat will cause hemorrhoids.

NOTES

1. "Coughing" here means coughing that has lasted for a relatively long time. (01-117)

CLAUSE 11-20

Question: What are the syndromes of Accumulation, Assemblage and *Guqi*?

Master: Accumulation (1) is a disease of the Viscera, which does not change its location. Assemblage (2) is a disease of the Bowels with sporadic attacks and changes of location. It is a curable disease. *Guqi* (3) is a pain which occurs in the costal regions. When pressed, it subsides but resumes later. Diagnosis of the Accumulation syndrome: The pulse is slender and appears as deep as if it were near a bone. If such pulse appears at the Inch, the Accumulation is in the chest; if the pulse is a bit above the Inch (nearer to the palm), the Accumulation is in the throat; pulse at the Bar indicates Accumulation near the navel; pulse above the Bar (between Bar and Inch) indicates Accumulation in the epigastrium; pulse located beneath the Bar (between Bar and Cubit) indicates Accumulation in the abdomen; pulse located in the Cubit indicates Accumulation at Qichong (ST 30) (4). When the pulse is sensed on the left wrist, the pathological condition is located on the right side and vice versa. If the pulse appears on both wrists, the Accumulation is located in the middle. Treat the syndrome according to its location.

NOTES

1. Accumulation (*Ji*): Tumor located in the Viscera with pain at a definite location generally caused by the accumulation of Yin Vital Essence (the Blood). (02-94)

2. Assemblage (*Ju*): Tumor located in the Bowels with sporadic attacks of pain at indefinite locations, caused by stagnation of the Vital Energy. (02-94)

3. *Guqi* is caused by indigestion. When the Cereal Vital Energy stagnates in the Spleen and the Stomach, the Liver is also affected, causing pains in the costal regions. (02-94)

4. An acupoint near the pubic hair. Accumulation at Qichong (ST 30) generally signifies abdominal pain caused by Cold. (01-118)

Remark: Chapter XI is incomplete with omissions and copying errors. Lin Yi wrote, "Since we are far from ancient times, these omissions and errors cannot be rectified."

CHAPTER XII

ON PULSE, SYMPTOM COMLEX AND TREATMENT OF *TANYIN* AND COUGHING

CLAUSE 12-1

Question: The Fluid-retention syndrome (1) can be divided into four categories. What are they?

Master: *Tanyin* Fluid-retention, *Xuanyin* Fluid-retention, *Yiyin* Fluid-retention, and *Zhiyin* Fluid-retention.

Question: How do they differ?

Master: A patient with a plump build loses weight and a splashing sound can be heard in his intestines. This is a *Tanyin* Fluid-retention syndrome.

After drinking water, the fluid flows and collects in the patient 's costal regions. A dragging pain occurs when the patient coughs or spits. This is *Xuanyin* Fluid-retention.

After drinking water, the fluid flows and collects in the extremities. The patient cannot sweat when he should, and feels pain and heaviness in his body. This is *Yiyin* Fluid-retention.

Zhiyin Fluid-retention syndrome may include symptoms and signs of coughing with adverse ascending gas and labored respiration, and shortness of breath that prevents the patient from lying quietly in bed.

NOTES

1. This chapter discusses symptoms, signs and treatment of *Tanyin* Fluid-retention and coughing. Coughing discussed here only refers to that caused by *Tanyin* Fluid-retention syndromes, not by other pathological conditions.

Tanyin Fluid-retention is a generalized term inclusive of four Fluid-retention syndromes of *Tanyin*, *Xuanyin*, *Yiyin* and *Zhiyin*. Thus *Tanyin* is both a general and a particular syndrome. The term has its broad and narrow senses. In addition, there are also Remaining Fluid-retention and Hidden Fluid-retention (*Liuyin* and *Fuyin*) syndromes. These terms are not independent of the four Fluid-retention syndromes above. They only indicate the seriousness and endurance of the above Fluid-retention syndromes. (02-97)

CLAUSE 12-2

When the pathogenetic Water collects in the Heart (1), a hard mass and jumping will appear in the epigastrium with shortness of breath. The patient will also feel disgust at the sight of water or when drinking water.

NOTES

1. The Heart here refers to the gastric region. (01-120)

CLAUSE 12-3

When the Water collects in the Lung, copious salivation and thirst will result.

CLAUSE 12-4

When the Water collects in the Spleen, shortness of breath and heaviness of movement will result.

CLAUSE 12-5

When the Water collects in the Liver, the patient will sense distention and fullness in the costal regions and a pain in the same area when sneezing.

CLAUSE 12-6

When the Water collects in the Kidney, palpitation beneath the Heart (1) will result.

NOTES

1. Palpitation beneath the Heart means a jumping movement in the epigastrium due to the adverse ascending of pathogenetic Water in the Kidney to the Heart (*Jinkui E*). According to Wu Qian, "beneath the Heart" should read "beneath the navel" (*Jinjian*).

Commentary: Clauses 12-2 to 12-6 refer to five different symptoms of Fluid-retention (or Water-retention) in the Five Viscera. The Five Viscera here are not the internal organs as known to modern anatomy. They should be understood as five different pathological reactions to different Fluid-retention syndromes. (01-120)

CLAUSE 12-7

When Remaining Fluid-retention occurs in the epigastrium the patient will feel cold in his back in an area the size of the palm. (1)

NOTES

1. This is a *Tanyin* Fluid-retention syndrome which has continued for a long period of time. (01-121)

CLAUSE 12-8

When the *Tanyin* Fluid-retention has continued for a long period of time, the patient will feel pain in the costal regions with dragging pains leading to the supraclavicular fossa. When the patient coughs, the pain will be aggravated.

CLAUSE 12-9

When the *Tanyin* Fluid-retention occurs in the chest, the patient feels a shortness of breath and thirst, and suffers arthralgia in all the joints of the body. A deep pulse is diagnosed. This is the Remaining Fluid-retention syndrome.

CLAUSE 12-10

When *Tanyin* Fluid-retention occurs in the cavity above the diaphragm, the following symptoms and signs will be observed: a sensation of fullness, wheezing, coughing and vomiting. With the onset of the syndrome, there will be fever and chill, pains in the back and lumbar region, fierce shaking of the body, and spontaneous tears. This is the Hidden Fluid-retention syndrome.

Commentary: This clause discusses the Hidden Fluid-retention syndrome. When *Tanyin* occurs in different places, different syndromes are caused. By referring to Clause 12-1, it can be understood that the Remaining Fluid-retention beneath the Heart (Clause 12-7) is actually a *Tanyin* Fluid-retention (in the narrow sense). Remaining Fluid-retention in the costal regions (Clause 12-8) is *Xuanyin* Fluid-retention. Hidden Fluid-retention above the diaphragm (Clause 12-10) and Remaining Fluid-retention in the chest (Clause 12-9) are actually *Zhiyin* Fluid-retention. (02-98)

CLAUSE 12-11

If the patient drinks too much water he will suffer a sudden attack of wheezing with sensation of fullness. When the patient eats little but drinks copiously the Water will collect in the epigastrium. An acute case will bring about palpitations, while a mild one will cause shortness of breath. (1)

Tight pulse in both wrists indicates a syndrome of a Cold nature, which is a deficient state caused by the administration of drastics. If tight pulse appears only in one wrist, it indicates a *Tanyin* Fluid-retention syndrome. (2)

NOTES

1. When the Spleen ceases its normal function of transmission, Body Fluid is not deployed evenly, and Water then stagnates in the Interior as *Tanyin* Fluid-retention. Pathological changes of the Lung and the Kidney may also cause *Tanyin* Fluid-retention syndromes. (01-99)

2. Wu Qian: When tight pulse appears only in one wrist, this is *Tanyin* Fluid-retention. A purgative may be adopted, but it should not be too powerful in its function. Otherwise, the patient will become so deficient and weak that the pulse in both wrists will become tight. Tight pulse is of a Yin nature, which is why a tight pulse in both wrists (a manifestation of overall pathological conditions) indicates a case of a Cold nature. This clause also teaches practitioners that not all tight pulses indicate Fluid-retention syndromes. (05-571)

CLAUSE 12-12

Fluid-retention in the Lung will not cause a tight pulse, but bring about panting and shortness of breath.

CLAUSE 12-13

Zhiyin Fluid-retention syndrome will make it difficult for the patient to lie in bed due to panting and severe shortness of breath. The pulse is even (quiet and moderate).

CLAUSE 12-14

Tanyin Fluid-retention syndromes (1) can be cured by warm drugs. (2)

NOTES

1. Zhao Yide: *Tanyin* Fluid-retention syndrome is caused by accumulation of pathogenetic Water. When Cold prevails, accumulation takes place. When Heat prevails, accumulation is dispersed. Circulation of Water largely depends on the movement of the Vital Energy. Warm drugs can stimulate Yang Vital Energy, open up the *Couli* and dredge through the channel to allow the Water to flow.

— *Synopsis of the Golden Chamber annotated by Zhao Yide*

2. *Jinkui E*: Warm drugs mentioned here are mainly those that can promote the functioning of the Yang Vital Energy to disperse the Humidity. Decoction of Lesser Rhizoma Pinelliae (Clause 12-26) and Decoction of Poria, Ramulus Cinnamomi, Rhizoma Atractylodis Macrocephalae and Radix Glycyrrhizae (Clause 12-15) are such prescriptions.

CLAUSE 12-15

Tanyin Fluid-retention in the epigastrium with distention and fullness in the chest and costal regions and vertigo can be treated with Decoction of Poria, Ramulus Cinnamomi, Rhizoma Atractylodis Macrocephalae and Radix Glycyrrhizae.

Decoction of Poria, Ramulus Cinnamomi, Rhizoma Atractylodis Macrocephalae and Radix Glycyrrhizae*
(*Ling Gui Zhu Gan Tang*)

Poria	4 *liang*
Ramulus Cinnamomi	3 *liang*
Rhizoma Atractylodis Macrocephalae	3 *liang*
Radix Glycyrrhizae	2 *liang*

Stew the drugs in six *sheng* of water until three *sheng* remain. Serve the lukewarm decoction in three doses. Urination will be normal.

*This prescription also appears in *Shanghan Lun*, Clause 74.

Explanation of the Prescription: This clause discusses the symptoms and treatment of *Tanyin* Fluid-retention (in the narrow sense). The Stomach is located in the epigastrium. When Water collects in the Stomach, distention and fullness in the chest and costal regions occur. When the Fluid-retention obstructs the passage of the Yang Vital Energy on its way to the Upper Portion, vertigo results. Decoction of Poria, Ramulus Cinnamomi, Rhizoma Atractylodis Macrocephalae and Radix Glycyrrhizae warms the Yang, disperses the Fluid-retention, tonifies the Spleen and eases Water circulation. Poria and Ramulus Cinnamomi, when given together, warm the Yang and eliminate the Water. Rhizoma Atractylodis Macrocephalae tonifies the Spleen and dries up the Humidity. Radix Glycyrrhizae harmonizes the Interior and tonifies the Vital Energy. (02-100)

CLAUSE 12-16

Treatment of shortness of breath caused by minor case of Fluid-retention syndrome should follow the principle of removing pathogenetic factors from urine. Decoction of Poria, Ramulus Cinnamomi, Rhizoma Atractylodis Macrocephalae and Radix Glycyrrhizae (prescription see Clause 12-15) can be adopted. Pills of Eight-Ingredients of the Kidney Vital Energy can also be adopted. (1) (See Appendix to Chapter V: Pills of Eight-Ingredients.)

NOTES

1. A slight case of Fluid-retention with shortness of breath but no other Exterior symptoms is nevertheless a mild case, though early treatment should be adopted. Although case is mild, it may become aggravated due to obstruction of Fluid-retention that hampers normal functioning of the Yang Vital Energy. Root cause of the syndrome is a disorder of either the Spleen or the Kidney.

If case is caused by debility of the Spleen Vital Energy, other symptoms such as a sensation of fullness and adverse ascending in the epigastrium, as well as vertigo experienced when the patient stands up can be observed. The case can be treated with Decoction of Poria, Remulus Cinnamomi, Rhizoma Atractylodis Macrocephalae and Radix Glycyrrhizae.

If syndrome is caused by Deficiency of the Kidney Yang Vital Energy, other symptoms and signs may include aversion to cold, cold in lower extremities, and pain and numbness in the abdomen. Pills of Eight-Ingredients of the Kidney Vital Energy can be adopted to warm the Kidney and disperse the Fluid-retention. (02-100)

CLAUSE 12-17

Pulse is hidden. The patient feels the urge to defecate. After the stool, he gains some relief. This indicates the dispersion of Fluid-retention. If after the stool, the patient still feels a sense of fullness and distention in the epigastrium, Decoction of Radix Euphorbiae Kansui and Rhizoma Pinelliae can be adopted.

Decoction of Radix Euphorbiae Kansui and Rhizoma Pinelliae
(*Gansui Banxia Tang*)

Radix Euphorbiae Kansui	3 big pcs.
Rhizoma Pinelliae (stew in one *sheng* of water until one half *sheng* remains, filter the decoction)	12 pcs.
Radix Paeoniae	5 pcs.
Radix Glycyrrhizae Praeparata	1 thumb-size pc.

Stew the drugs in two *sheng* of water until one half *sheng* remains. Filter the decoction and blend with one half *sheng* of honey. Stew again until eight *ge* remain. Serve the decoction at one draft.

Explanation of the Prescription: This prescription disperses Fluid-retention in the epigastrium. Radix Euphorbiae Kansui is a strong Water-expellent. Honey, Radix Glycyrrhizae and Radix Paeoniae are adopted to slow down the powerful effect of the drug. It is said that Radix Euphorbiae Kansui and Radix Glycyrrhizae are incompatible. But in this prescription, efficacy of the two drugs is actually enhanced by each other. (01-124)

CASES

Case 1 (64-422): Case Recorded in Journal of *Jiangxi Chinese Medicine*, 3:45, 1982

Jiang, 32, female, first treatment in May 1969. The patient's abdomen was enlarging, resembling that of 8-month pregnancy. When palpitated, it was soft. The patient felt distended, had general fatigue and lassitude with a tendency to sleep. Anorexia and loose stool also reported. There had been no menses for three months but profuse leukorrhea with clear and smelly discharge. Urination was sufficient. Tongue was pale, covered with white, greasy coating. Pulse was deep-slippery.

Diagnosis: Syndrome caused by Spleen too deficient to circulate the Fluid, causing Fluid-retention. Decoction of Euphorbiae Kansui and Rhizoma Pinelliae was given:

Euphorbiae Kansui	9 grams
Rhizoma Pinelliae	9 grams
Radix Glycyrrhizae Praeparata	9 grams
Radix Paeoniae Alba	9 grams
Rhizoma Atractylodis Macrocephalae	12 grams
Poria	18 grams

Second treatment: Three doses of the decoction were served, which reduced symptoms. Watery stool was still aggravated. Three more doses of the same decoction were given.

Third treatment: Abdominal distention reduced by two-thirds. Stool was still greasy. Pulse was deep-slippery. The same decoction was given for another three doses.

Two years later the patient gave birth to a baby, she reported that nine doses cured the ailment, leukorrhea subsided and menstruation resumed.

Case 2 (02-101): Case Recorded in Journal of *Bare-foot Doctor*, Compiled in Changwei, Shandong, 1:48, 1978

Mr. Li, 29, began to cough in early winter 1976.

First treatment on February 3, 1977. Cough was aggravated. Asthma occurred, with spitting of phlegm when coughing. There was pain in the right flank, chill and fever. Pulse was deep-excessive.

Diagnosis: Cough caused by accumulation of phlegm and stagnation of Vital Energy. Ordinary expectorant could not disperse the syndrome. Decoction of Euphorbiae Kansui and Rhizoma Pinelliae was the cure:

Euphorbiae Kansui (powdered, blend into the already-stewed decoction before service)	6 grams
Rhizoma Pinelliae	15 grams

Radix Paeoniae Alba	15 grams
Radix Glycyrrhizae	9 grams

Second treatment on February 5. All symptoms were subsiding after one dose of the decoction was served. Another dose of the same decoction was given.

Third treatment on February 7. The patient needed no more drugs.

Case 3 (52-745): Case Recorded in *Supplement to Classified Case Studies of Famous Doctors*

Mr. Wang, merchant, was stout and suffered from Fluid-retention. When he had a loose stool, he felt better. Fullness and distention were sensed in epigastrium. Pulse was deep. Complexion around nose was bright. This was Fluid-retention syndrome. Decoction of Euphorbiae Kansui and Rhizoma Pinelliae served together with honey worked effectively.

CLAUSE 12-18

Floating and slender-slippery pulse indicates the onset of a Fluid-retention syndrome. (1)

NOTES

1. Li Wen: The pulse corresponding to Fluid-retention syndrome is a deep pulse. But in this clause, floating pulse is given. This indicates that the Fluid-retention is in the Lung. (05-562)

CLAUSE 12-19

The pulse corresponding to Fluid-retention of a Cold nature is tight-speedy. Such a case will be difficult to treat in summer or winter. (1)

NOTES

1. This clause describes a syndrome with contradictory symptoms in the pulse. When the weather is cold in winter, hot drugs should be adopted, but this will speed up the pulse. In summer, drugs with cold or cool qualities should be prescribed. This is contradictory to Fluid-retention of a Cold nature. Thus the text describes it as a case difficult to treat in summer and winter. (01-124)

CLAUSE 12-20

Deep-tight pulse (1) indicates a case of *Xuanyin* Fluid-retention with pains (in the chest and costal regions). Decoction of Ten Pieces of Fructus Ziziphi Jujubae will provide a cure (2).

NOTES

1. Deep pulse indicates that the syndrome is located in the Interior. Tight pulse generally signifies Fluid-retention and presence of pain. *Xuanyin* Fluid-retention is located in the chest and costal regions. Thus the pulse is deep-tight. (02-99)

2. Wu Qian: Decoction of Ten Pieces of Fructus Ziziphi Jujubae is applicable to those with a strong constitution. For patients with weak constitution, administer medicine with care. (05-566)

Decoction of Ten Pieces of Fructus Ziziphi Jujubae*
(*Shi Zao Tang*):

Flos Genkwa (stewed)
Radix Euphorbiae Kansui
Radix Euphorbiae Pekinensis

Pound the drugs in equal doses into powder. Stew ten large dates (Fructus Ziziphi Jujubae) in one and a half *sheng* of water until eight *ge* remain. Filter the decoction and add one and a half *qianbi* of the powder for a strong patient and one half *qianbi* for a weak patient. Serve the lukewarm decoction during the day. If there is no stool, increase dose by one half of a *qianbi* on the next day. Once a loose stool is observed, serve the patient porridge to complete recovery.

*This prescription also appears in *Shanghan Lun* (Clause 152).

Explanation of the Prescription: Li Wen: The three drugs in this prescription are all bitter in taste, and serve to purge the Fluid-retention. But they function with great strength. Ten pieces of Fructus Ziziphi Jujubae are added to the decoction to protect the Body Resistance and slow down the drug's action. Fructus Ziziphi Jujubae tonifies the Spleen, so that when the Earth (the Spleen) is enhanced, Water will be easier to control. (05-567)

CLAUSE 12-21

Diaphoresis should be practiced for *Yiyin* Fluid-retention syndromes. Decoction of Greater *Qinglong* will provide a cure. Decoction of Lesser *Qinglong* can also be adopted. (1)

NOTES

1. This clause discusses the symptoms and treatment of *Yiyin* Fluid-retention syndromes. In this syndrome, Fluid-retention occurs in the muscle and the Exterior due to the etiology of a patient being unable to perspire when perspiration is physiologically necessary. Fluid collects in the muscle and the Exterior, causing pains and heaviness throughout the body. Since the Fluid-retention occurs at the Exterior, diaphoresis is adopted to disperse the pathological condition from the Exterior. There are two types:

a) *Yiyin* Fluid-retention with condensed Heat. Symptoms and signs include floating-tense pulse, fever with aversion to cold, bodily pain, wheezing without perspiration, and restlessness. Treat with Decoction of Greater *Qinglong*.

b) *Yiyin* Fluid-retention with Exterior Cold. Symptoms and signs include fever with aversion to cold, Vital-energy Stagnation in the chest, nausea, coughing and wheezing. Treat with Decoction of Lesser *Qinglong*. (02-107)

Decoction of Greater *Qinglong** (*Da Qinglong Tang*):

Herba Ephedrae	6 *liang*
Ramulus Cinnamomi	2 *liang*
Radix Glycyrrhizae Praeparata	2 *liang*
Semen Armeniacae Amarum	40 pcs.
Rhizoma Zingiberis Recens	3 *liang*
Fructus Ziziphi Jujubae	12 pcs.
Gypsum Fibrosum	1 pc.**

Stew Herba Ephedrae in nine *sheng* of water until seven *sheng* remain. Skim off the foam and add the remaining drugs. Stew the decoction again until three *sheng* remain. Filter the decoction and serve one *sheng* lukewarm decoction per dose to induce a light perspiration. If there is a profuse perspiration, the sweat can be absorbed with *Wenfen* Powder.*** (01-126)

*The prescription also appears in Clause 38 of *Shanghan Lun*.

**The size of an egg, crushed into small pieces.

***According to *Qianjin*, *Wenfen* powder is a mixture of powdered Os Draconis Ustem, Concha Ostreae Usta, Radix Astragali, and Semen Oryzae Nonglutinosae.

Explanation of the Prescription: This prescription is applicable to Fluid-retention syndromes with condensed Heat and moderate Fluid-retention. (01-126)

Decoction of Lesser *Qinglong**
(*Xiao Qinglong Tang*):

Herba Ephedrae	3 *liang*
Radix Paeoniae	3 *liang*
Fructus Schisandrae	0.5 *sheng*
Rhizoma Zingiberis	3 *liang*
Radix Glycyrrhizae Praeparata	3 *liang*
Herba Asari	3 *liang*
Ramulus Cinnamomi	3 *liang*
Rhizoma Pinelliae	0.5 *sheng*

Stew Herba Ephedrae in one *dou* of water until eight *sheng* remain. Skim off the foam and add remaining drugs. Stew until three *sheng* remain. Filter the decoction and serve one *sheng* lukewarm decoction per dose.

*This prescription also appears in Clause 40 of *Shanghan Lun*.

Explanation of the Prescription: This prescription is applicable to Fluid-retention syndromes with serious Fluid-retention and coughing. (01-126)

CLAUSE 12-22

Zhiyin Fluid-retention in the diaphragm region is accompanied by the following symptoms and signs: Wheezing, sensation of fullness, Vital-energy Stagnation and formation of a hard mass in the epigastrium, dark complexion, and deep-tense pulse. The syndrome lasts many weeks. Emetics and purgatives have been prescribed, but there is no improvement. Decoction of Radix Stephaniae Tetrandrae can then be adopted. If the syndrome is of a deficient nature, the decoction will bring a recovery. If it is a case of an excessive nature, a recurrence will occur within three days. If further doses of Decoction of Radix Stephaniae Tetrandrae are ineffective, Decoction of Radix Stephaniae Tetrandrae subtracting Gypsum Fibrosum adding Poria and Natrii Sulfas can be prescribed.

Decoction of Radix Stephaniae Tetrandrae
(*Mufangji Tang*):

Radix Stephaniae Tetrandrae	3 *liang*
Gypsum Fibrosum	12 egg-sized pcs.*
Ramulus Cinnamomi	2 *liang*
Radix Ginseng	4 *liang*

Stew the drugs in six *sheng* of water until two *sheng* remain. Serve the decoction in two doses.

*According to *Waitai*, the dosage should be three egg-sized pieces.

Explanation of the Prescription: This prescription simultaneously tonifies the Body Resistance and eliminates the pathogenetic factors. Radix Stephaniae Tetrandrae disperses the Fluid-retention. Gypsum Fibrosum clears away the Heat in the Lung. Ramulus Cinnamomi facilitates the normal flow of the Yang Vital Energy and disperses the Water. Radix Ginseng warms the Interior and tonifies the Vital Energy. Once the Body Resistance regains its normal functioning, Fluid-retention will disperse spontaneously. (01-127)

Decoction of Radix Stephaniae Tetrandrae subtracting
Gypsum Fibrosum adding Poria and Natrii Sulfas
(*Mufangji Qu Shigao Jia Fuling Mangxiao Tang*):

Radix Stephaniae Tetrandrae	2 *liang*
Ramulus Cinnamomi	2 *liang*

Radix Ginseng	4 *liang*
Poria	4 *liang*
Natrii Sulfas	3 *ge*

Stew first four drugs in six *sheng* of water until two *sheng* remain. Add Natrii Sulfas and stew again for a short while. Serve the decoction in two doses. When mild diarrhea appears, the syndrome disappears.

Explanation of the Prescription: If after taking Decoction of Radix Stephaniae Tetrandrae, the Vital-energy Stagnation and hard mass disappears, this is evidence of the dispersion of Fluid-retention and the resumption of the normal flow of the Vital Energy. If the Vital-energy Stagnation and hard mass remain as before, this shows syndrome is still present, and that the syndrome is a complicated case. Thus adoption of the original prescription will have no effect. Gypsum Fibrosum, not effective in treating Fluid-retention, is subtracted, and Poria is used to lead the Water downward. Natrii Sulfas softens the hard mass and disperses the retention. Thus it is more effective in treating the syndrome. (02-104)

CASES

Case 1 (52-448): Case Recorded in *Memoirs of Clinical Experience of Dr. Zhao Shouzhen*

Old Liu, in his seventies, plump and stout build, was addicted to alcohol. He was happy until his elder son died and the family situation changed. He had distended feeling in chest and began to cough. Every morning he spit several mouthful of greasy phlegm, which gave him relief. He still drank heavily to forget his sorrow. One evening, after drinking he vomited profusely, with pain and stagnation feeling in chest and epigastrium, and copious salivation.

Examination: Complexion was dark-black. He was panting with irritation. The patient was losing weight, with anorexia and depression. Pulse was deep-tight and strengthless. Restlessness, parched feeling in mouth and insomnia were reported.

Diagnosis: Excessive drinking of wine resulted in accumulation of Humidity, which evolved into Heat.

First treatment: Decoction of Radix Stephaniae Tetrandrae was given as the cure. Poria was added to strengthen the Water-expellent function.

Prescription:

Radix Stephaniae Tetrandrae	12 grams
Radix Codonopsis Pilosulae	12 grams
Gypsum Fibrosum	18 grams
Ramulus Cinnamomi	6 grams
Poria	15 grams

Second treatment: Three doses were served, worked effectively. The patient had no appetite. The next prescription with alterations was made:

Subtract: Gypsum Fibrosum.

Add: Fructus Citri Sarcodactylis, Fructus Amomi, Endothelium Corneum Gigeriae Galli.

Third treatment: Four doses of the decoction reduced symptoms. Decoction of Poria (*Fu Ling Yin** of *Waitai*) was given to harmonize the Interior, and to bring full recovery.

**Fu Ling Yin*: Poria, Radix Ginseng, Fructus Aurantii Immaturus, Rhizoma Atractylodis Macrocephalae, Pericarpium Citri Reticulatae, Rhizoma Zingiberis Recens.

Case 2 (46-213):

Mr. Xie, 48, suffered from pulmonary heart disease with concurrent infection. Chill and fever occurred, with temperature of 39 ℃. The patient could not lie flat because of panting and chest distress. Other symptoms: pallid, gray face, thirst, yellow tongue coating, dropsy in both legs, scanty urination and deep-tense pulse.

Diagnosis: *Zhiyin* Fluid-retention syndrome complicated with contraction of Exterior syndrome. Cold and Heat, Deficiency and Excess intermingled.

First treatment: Decoction of Radix Stephaniae Tetrandrae was given to regulate Heat and Cold, tonify the Deficiency and purge the Excess:

Radix Stephaniae Tetrandrae	10 grams
Lignum Cinnamomi	10 grams
Gypsum Fibrosum	10 grams
Radix Ginseng (stewed separately and blend into the decoction before service)	10 grams
Herba Houttuyniae	15 grams
Semen Coicis	12 grams
Semen Benincasae	15 grams
Rhizoma Phragmitis	15 grams

Second treatment: After three doses of the decoction, chill and fever subsided. Tongue coating turned white and greasy. Another ten doses were given before full recovery achieved.

Prescription:

Radix Glehniae
Semen Armeniacae Amarum
Semen Coicis
Semen Cardamomi Rotundi
Cortex Magnoliae Officinalis
Rhizoma Pinelliae Praeparata
Poria
Pericarpium Citri Reticulatae
Fructus Perillae
Semen Lepidii seu Descurainiae
Cortex Mori Radicis
Pericarpium Arecae
Cortex Zingiberis

After taking the decoction, chest distress and panting subsided and dropsy disappeared.

Case 3 (48-158): Exudative Pleurisy

A peasant woman suffered from exudative pleurisy with fever, cough and chest pain. X-ray diagnosis showed exudative pleurisy at lower left position. Temperature was 38 ℃. The patient had flushed face, profuse perspiration, white-slippery tongue coating, slender-tight pulse.

First treatment: Decoction of Lesser Radix Bupleuri (see Clause 17-15) with following added drugs was given:

Herba Artemisiae Chinghao
Carapax Trionycis
Semen Sinapis Albae

Second treatment: Five doses were served. Body temperature dropped gradually, still cough and panting, perspiration, chest distress, parched feeling in mouth. Tongue was covered with white-slippery coating, with a red fringe. Pulse was slightly tight. Decoction of Radix Stephaniae Tetrandrae was prescribed:

Ramulus Cinnamomi	9 grams
Radix Stephaniae Tetrandrae	12 grams
Gypsum Fibrosum	15 grams
Radix Codonopsis Pilosulae	12 grams
Radix Stellariae	9 grams
Radix Curcumae	9 grams
Semen Sinapis Albae	9 grams
Herba Artemisiae Chinghao	30 grams

Carapax Trionycis	30 grams
Radix Scutellariae	9 grams

The syndrome was gone after several doses of the decoction were consumed.

CLAUSE 12-23

Zhiyin Fluid-retention in the epigastrium will cause vertigo (1). Decoction of Rhizoma Alismatis can be prescribed.

NOTES

1. When the Fluid-retention is in the epigastrium, the lucid Yang cannot ascend as it should, while the turbid Yin ascends irregularly, resulting in vertigo. This symptom frequently occurs in *Tanyin* Fluid-retention syndromes. (02-106)

Decoction of Rhizoma Alismatis
(*Zexie Tang*):

Rhizoma Alismatis	5 *liang*
Rhizoma Atractylodis Macrocephalae	2 *liang*

Stew the drugs in two *sheng* of water until one *sheng* remains. Serve the lukewarm decoction in two doses.

Explanation of the Prescription: Rhizoma Alismatis functions on the Kidney, drawing out pathogenetic Fluid with the urine. Rhizoma Atractylodis Macrocephalae tonifies the Earth (Spleen) to better control the Water. This prescription is applicable to mild cases of *Zhiyin* Fluid-retention. (01-128)

CASES

Case 1 (64-434): Case Recorded in *Case Studies of Dr. Wu Jutong*

Mr. Chen, 51, was impotent for many years. He had vertigo, mental confusion and an uneasy feeling in chest. Whenever he drank much water, he had discomfort. Vertigo was caused by Hidden Fluid-retention. Treatment should be directed to retention, then impotence could be treated.

Decoction of Rhizoma Alismatis was given to alleviate Fluid-retention:

Rhizoma Atractylodis Macrocephalae	2 *liang*
Rhizoma Alismatis	2 *liang*

The decoction produced results but more doses were needed. The syndrome was gone after more than a dozen doses were taken.

Case 2 (64-434): Meniere's Disease, Case Recorded in Journal of *Henan Chinese Medicine*, 2:25, 1982

Mr. Liu, 49, suffered from repeated vertigo for almost twenty years which was diagnosed as Meniere's disease. In recent weeks the syndrome became aggravated and the patient consulted a doctor of Chinese medicine. When vertigo attacked, the patient had blurred vision, tinnitus, nausea and vomiting, a feeling as if everything around him was moving. He could not move his body, for fear the vertigo could become bad. Accompanying symptoms: chest distress, anorexia, general fatigue, yellow and puffy face, swollen tongue and slow pulse.

Diagnosis: Spleen failed to function when Humidity was prevalent.

First treatment: Decoction of Rhizoma Alismatis was given to drain excessive Humidity:

Rhizoma Alismatis	15 grams
Rhizoma Atractylodis Macrocephalae	15 grams
Poria peel	15 grams

Second treatment: Five doses of the decoction were served. Vertigo reduced. In next decoction, Poria peel was reduced to nine grams.

Third treatment: All symptoms were subsiding. Decoction of Rhizoma Alismatis was prescribed:

Rhizoma Alismatis	12 grams
Rhizoma Atractylodis Macrocephalae	18 grams

Thirty to forty doses of Decoction of Rhizoma Alismatis were taken in one month. The syndrome was gone, no recurrence was reported in the next three years.

Case 3 (65-335): Case Recorded in Journal of *Chinese Medicine*, 7:16, 1980

Mr. Xu, 45, first treatment on December 2, 1975. When the patient was young, he had otitis media. In the last few years, he suffered from repeated vertigo. When vertigo became aggravated, he had to lie in bed, with eyes closed. When he opened his eyes, vertigo was worse. Other symptoms: plump build, pallid face, thin, greasy tongue coating, soft pulse and frequent loose stool. Decoction of Rhizoma Alismatis was given:

Rhizoma Atractylodis Macrocephalae	12 grams
Rhizoma Alismatis	25 grams

Four doses of the decoction were effective. More doses were given to complete treatment.

CLAUSE 12-24

Zhiyin Fluid-retention with fullness in the chest (1) can be treated with Decoction of Cortex Magnoliae Officinalis and Radix et Rhizoma Rhei.

NOTES

1. Wu Qian: "In the chest" here should read "in the abdomen." This is a copying mistake, otherwise how could purgative be used? (05-564)

Decoction of Cortex Magnoliae Officinalis and
Radix et Rhizoma Rhei
(*Houpo Dahuang Tang*):

Cortex Magnoliae Officinalis	1 foot-long pc.
Radix et Rhizoma Rhei	6 *liang*
Fructus Aurantii Immaturus	4 pcs.

Stew the drugs in five *sheng* of water until two *sheng* remain. Serve the lukewarm decoction in two doses.

Explanation of the Prescription: Cortex Magnoliae Officinalis and Radix et Rhizoma Rhei are heavily dosed to strengthen their efficacy in dispersing the Fluid-retention, dredging through the Vital-energy Stagnation and loosening the bowels. Except for a sense of fullness in the abdomen, other symptoms and signs may include sporadic pains in the epigastrium, and constipation. (02-102)

CASES

Case 1 (52-598): Bronchitis with Concurrent Infection

Han, 60, female, first treatment on November 28, 1962. The patient suffered from cough and asthma for twenty years. The syndrome was aggravated in winter. Ten days before the patient came to consult the doctor, she had a cold sweat, which caused an attack of cough and asthma with spitting of clear phlegm. In the last two or three days, volume of phlegm increased. There was chest distress, abdominal distention, anorexia, and no stool for three days. She could not lie flat because of severe coughing and asthma. The patient had puffy face, tongue was covered with thin, yellow coating, pulse was tight-slippery and mighty. This was a *Tanyin* Fluid-retention syndrome with abdominal excess. Decoction of Cortex Magnolicae Officinalis and Radix et Rhizoma Rhei was given with additions:

Cortex Magnoliae Officinalis	18 grams
Radix et Rhizoma Rhei	10 grams
Fructus Aurantii Immaturus	10 grams
Poria	14 grams
Radix Glycyrrhizae	6 grams
Fructus Schisandrae	10 grams
Rhizoma Zingiberis	6 grams
Herba Asari	5 grams
Rhizoma Pinelliae	12 grams
Semen Armeniacae Amarum	10 grams

Second treatment: After taking one dose of the decoction, there was a loose stool and other symptoms reduced. Another three doses were given. Chest distress and abdominal distention subsided, cough and asthma reduced. The patient could lie flat. Tongue coating was thin and white, pulse was still slippery.

Third treatment: Decoction of *Erchen* was given to eliminate the phlegm:

Rhizoma Pinelliae Praeparata
Pericarpium Citri Reticulatae
Poria
Radix Glycyrrhizae Praeparata
Rhizoma Zingiberis Recens
Fructus Mume

Case 2 (65-336): *Zhiyin* Fluid-retention with Heat

Mr. Yang, 32-year-old farmer, first treatment on June 10, 1968.

Examination: Fever lasted for twenty days. Accompanying symptoms: distention and pain in chest and costal regions, pallid and yellow complexion, cough with dyspnea made it impossible for him to lie flat. There was spontaneous perspiration with low fever, headache and heaviness all over body, parched lips and oral cavity, anorexia, epigastric distress, constipation, yellow, turbid urine, deep-tight and speedy pulse, red tongue covered with thick yellow, greasy coating.

Diagnosis: Pathological condition of Fluid-retention stagnating in chest and epigastrium, complicated by pathogenetic Heat in Stomach and Intestine. Purgative should be served to facilitate the down-flow of pathological conditions. Decoction of Cortex Magnolicae Officinalis, Radix et Rhizoma Rhei was used:

Radix et Rhizoma Rhei	12 grams

gas rushing from the abdomen to the chest and throat, numbness in the extremities, with flushed and hot face as if he were drunk. When the patient feels gas flowing down to the genitals, dysuria will result. Vertigo is also observed. Decoction of Poria, Ramulus Cinnamomi, Fructus Schisandrae and Radix Glycyrrhizae can be adopted to stop the adverse ascending.

Decoction of Poria, Ramulus Cinnamomi, Fructus Schisandrae and Radix Glycyrrhizae
(*Gui Ling Wuwei Gancao Tang*):

Poria	4 *liang*
Ramulus Cinnamomi	4 *liang*
Radix Glycyrrhizae Praeparata	3 *liang*
Fructus Schisandrae	0.5 *sheng*

Stew the drugs in eight *sheng* of water until three *sheng* remain. Filter the decoction and serve lukewarm in three doses.

Explanation of the Prescription: This prescription treats the complications arising from the adoption of Decoction of Lesser *Qinglong*. In that prescription, drugs of pungent taste and warm quality, such as Herba Ephedrae and Herba Asari, are dispersive and therefore injure the Yin and Yang (pungent and warm quality injures the Yin; dispersive quality injures the Yang), and the symptoms and signs described in the text appear. This decoction is adopted to stimulate the flow of the Yang Vital Energy, harmonize the Yin, reverse the adverse ascending and disperse the Fluid-retention. (01-133)

CASES

Case 1 (64-456): Case Recorded in *Collection of Case Studies of Doctors in Hunan Province*

Mr. He suffered from *Tanyin* Fluid-retention a long time and had contracted a cold. He began to cough, had dyspnea and severe dropsy on both feet. The patient could not lie flat in bed but curled up and panted hard. Decoction of Lesser *Qinglong* and Decoction of *Zhenwu* (prescription see *Shanghan Lun*, Clause 316. Ingredients: Poria, Radix Paeoniae, Rhizoma Atractylodis Macrocephalae, Rhizoma Zingiberis Recens and Radix Aconiti

Praeparata) did not seem help. *Pills of Ji Sheng Shen Qi** were given to tonify the Kidney, which did not work.

Finally, Decoction of Poria, Ramulus Cinnamomi, Fructus Schisandrae and Radix Glycyrrhizae adding Ochra Haematitum and Fructus Perillae was given, which was effective.

After four doses taken, the patient was then able to sleep quietly and dropsy began to subside.

In the next treatment, the following decoction was prescribed:

Poria
Ramulus Cinnamomi
Rhizoma Atractylodis Macrocephalae
Radix Glycyrrhizae
Fructus Schisandrae

Adoption of the above decoction completed the treatment.

**Pills of Ji Sheng Shen Qi*: Radix Rehmanniae, Rhizoma Dioscoreae, Fructus Corni, Rhizoma Alismatis, Poria, Cortex Moutan Radicis, Ramulus Cinnamomi, Radix Aconiti Praeparata, Radix Achyranthis Bidentatae, Semen Plantaginis.

Case 2 (64-456):

A gentleman suffered from emission for a long time, which made him weak and cough. In autumn and summer, cough was aggravated and ascending gas in the body cavity made him unable to sleep. He had aversion to cold and coldness on extremities. It was syndrome caused by stagnation of phlegm resulting from accumulation of Fluid. Treatment should be directed to retention, not to Lung condition. Decoction of Poria, Ramulus Cinnamomi, Fructus Schisandrae and Radix Glycyrrhizae was given.

Ramulus Cinnamomi
Poria
Fructus Schisandrae
Radix Glycyrrhizae Praeparata
Radix Paeoniae Alba
Rhizoma Zingiberis

Case 3 (65-354): Fluid-retention with Ascending Gas, Case Recorded in *A Guide to Clinical Practice with Medical Records*

Mr. Cheng, 57, had been plump but became thin recently. Pulse was deep-tight, indicating Fluid-retention syndrome. Man of old age generally had Deficiency in Kidney, with loss of Vital Energy. The ascending phlegm and Vital Energy appeared as cough and asthma. Doctors tend to cure cough with drugs to bring down the adverse ascending and eliminate phlegm. This did not cure all cases of coughing. As this failed, drugs to moisten the Yin were given (presuming that cough was caused by the Dryness), which made the syndrome worse. This was a case with Fluid-retention (in Yin nature), when moist drugs (also in Yin nature) were given, syndrome was aggravated. Correct therapy for this syndrome was to disperse the retention by giving warm drugs. Decoction of Poria, Ramulus Cinnamomi, Fructus Schisandrae and Radix Glycyrrhizae was given, adding Radix Aconiti Praeparata and Semen Juglandis. The decoction helped.

CLAUSE 12-35

After taking Decoction of Poria, Ramulus Cinnamomi, Fructus Schisandrae and Radix Glycyrrhizae, coughing becomes more acute with a sensation of fullness in the chest. Subtract Ramulus Cinnamomi, add Rhizoma Zingiberis and Herba Asari to the prescription in order to treat syndrome of coughing and fullness.

Decoction of Poria, Radix Glycyrrhizae, Fructus Schisandrae, Rhizoma Zingiberis and Herba Asari
(*Ling Gan Wuwei Jiang Xin Tang*):

Poria	4 *liang*
Radix Glycyrrhizae	3 *liang*
Rhizoma Zingiberis	3 *liang*
Herba Asari	3 *liang*
Fructus Schisandrae	0.5 *sheng*

Stew the drugs in eight *sheng* of water until three *sheng* remain. Filter the decoction. Serve one half *sheng* of the lukewarm decoction per dose three times a day.

Explanation of the Prescription: Decoction of Poria, Ramulus Cinnamomi, Fructus Schisandrae and Radix Glycyrrhizae eliminates adverse ascending gas, though coughing and sensation of fullness become acute. This is an indication of an attack by Fluid-retention. Treatment is to eliminate the Fluid-retention and reduce the coughing. As there is no feeling of ascending, Ramulus Cinnamomi is subtracted, and Rhizoma Zingiberis and Herba Asari are added to disperse the fullness and warm the inner Cold. Together with

Fructus Schisandrae, they eliminate the Fluid-retention and suppress the coughing. (02-109)

CASES

Case 1 (65-355): Cough, Case Recorded in *Dr. Chen Yaogeng's Case Studies*

Mr. Zhou, 36-year-old farmer, suffered from a cough and spitting phlegm more than a year. While gathering firewood in the mountain a few days before, he was caught in the rain. As soon as he was home, he began to cough, and spat phlegm. This did not stop till the next morning. Headache, palpitation and general fatigue were accompanied the symptom. Decoction of *Liu Jun Zi** was given, but did not work.

Then the decoction in Clause 12-35 was prescribed:

Poria
Ramulus Cinnamomi
Rhizoma Atractylodis Macrocephalae
Radix Glycyrrhizae
Rhizoma Zingiberis
Herba Asari
Fructus Schisandrae

One dose was effective in reducing the cough. More doses were given successfully.

*Decoction of *Liu Jun Zi*: Pericarpium Citri Reticulatae, Rhizoma Pinelliae, Poria, Radix Glycyrrhizae, Radix Ginseng, Rhizoma Atractylodis Macrocephalae.

CLAUSE 12-36

When coughing and fullness are eliminated, the patient has a great thirst and adverse ascending recurs. This is due to the hot quality of Herba Asari and Rhizoma Zingiberis, which causes thirst. If the patient is not thirsty, it is a case of *Zhiyin* Fluid-retention. *Zhiyin* Fluid-retention usually has vertigo as a symptom accompanied by nausea and vomiting, which can be eliminated by Rhizoma Pinelliae. Add Rhizoma Pinelliae to disperse the Water.

Decoction of Poria, Ramulus Cinnamomi, Fructus Schisandrae and Radix Glycyrrhizae subtracting Ramulus Cinnamomi adding Rhizoma Zingiberis, Herba Asari and Rhizoma Pinelliae
(*Gui Ling Wuwei Gancao Qu Gui Jia Ganjiang Xixin Banxia Tang*):

CHAPTER XIII

ON PULSE, SYMPTOM COMPLEX AND TREATMENT OF *XIAOKE* (DIABETES), DYSURIA AND URINARY DISTURBANCE

CLAUSE 13-1*

Greater Yin syndrome has the following symptoms and signs: Great thirst with frequent urination (1), uncomfortable feeling of ascending air rushing up from beneath the epigastrium, heat and pain in the Stomach, hunger with inability to eat. When food is eaten, ascarides will be vomited out. If purgative is given, there will be continuous diarrhea.

NOTES

1. Great thirst with frequency of urination: The original Chinese is *Xiaoke*, which means, 1) diabetes; 2) a range of diseases with symptoms of constant thirst, and frequent urination and defecation, including diabetes, mellitus and insipidus.

*This clause also appears in Clause 326 of *Shanghan Lun*.

CLAUSE 13-2

Pulse in the wrist is floating and slow. Floating pulse indicates a deficient case; slow pulse signifies a consumptive disease. Deficiency causes the Vital Resistance to become insufficient. Consumptive disease exhausts the Nutrient Essence. (1)

NOTES

1. Wu Qian: This clause should be in the chapter concerning "consumptive diseases." It is here due to an error. (05-575)

CLAUSE 13-3

Fuyang pulse is floating and speedy. Floating pulse indicates Excess of the Vital Energy (1). Speedy pulse indicates good digestion accompanied by constipation. Excessive Vital Energy causes frequent urination, which leads to constipation. The conflicting frequency of urination and constipation bring about a case of *Xiaoke* (diabetes).(2)

NOTES

1. Excess of Vital Energy means excessive Heat in the Stomach. (01-138)

2. Wu Qian: *Fuyang* pulse evinces pathological conditions in the Stomach. Floating and speedy pulse indicates the presence of pathogenetic Heat in the Stomach. When Heat prevails in the Stomach, digestion is good but the stool becomes hard; Excessive Vital Energy consumes the Water, and urination is frequent. When frequent urination and constipation occur simultaneously, it is a case of *Xiaoke* (diabetes). (05-575)

CLAUSE 13-4

Xiaoke (diabetes) in male patients (1): The patient has frequent urination (2). When he drinks one *dou* of water, he passes as much as one *dou* of urine. Pills of Eight-Ingredients of the Kidney Vital Energy can be adopted (3).

(For prescription, see Chapter V, Appendix.)

NOTES

1. The case does not only occur in male patients, but in female patients as well. (02-113)

2. The patient has frequent urination: When the patient is extremely thirsty due to exhaustion of the Body Fluid in an acute febrile disease, urination should not be frequent. But the pathology of the case is failure of the deficient Kidney Yang Vital Energy to evaporate the Body Fluid, resulting in a failure to bring the Fluid upward, which in turn causes great thirst and an inability to control urination due to poor circulation of the Vital Energy. (02-113)

3. Syndromes in Clauses 13-3 and 13-4 are cases of true *Xiaoke* (diabetes). Clause 13-3 gives a case caused by accumulation of pathogenetic Heat in the Middle Portion (the Stomach), thus it is called Middle *Xiaoke* (*Zhong xiao*). Clause 13-4 states that it is a male disease, indicating that its cause lies in sexual intemperance that has weakened the Kidney Vital Energy. Thus it is called Lower *Xiaoke* (*Xia xiao*). Pills of Eight-Ingredients of the Kidney Vital Energy is prescribed as the remedy. This is the principle set down by Master Zhang

Zhongjing for the treatment of Lower *Xiaoke*. In clinical practice, three *Xiaoke* syndromes can be observed as follows:

Syndrome	*Cause of Disease*
Upper *Xiaoke*	Disorder of the Lung
Middle *Xiaoke*	Disorder of the Stomach
Lower *Xiaoke*	Disorder of the Kidney

(01-138)

CLAUSE 13-5

Xiaoke syndrome with floating pulse, dysuria and a low fever should be treated with *Wuling* Powder which acts as a diuretic as well as a diaphoretic (1).

(For prescription, see Clause 12-29.)

NOTES

1. Wu Qian: Floating pulse indicates Exterior syndrome. Dysuria indicates that the Fluid is stagnating in the Interior. *Wuling* Powder is the only medicine that can simultaneously disperse the Exterior syndrome, drain the Fluid, quench the thirst and produce the Body Fluid. (05-576)

CLAUSE 13-6*

Though thirsty, the patient will vomit the water he is drinking. This is known as "Water Regurgitation (1)." *Wuling* Powder will provide the cure.

Febrile disease caused by Wind: In both Exterior and Interior syndromes, the patient has fever and experiences general anxiety for six to seven days. Though he is thirsty, he will vomit the water he is drinking. This is known as "Water Regurgitation." *Wuling* Powder will provide the cure.

*This clause also appears in Clause 74 of *Shanghan Lun*.

NOTES

1. Wu Qian: Water Regurgitation occurs when there is a slight Interior Heat and a strong pathogenetic Water. A slight Heat compels the patient to drink water, but the strong Water stagnation will cause the patient to reject the intake of water. (05-577)

CLAUSE 13-7

The patient is thirsty. He drinks great quantities of water but his thirst is still not quenched. *Wenge* Powder will provide a cure.

Wenge Powder
(*Wenge San*):

*Wenge** 5 *liang*

Pound the drug into powder. Place one *fangcunbi* of powder into five *ge* of boiling water. Serve the medicine when lukewarm.

**Wenge*: This substance has been variously interpreted as Concha Meretricis seu Cyclinae or Galla Chinensis.

CLAUSE 13-8

Urinary disturbance (gonorrhea) (1) will bear the following symptoms and signs: Dripping urine, acute pain and contraction in the abdomen with dragging pain in the navel.

NOTES

1. Urinary disturbance (*Lin zheng*) includes pains during urination, pollakiuria, dysuria and dripping urine.

CLAUSE 13-9

Speedy *Fuyang* pulse indicates Heat in the Stomach, which will bring about good digestion and a good appetite. Constipation and frequent urination are the necessary consequences. (1)

NOTES

1. This clause should follow Clause 13-3. It is a Middle *Xiaoke* syndrome. (01-140)

CLAUSE 13-10*

Diaphoresis is prohibited when the patient experiences urinary dripping (urinary disturbance). If it is adopted, hematuria will result.

*This clause also appears in Clause 84 of *Shanghan Lun*.

CLAUSE 13-11

Dysuria is a sign of stagnant Water. When thirst is observed, Pills of Radix Trichosanthis and Herba Dianthi can be adopted.

Pills of Radix Trichosanthis and Herba Dianthi
(*Gualou Qumai Wan*)::

Radix Trichosanthis	2 *liang*
Poria	3 *liang*
Rhizoma Dioscoreae	3 *liang*
Radix Aconiti Praeparata	1 pc.
Herba Dianthi	1 *liang*

Pound the drugs into powder. Form pills the size of Chinese parasol seeds with honey. Take three pills per dose three times a day. If this is not effective, increase dosage to seven or eight pills. When the urination becomes normal and warmness in the abdomen is felt, the cure can be considered effective.

Explanation of the Prescription: This clause discusses syndromes of dysuria, Cold at the Lower Portion, and Dryness at the Upper Portion. The Kidney controls Water circulation and the functioning of the Vital Energy. When the Vital Energy no longer functions normally, dysuria results, and Water stagnates in the Interior. When the Vital Energy cannot carry the Water up to the Upper Portion, the patient feels thirsty. Treatment of the disease aims to facilitate normal functioning of the Vital Energy, drain the stagnant Water and moisten the Dryness. Pills of Radix Trichosanthis and Herba Dianthi are the correct curative.

Radix Trichosanthis and Rhizoma Dioscoreae stimulate production of Body Fluid and moisten the Dryness. Herba Dianthi and Poria drain the stagnant Water and circulate the Fluid, thus easing urination. Radix Aconiti Praeparata warms the Yang Vital Energy and facilitate its normal functioning. This therapy follows the same principle as that of Pills of the Eight-Ingredients of the Kidney Vital Energy. When Radix Aconiti Praeparata is used, no symptoms of a Heat nature should be observed, and the pulse should be deep.

The statement "When urination is normal and warmness in the abdomen is felt" in the prescription is evidence that this is a case of Deficiency of the Interior Yang Vital Energy. From this, it can be inferred that Radix Aconiti Praeparata is the principal ingredient of the prescription. (02-115)

CASES

Case 1 (65-374): Case Recorded in *Collection of Cases Studies of Doctors in Hunan Province*

Mr. Cheng suffered from stranguria, then anuresis occurred. Pulse was deep-moderate on the left wrist. Pills of Radix Trichosanthis and Herba Dianthi were prescribed, adding:

Semen Plantaginis
Radix Achyranthis Bidentatae

When three doses were served, urine returned to normal.

Case 2 (62-289):

Liu, 40, female, first treatment on December 20, 1964. The patient had thirst, dysuria and dropsy for about one year.

Examination: Puffiness all over the body, great thirst (she brought with her a big mug even when consulting the doctor. Twenty-four mugs of water, or twenty-four pounds, were consumed each day), cold feeling in lumbar region, flabby legs, anorexia, dysuria (scanty urine of yellow color, but no hot feeling during urination), pallid face, pale lips, tongue free from coating, deep-slender pulse and depression. The condition had been diagnosed chronic glomerular nephritis.

Diagnosis: Syndrome of dysuria and dropsy caused by Deficiency of Kidney Yang, which failed to control the Water circulation. Prescription of Pills of Radix Trichosanthis and Herba Dianthi with alterations was given.

Prescription (in decoction form):

Radix Trichosanthis	30 grams
Rhizoma Dioscoreae	30 grams
Poria	15 grams
Herba Dianthi	15 grams
Radix Aconiti Praeparata (stewed two hours earlier than other drugs)	15 grams
Colla Cornus Cervi (steamed to melt, blend into the decoction before service)	12 grams

Second treatment: Two doses of the decoction were served. Thirst and dropsy were reduced. She only drank twelve pounds of water a day. Urination was smooth. Since the decoction was effective, another two doses were given.

Third treatment: After second treatment, drinking of water reduced to four pounds per day. Dropsy and dysuria disappeared.

Ten doses of the decoction were served before final recovery was achieved.

Case 3 (64-485): Case Recorded in Journal of *Shandong Chinese Medicine*, 2:8, 1983

Mr. Yu, 72, suffered from anuresis. Treatment of Chinese and Western medicines did not help him urinate. The patient refused surgery.

Examination: He had thirst but did not want to drink water, so was having fruits to quench thirst. There was no urination, resulting in distention in lower abdomen, with coldness on hands and feet. Tongue was fat, with teeth marks on edge, covered with dry, yellow coating. Pulse was deep-slender and speedy. Pills of Radix Trichosanthis and Herba Dianthi were given:

Radix Trichosanthis	12 grams
Herba Dianthi	10 grams
Poria	10 grams
Rhizoma Dioscoreae	12 grams
Radix Achyranthis Bidentatae	12 grams
Semen Plantaginis	12 grams
Radix Aconiti Praeparata	10 grams

One dose of the decoction enabled the patient to urinate and distention was reduced. Three more doses completed the treatment.

CLAUSE 13-12

Dysuria can be treated with the following prescriptions:
Powder of Ash of Pollen Typhae;
Powder of Talcum and *Baiyu*;
Decoction of Poria and Halitum.

Powder of Ash of Pollen Typhae
(*Pu Hui San*):

Ash of Pollen Typhae	7 *fen*
Talcum	3 *fen*

Pound the drugs into powder. Take one *fangcunbi* with water per dose three times a day.

Explanation of the Prescription: Ash of Pollen Typhae drains the Humidity and eases urination. Talcum eliminates the Heat, drains the Humidity and eases urination. (01-141)

Ash of Pollen Typhae: *Qianjin* contains a recipe composed of Pollen Typhae and Talcum, which is effective for dysuria, pain in the penis, pain and contractions in the abdomen. From this it can be inferred that Ash of Pollen Typhae mentioned in the prescription should be Pollen Typhae, but not the ash. (02-116)

Powder of Talcum and *Baiyu**
(*Huashi Baiyu San*):

Talcum	2 *fen*
Ash of human hair**	2 *fen*
Baiyu	2 *fen*

Pound the drugs into powder. Take one *fangcunbi* of the powder with water per dose three times a day.

**Baiyu*: According to *Shen Nong's Herbal and Compendium of Materia Medica, Baiyu* may either refer to a particular fish (*Compendium of Materia Medica*, p. 2432) or a particular moth (*Shen Nong's Herbal*, p. 127).
**Or human hair.

Decoction of Poria and Halitum
(*Fuling Rongyan Tang*):

Poria	0.5 *jin*
Rhizoma Atractylodis Macrocephalae	2 *liang*
Halitum	1 bullet-size pc. (size of an egg yolk)

Explanation of the Prescriptions: The three prescriptions above are all effective in cases of dysuria, urinary disturbances (gonorrhea) and hematuria. In the above three cases, the diseases are caused by pathogenetic Heat in the Kidney and the Urinary Bladder, which is completely different from that given in Clause 13-11. However, the prescriptions still have different effects: Powder of Ash of Pollen Typhae and Powder of Talcum and *Baiyu* have a strong effect in easing urination, removing the stasis, and eliminating the Heat, whereas Decoction of Poria and Halitum tonifies the Kidney and Spleen and drains the Humidity; it is a prescription with both tonifying and eliminating effects. The three prescriptions given in this clause are for different cases. Although the clause is quite simple and records no specific symptoms or signs, efficacy of the prescriptions cannot be overlooked. (02-116)

CASES

Case 1 (02-117): Case Recorded in Journal of *Jiangxi Chinese Medicine and Pharmacology*, 10:30, 1959

Mr. Wen, 49-year-old farmer, first treatment on June 1958. Last March he began to have urinary dripping. In April, he experienced urodynia. Pulse was moderate but slender-speedy at Cubit position. The classic said dysuria with thirst could be treated with Pills of Radix Trichosanthis and Herba Dianthi. In this case, there was not thirst. Clause 13-12 discussed the treatment of dysuria: Powder of Talcum and *Baiyu*, and Decoction of Poria and Halitum combined to make the prescription:

Poria	8 *qian*
Rhizoma Atractylodis Macrocephalae	2 *qian*
Halitum	2 *qian*
Talcum	6 *qian*
Endothelium Corneum Gigeriae Galli	2 *qian*
Fructus Malvae Verticillatae	3 *qian*

Eight doses were served and worked effectively.

Second treatment: Pulse in the Cubit position was tight-speedy, showing a Yin-deficiency. Decoction of Polyporus Umbellatus (Clause 13-14) with the following additions was given to complete the cure:

Radix Paeoniae
Radix Glycyrrhizae Praeparata

Case 2 (65-375): Case Recorded in Journal of *Liaoning Chinese Medicine*, 7:1, 1980

Mr. Zheng, 32, suffered from stranguria with complication of hematuria for five days. The patient had fever (38.3 °C), thirst of water, dysuria with hematuria and urodynia, frequent urination and abdominal distention. Pulse was slippery-speedy. Tongue was covered with yellow-greasy coating.

Diagnosis: Syndrome caused by downflowing of Humidity-Heat with pathogenetic factors in the Blood. Powder of Ash of Pollen Typhae with additions were prescribed:

Pollen Typhae	3 grams
Talcum	12 grams
Radix Rehmanniae	20 grams
Caulis Akebiae	5 grams
Folium Bambusae	10 grams
Radix Glycyrrhizae	5 grams
Herba Cephalanoploris	15 grams

Four doses were served. Fever went down and stranguria with hematuria subsided.

Second treatment: Three more doses were given, with alterations:

Subtract: Caulis Akebiae.

Add: Nodus Nelumbinis Rhizomatis.

The syndrome was cured.

CLAUSE 13-13*

Decoction of *Baihu* adding Radix Ginseng is effective in cases with symptoms and signs of parched tongue and throat and thirst of water.

(For prescription, see Clause 2-26.)

CLAUSE 13-14**

Decoction of Polyporus Umbellatus can be prescribed for a syndrome with the following symptoms and signs: Floating pulse, fever, thirst and dysuria.

Decoction of Polyporus Umbellatus
(*Zhuling Tang*):

Polyporus Umbellatus	1 *liang*
Poria	1 *liang*
Talcum	1 *liang*
Rhizoma Alismatis	1 *liang*
Colla Corii Asini	1 *liang*

Stew the first four drugs in four *sheng* of water until two *sheng* remain. Filter the decoction. Add Colla Corii Asini until it melts. Serve seven *ge* of the lukewarm decoction per dose three times a day.

*This clause also appears in Clause 222 of *Shanghan Lun*.
** This clause also appears in Clause 223 of *Shanghan Lun*.

Explanation of the Prescription: This prescription treats dysuria caused by the intermingling of Water and Heat that has injured the Yin. Decoction of Polyporus Umbellatus drains the Water and moistens the Yin Vital Essence. Polyporus Umbellatus, Poria, Rhizoma Alismatis and Talcum drain the Water and eliminate the Heat. Colla Corii Asini tonifies the Yin and moistens the Dryness. When Water is drained, Heat can no longer remain as there are no pathogenetic factors for it to attach itself to. When Body Fluid returns, thirst of water disappears. (02-115)

CHAPTER XIV

ON PULSE, SYMPTOM COMPLEX AND TREATMENT OF EDEMA

CLAUSE 14-1

Master: Edema can be classified into five categories: Wind-edema; Skin-edema; *Zheng*-edema; Stone-edema; and Yellow-sweat.

Wind-edema (1) has the symptoms and signs of floating pulse, arthritis and aversion to cold;

Skin-edema (2) has the symptoms and signs of floating pulse, acute dropsy wherein the doctor's finger will disappear in a fold of skin when the skin is pressed. The abdomen is distended as tight as a drum. The patient is not thirsty and has no aversion to cold. Treatment should be diaphoresis;

Zheng-edema (3) has the symptoms and signs of deep-slow pulse and wheezing;

Stone-edema (4) has the symptoms and signs of deep pulse and abdominal distention without wheezing;

Yellow-sweat (5) has the symptoms and signs of deep-slow pulse, fever, fullness in the chest, dropsy in the extremities, head and face. Carbuncle may appear if the syndrome lasts a long time.

NOTES

1. Wind-edema, (*Feng shui*): edema caused by Wind-evil; closely related to the Lung. As the Lung controls the skin and hair, when pathogenetic Wind invades the Exterior, floating pulse and aversion to cold will result. When the pathogenetic Humidity flows through the joints, arthritis results. When the skin is affected, the Lung ceases its normal processing of Humidity, thus Humidity collects in the Exterior. Other symptoms may include dropsy in the head and face as well as fever. (02-119)

2. Skin-edema (*Pi shui*) is closely related to the Spleen and the Lung. The Spleen controls the extremities and the muscles. When the Spleen ceases its normal functioning, Humidity will obstruct the channel of the Spleen, causing the abdomen to become distended as tight as a drum, with no sensation of thirst.

When Water stagnates at the lower extremities, dropsy in condyles is so serious that the doctor's finger will disappear when the patient's skin is pressed. When the Water moves under the skin, a floating pulse is observed. Since there is no Wind-evil, there is no aversion to cold. Since the pathological condition of the Skin-edema is located in the Exterior, diaphoresis can disperse the pathogens from the skin. (02-119)

3. & 4. Both *Zheng*-edema and Stone-edema are related to the Kidney. *Zheng* edema (*Zheng shui*) is caused when the Kidney Yang Vital Energy is in a deficient state and fails to circulate the Water. When Water stagnates, pulse is deep-slow. Stone-edema (*Shi shui*) is caused by an accumulation of Yin and Cold at the Lower Portion. The corresponding pulse is deep. Since both the syndromes are located in the Interior, abdominal distention is the principal symptom of both cases. Water-evil of *Zheng*-edema follows the Kidney Channel of Foot-Lesser Yin and ascends to the Lung, bringing about the syndrome of wheezing. Stone-edema is a case of Water-stagnating in the abdomen thus the abdomen is distended and is as hard as a rock. (02-119)

5. Yellow-sweat (*Huang han*) is closely related to the Spleen. Pathology of the case is as follows: When Humidity stagnates in the Interior, the Blood is affected and deep-slow pulse is observed. Fullness in the chest is caused by the abnormal functioning of the Lung Vital Energy, which is affected by a deficient Spleen which cannot circulate the Water normally. Physiological activity of the Vital Resistance is restricted and the Blood is affected by Heat; thus fever and dropsy in the extremities, head and face occur. As the sweat is yellowish in color, the case is termed Yellow-sweat. (02-119)

CLAUSE 14-2

The pulse is floating and grand. A floating pulse indicates the existence of pathogenetic Wind, whereas a grand pulse indicates strong Vital Energy (1). Wind and Vital Energy intermingle with each other. When Wind prevails, urticaria appears on the skin and causes itching; this is called "Wind-leading." If the case lasts a long time, scabs and tinea will appear. When Vital Energy prevails, edema will result and the patient will have difficulty moving his body. Conflict between the Wind and the Vital Energy results in serious edema throughout the body. Diaphoresis will provide a cure. Aversion to cold is an indication of a deficient state. Wind is the cause of the disease. The Yellow-sweat syndrome will not have the symptom of aversion to cold. Other symptoms include normal urination and copious salivation. This is a case of Yellow-sweat with pathogenetic Cold resting in the Upper Portion of Body Cavity. (2)

NOTES

1. Strong Vital Energy: According to *Jinkui E*, Vital Energy should read "Water stagnation." (01-144)

2. You Yi: Wind is the Vital Energy of nature; the Vital Energy in this clause refers to that of human beings. The Vital Energy of both nature and human beings loses its normal function and causes the disease. Wind and Humidity are in conflict with each other. When Wind prevails, Vital Energy will follow the Wind and invade the skin, causing scabs and tinea. When Vital Energy prevails, Wind will follow the Vital Energy and stimulate the pathogenetic Water, causing an edema syndrome. When both the Vital Energy and Wind are strong, Water will follow them and cause Wind-edema. When diaphoresis is adopted, Wind will be dispersed and Water will resume its normal flow. Aversion to cold is an indication of an Exterior Deficiency. No aversion to cold accompanied by normal urination indicates prevalence of pathogenetic Cold in the Upper Portion and failure to control the Body Fluid. Consequently, copious salivation occurs.

CLAUSE 14-3

Deep-slippery pulse in the wrist indicates an edema syndrome. Wind-edema syndrome will have the symptoms and signs of a swollen face and fever. In other cases of Wind-edema, the following symptoms and signs may be observed: Puffiness of the eyelids resembling a dormant silkworm coming awake, (1) and jumping movement in the vessels on the neck. The patient coughs frequently. Edema on hands and feet is so severe that when pressed with a finger, skin will not immediately resume its original appearance. (2)

NOTES

1. Puffiness of the eyelids resembling a dormant silkworm coming awake: According to *The Pulse Classic*, this should read, "The eyelids are puffy, as if the patient has just woken up." (02-120)

2. Pulse corresponding to Wind-edema is floating. When deep-slippery pulse is observed in the wrist, it indicates that the Water is stagnated in the Interior and edema is becoming aggravated. When edema occurs above the chest and neck, flow of the Vital Energy is obstructed, and swelling of face and fever occur. While the Water soaks into the Lung, the Lung Vital Energy cannot flow normally, and coughing results. Other symptoms described in the text indicate aggravated condition of the Wind-edema. A jumping movement in the vessels on the neck becomes visible when the Water invades the Lung and the

Stomach. (02-120)

CLAUSE 14-4

Initial Yang syndrome: Floating and tense pulse usually indicates arthralgia, but the patient does not have arthralgia. He feels heavy and limp when moving any part of the body and does not experience thirst. This is a Wind-edema syndrome. One dose of a diaphoretic will cure the disease. If the patient has chills, this is due to adopting diaphoresis when the patient's health is in an extremely deficient state (1).

If the patient is thirsty but has no aversion to cold, then it is a Skin-edema syndrome.

Yellow-sweat syndrome has the following symptoms and signs: edema throughout the body, aversion to cold, symptoms resembling that of a General Obstruction syndrome (2) with suffocation in the chest, anorexia, concentrated pains in the joints, and restlessness at night that prevents the patient from falling asleep.

Coughing and wheezing without thirst is a case of Spleen-distention (3), with edema throughout the body. Treat by diaphoresis.

For the above syndromes, diaphoresis is prohibited when the following symptoms are observed: Thirst with diarrhea and frequent urination (4).

NOTES

1. Edema syndromes are generally accompanied by Deficiency of the Yang Vital Energy. If diaphoresis is adopted in an inappropriate way, the Yang Vital Energy will be further consumed. The patient's health will be further threatened, and aversion to cold will be present. (02-120)

2. General Obstruction syndrome (*Zhou bi*): A syndrome with pathogenetic factors in the Blood which causes a wandering pain throughout the body. (01-146)

3. Spleen-distention: Wu Qian wrote in *Jinjian* (p. 593) that this should read "Lung-distention." It must be a copying mistake.

4. Diaphoresis is prohibited when thirst, diarrhea and frequent urination are observed. If the Body Fluid has been exhausted by the above-mentioned symptoms, it would be dangerous to adopt diaphoretic again, which would only further exhaust the Body Fluid. (02-121)

CLAUSE 14-5

Interior-edema (1) has the symptoms of severe edema (2) throughout the entire body and the face, with deep pulse and dysuria. Dysuria is the cause of edema. Decoction of *Yuebei* adding Rhizoma Atractylodis Macrocephalae can be adopted to provide a cure.

If urination is normal, then the case is caused by loss of Body Fluid, which will in turn cause thirst.

NOTES

1. Interior-edema should be "Skin-edema," according to *The Pulse Classic*.

2. Severe edema: According to the original text, this should read "Yellow-edema." But *The Pulse Classic* records the text as "severe edema" (*Hong zhong*).

Decoction of *Yuebei* adding Rhizoma Atractylodis Macrocephalae (*Yuebei Jia Zhu Tang*):

Herba Ephedrae	6 *liang*
Gypsum Fibrosum	0.5 *jin*
Rhizoma Zingiberis Recens	3 *liang*
Radix Glycyrrhizae	2 *liang*
Rhizoma Atractylodis Macrocephalae	4 *liang*
Fructus Ziziphi Jujubae	15 pcs.

Stew briefly Herba Ephedrae in six *sheng* of water. Skim off the foam and add the remaining drugs. Stew the decoction again until three *sheng* remain. Serve the lukewarm decoction in three doses. Add one piece of Radix Aconiti Praeparata when the patient experiences an aversion to cold.

Explanation of the Prescription: This clause discusses the symptoms and treatment of Skin-edema. As the Spleen is deficient and therefore fails to move the Humidity, and because the Lung Vital Energy ceases its normal function of dredging the channels of Water flowing to the Urinary Bladder, Water stagnates in the Interior, causing severe edema throughout the entire body and face, deep pulse and dysuria. As the Lung controls the skin and hair, when its physiological activities are disturbed, Humidity cannot escape through the skin, nor can the Humidity leave the body along with the urine. Then Humidity stagnates in the Spleen and the Stomach, and pathogenetic Heat is also produced. Decoction of *Yuebei* is adopted to induce perspiration, stimulate the flow of Water and eliminate the accumulated Heat. Rhizoma Atractylodis Macrocephalae is added to disperse the Humidity in the muscles and the skin. If urination is normal, this indicates that the Body Fluid has been exhausted, rendering this prescription unnecessary. (02-126)

CASES

Case 1 (55-143):

Han, 32, female patient. After giving birth to the third baby, the patient had slight dropsy on both legs. She did not take this seriously until the syndrome was aggravated two years later. She began to feel flabby legs and could not stand. She needed help in moving only a few steps.

Examination: The patient was emaciated, depressed and thirsty. Appetite was good. When she moved, she sweat. Legs were puffy and finger print remained when they were pressed. Legs were cold and could not support the body. Pulse was huge and speedy. Tongue was red covered with greasy coating.

First treatment: Decoction of *Yuebei* adding Rhizoma Atractylodis Macrocephalae was prescribed:

Herba Ephedrae	10 grams
Gypsum Fibrosum	15 grams
Radix Glycyrrhizae	15 grams
Rhizoma Atractylodis Macrocephalae	15 grams
Poria	30 grams
Radix Stephaniae Tetrandrae	15 grams
Rhizoma Zingiberis Recens	6 grams
Fructus Ziziphi Jujubae	5 pcs.

Five doses were served. Dropsy subsided and the patient could move by herself. Urination was smooth.

Second treatment: Another five doses were given, which effectively eliminated dropsy. The patient could walk twenty to thirty steps by herself. Drugs to harmonize and tonify were given to help the patient resume activity. Also they worked.

Case 2 (64-509): Case Recorded in *Journal of Chengdu College of Chinese Medi-*

cine, 2:42, 1959

Mr. Chen, 51, first treatment on January 29. The patient had been sick for half a month.

Symptoms: Puffy face, coldness on the back, fever, perspiration, epistaxis, cough with dyspnea, chest pain, vertigo, a feeling of unsteadiness when standing, yellow-white and greasy tongue coating, tight-speedy pulse. Decoction of *Yuebei* adding Rhizoma Atractylodis Macrocephalae and others was given:

Herba Ephedrae	2 *qian*
Gypsum Fibrosum	3 *qian*
Radix Glycyrrhizae	2 *qian*
Rhizoma Atractylodis Macrocephalae	3 *qian*
Rhizoma Zingiberis Recens	3 *qian*
Poria	3 *qian*
Radix Stephaniae Tetrandrae	3 *qian*

After one dose of the decoction, dropsy began to subside. Several doses completed the treatment.

Case 3 (49-187):

Mr. Zhang, 26-year-old worker, first treatment on July 18, 1975. The patient's right arm was burned by high-pressure steam, with an affected area as large as a palm. Blisters were as big as soya-beans. There was pain, restlessness and thirst. Decoction of *Yuebei* adding Rhizoma Atractylodis Macrocephalae was prescribed:

Herba Ephedrae	10 grams
Gypsum Fibrosum	30 grams
Rhizoma Zingiberis Recens	3 slices
Radix Glycyrrhizae	6 grams
Fructus Ziziphi Jujubae	7 pcs.
Rhizoma Atractylodis Macrocephalae	12 grams
Poria	12 grams

After three doses of the decoction, the patient had smooth urination and blisters began to merge. Another three doses were given effectively.

Case 4 (49-187): Case Recorded in *Dr. Wu Jutong's Case Studies*

A female of fourteen had puffiness from head to toe. Pulse was speedy. Decoction of *Yuebei* adding Rhizoma Atractylodis Macrocephalae was prescribed:

Herba Ephedrae	5 *qian*

Rhizoma Atractylodis Macrocephalae	3 *qian*
Semen Armeniacae Amarum	5 *qian*
Gypsum Fibrosum	6 *qian*
Ramulus Cinnamomi	3 *qian*
Radix Glycyrrhizae Praeparata	1 *qian*

The decoction worked effectively.

CLAUSE 14-6

The *Fuyang* pulse, normally hidden, is now tense. This indicates the prevalence of pathogenetic Cold. *Shanjia* (1) and abdominal pain will occur. After the doctor prescribes a dose of purgative, the patient will suffer sensation of fullness in the chest and shortness of breath.

The *Fuyang* pulse, normally hidden, is now speedy. This indicates the prevalence of pathogenetic Heat. The patient will have a good digestion and frequent urination. In case dysuria is observed, edema will follow. (2)

NOTES

1. *Shanjia*: The term has two meanings. First, it refers to a case with a feeling of heat and pain in the abdomen, with a white urethral discharge. Second, it may refer to two diseases: *Shan* and *Jia*. *Shan*: acute pain in the testes with a dragging pain in the abdomen; *Jia*: abdominal mass which accumulates and disperses sporadically. (01-147)

2. Wu Qian: This clause discusses an improper treatment consisting of the application of purgatives to an edema syndrome with complications of pathogenetic Heat or Cold. The hidden pulse of the edema syndrome mentioned here is not the hidden pulse in the various positions of the wrist pulses (Inch, Bar and Cubit), but rather the hidden pulse at *Fuyang*, the Stomach pulse. If the pulse is not hidden but tense, it is due to the prevalence of pathogenetic Cold. When Water and Cold intermingle with each other, there will be abdominal pain and *Shanjia*. The doctor understood it as a case of Interior Water stagnation, and a purgative was given to disperse the Water. Once the Water is dispersed, Cold remains, and the Interior Deficiency will become more acute. That is why the patient experiences a feeling of fullness in the chest and shortness of breath. A speedy pulse indicates the prevalence of Heat. When Water and Heat intermingle, good digestion and frequent urination will occur. This is not edema. When dysuria is observed, edema will result.

CLAUSE 14-7

Pulse in the wrist is floating and slow. Floating pulse indicates existence of pathogenetic Heat. Slow pulse signifies the descent of the syndrome. When Heat and the descending pathological condition conflict with each other, this is called *Deep* (pulse).

Fuyang pulse is floating and speedy. Floating pulse indicates existence of Heat. Speedy pulse signifies a *Stop*. When Heat and *Stop* conflict with each other, this is called *Hidden* (pulse). When *Deep* and *Hidden* conflict with each other, edema results. *Deep* (pulse) indicates the Deficiency of the Collaterals; *Hidden* (pulse) indicates dysuria. When Deficiency and dysuria intermingle, edema moves to the skin. This is a case of edema. (1)

NOTES

1. Wu Qian: This clause contains many contradictions without a sufficient explanation. (05-600)

CLAUSE 14-8

Pulse on the wrist is tight and tense. Tight pulse indicates the stagnating Vital Resistance. Then aversion to cold is observed. The Water flows in the intestines. (1)

NOTES

1. Wu Qian: This clause has several omissions. No explanation is given. (05-600)

CLAUSE 14-9

Pulse of the Lesser Yin is tense and deep. Tense pulse indicates pain; deep pulse signifies a case of edema. Dysuria will result. (1)

NOTES

1. Wu Qian: This clause contains many contradictions and omissions. No explanation is given. (05-580)

CLAUSE 14-10

Deep pulse appearing at different pulse positions with edema throughout the body is a pathological condition caused by Water (1). When the pulse is evanescing (2), case will be fatal (3).

NOTES

1. Coughing and wheezing without edema and distention is a syndrome of *Tanyin* Fluid-retention. Edema without coughing and wheezing is a syndrome of Water-evil (edema). When deep pulse is sensed at different pulse positions without edema throughout the body, this is a pathological condition caused by the disorder of the Vital Energy. If edema is observed, Water-evil is the cause. As the Water stagnates in the Interior, the pulse is correspondingly deep when the Water overflows to the Exterior, resulting in edema all over the body. (05-580)

2. The pulse is evanescing: Pulse is floating and rootless which can be felt when pressed lightly and evanesces when pressed deeply. (01-147)

3. Shen Mingzong: Deep pulse indicates stagnating Vital Energy which cannot flow to the Exterior. This causes Deficiency in the Collaterals and, consequently, the Water overflows to the skin and muscles, leading to edema all over the body. This is a *Zheng*-edema syndrome, a case with excessive Yin and condensed Yang. The pulse must be extremely deep. When the pulse suddenly floats to the surface, it indicates the evanescence of the Body Resistance, indicating a fatal case. This principle is not applicable to Skin-edema and Wind-edema, as their corresponding pulses are grand and floating. (05-580)

CLAUSE 14-11

Lower eyelids of a patient suffering from a syndrome of edema are as puffy as if a silkworm were sleeping under the skin. His facial complexion is fresh and lustrous. The pulse is hidden. Other symptoms and signs are: *Xiaoke* (diabetes), enlarged and swollen abdomen caused by edema, dysuria and a deep pulse that is hardly palpable, all which indicate a case of prevalent Water. Purgative can be adopted to eliminate the Water (edema). (1)

NOTES

1. This clause discusses a case of edema, treatment of which is the adoption of a purgative. Spleen and Stomach of patients suffering from edema are generally affected by Water-Humidity. Stomach pulse passes through lower eyelids, thus when Water stagnates, eyelids will become puffy as if silkworms were sleeping there. As the skin is filled with Water, the complexion appears fresh and lustrous. Pulse of edema syndrome is generally deep; in acute cases, it is

hidden. Hidden pulse is evidence that case is worsening, and Yang Vital Energy will fail to produce the Body Fluid. *Xiaoke* (diabetes) occurs. *Xiaoke* creates great thirst, but copious drinking aggravates Water stagnation. Water stagnation in the abdomen makes the abdomen become enlarged and swollen. Yang Vital Energy cannot circulate the Water downward, and dysuria results. Patients suffering from edema with distended abdomen, dysuria and extremely deep pulse can be treated with purgatives and Water-expellent if their Body Resistance is not yet exhausted. (02-122)

Commentary: Edema can be treated with purgative and Water-expellent. But the pulse and symptoms should be observed carefully. This clause says, "Purgative *can* be adopted," indicating that it is not the only possibility. If edema is serious accompanied by abdominal distention, dysuria and extremely deep pulse, Decoction of Ten Pieces of Fructus Ziziphi Jujubae (*Shi Zao Tang*, see Clause 12-20) and Pills of Radix Stephaniae Tetrandrae, Semen Zanthoxyli, Semen Lepidii seu Descurainiae and Radix et Rhizoma Rhei (*Ji Jiao Li Huang Wan*, see Clause 12-27) can be adopted respectively. But to those cases with strong pathogenetic factors acting against weak Body Resistance, purgatives and Water-expellent cannot be tolerated by the patient. Treatment should follow the principle of warming the Yang to disperse the Water. One example of such practice is the adoption of Decoction of *Zhenwu* (see Clause 82 of *Shanghan Lun*. Ingredients are Poria, Radix Paeoniae, Rhizoma Zingiberis Recens, Rhizoma Atractylodis Macrocephalae and Radix Aconiti Praeparata) with addition of Caulis Akebiae, Radix Stephaniae Tetrandrae, and Semen Zanthoxyli. (02-122)

CLAUSE 14-12

Question: After the patient suffers a bout of diarrhea, he becomes thirsty. Other symptoms include dysuria, abdominal fullness and edema (1). Why does this happen?

Master: This is a case of edema. If urination is normal, or if perspiration is present, the patient will recover by himself (2).

NOTES

1. According to *The Pulse Classic*, "swelling of ventral genitalia" should

be added as one of the symptoms.

2. Cheng Lin: When the patient suffers from a case of diarrhea, the Spleen Vital Energy will be thoroughly exhausted and the Body Fluid seriously drained. Thus the patient becomes thirsty. When the Earth (Spleen) is weak, it loses control of the Water and dysuria results. As the Spleen is antagonistic to the Humidity, abdominal fullness results. As the Kidney dominates the Water, when it ceases its normal control, swelling of ventral genitalia is observed. This is no doubt a case of edema. When the urination returns to normal, the Water will find its way out. When the patient perspires, the Water can also be dispersed with the perspiration, which will lead to a self-cure.

CLAUSE 14-13

Edema caused by Heat-evil has the following symptoms and signs: Heaviness of bodily movement (1), shortness of breath, restlessness and irritability (2) that prevents the patient from lying quietly in bed, and swelling genitalia (3).

NOTES

1. Heaviness of bodily movement: According to *Qianjin*, this should read "edema throughout the body." (02-122)

2. Restlessness and irritability: "Restlessness and palpitation" are perhaps the correct term. (02-122)

3. You Yi: The Heart is a Viscus of a Yang nature. When it is endangered by Water, the Yang Vital Energy becomes weary and the patient experiences heaviness of bodily movement and shortness of breath. Swelling genitalia is caused by the descension of the Water following the Heart Vital Energy in its movement to join the Kidney Vital Energy (Kidney controls the genitalia).

CLAUSE 14-14

Edema caused by Liver illness has the following symptoms and signs: Edema enlarges the abdomen such that the patient experiences difficulty in moving his body and feels pain in the costal regions and abdomen. Occasionally there is secretion of saliva in his mouth and urination may return to normal. (1)

NOTES

1. You Yi: Liver illness tends to be transmitted to the Spleen. When the Spleen receives the Water from the Liver and is unable to transform it, the Water stagnates in the abdomen, swelling it so as to hinder normal movement.

As the Liver is located in the costal regions with its Vital Energy associated with the abdomen, pains in the costal regions and in the abdomen result. The Liver is characterized by rushing about and by transmission: when it rushes upward, secretion of saliva occurs; the moment it descends, urination temporarily returns to normal. (02-123)

CLAUSE 14-15

Edema caused by Lung illness has the following symptoms and signs: Edema throughout the body, dysuria and watery stool resembling duck excrement. (1)

NOTES

1. Xu Bin: The Lung dominates the circulation of the Vital Energy. When the Lung is damaged, it fails to stimulate the normal circulation and deployment throughout the body of the Vital Energy, and thus edema occurs. Urination will be normal when the Vital Energy functions normally. When the Vital Energy is not functioning smoothly, urination is no longer normal. The Lung and the Spleen are interrelated. When Spleen is not functioning normally, watery stool results. Watery stool resembles duck excrement.

CLAUSE 14-16

Edema caused by Spleen disease has the following symptoms and signs: Edema that enlarges the abdomen and makes it swell, sense of heaviness in moving the four limbs, shortness of saliva in the mouth (parched mouth), shortness of breath and dysuria. (1)

NOTES

1. You Yi: Pathological condition in the abdomen reflects pathological changes in the Spleen. The Vital Energy circulates among the extremities. When the Spleen is inhibited by Water, abdominal edema and sense of heaviness in moving the extremities will occur. Saliva (the Body Fluid) is produced by the Cereal Vital Energy. Cereal Vital Energy is determined by the Spleen. When the Spleen is weakened, the Cereal Vital Energy fails to produce Body Fluid and Vital Energy, and the patient feels parched in his mouth and short of breath. Stagnation of the Humidity causes dysuria.

CLAUSE 14-17

Edema caused by Kidney disease has the following symptoms

and signs: Edema that has caused the abdomen to enlarge and become swollen, puffy umbilicus, lumbago, dysuria, genitalia as damp as a bull's sweating nose, cold feet and leanness in the face. (1)

NOTES

1. You Yi: Region below the waist is controlled by the Kidney. When the Water invades the Kidney, lumbago, puffy umbilicus and abdominal swelling occur. Symptoms of dysuria with genitalia as damp as a bull's sweating nose and cold feet are indications of the prevalence of Yin, which is due to the fact that both the Kidney and the Humidity are of a Yin nature, leaving no room for Yang. The patient's lean face reflects the excessive activity of Yin in the lower part of the body and the evanescence of the Yang in the upper part of the body.

Commentary: Clauses 14-13 to 14-17 deal with cases of edema caused by a disorder of the Five Viscera. Considering the location and symptoms of the disease, the Liver, the Spleen and the Kidney all belong to the Yin Viscera. As they are all located in the abdomen, the pathological changes generally take place in the lower part of the body and the Interior. Thus symptoms of all three cases include abdominal edema. As the Heart and the Lung are Yang Viscera located in the chest, pathological changes generally take place in the upper part of the body and Exterior. That is why symptoms of edema throughout the body, heaviness of movement, restlessness and irritability are observed in both cases. (02-123)

CLAUSE 14-18

For all edema syndromes, when edema is observed in the region below the waist, a diuretic should be adopted; when edema only appears above the waist, diaphoretic should be adopted. (1)

NOTES

1. This clause gives the general principle of treating all edema syndromes. When edema is observed below the waist, it indicates that the Water-evil is located in the lower part of the body and in the Interior, both of a Yin nature. A diuretic should be adopted to lead the stagnant Water out with the urine. When edema is located above the waist, pathological condition is located in the upper part and the Exterior, which is Yang in nature. Diaphoretic is adopted to have the Water excreted together with the perspiration.

The principle for treating edema set down by Master Zhang Zhongjing has been proven correct. But this principle cannot be applied to the treatment of every individual case. This is due to the various interrelationship among the Viscera and the Bowels, the Exterior and the Interior, the upper part and the lower part of the body, and the influence of the affected Viscera and the Bowels on other related Viscera and Bowels. Thus it is hard to draw a clear line between adopting a diuretic or a diaphoretic. Moreover, this principle only applies to cases of an excessive nature. In sum; this principle can be put into practice on the condition that careful consideration of the specific case has been made. (02-124)

Commentary: According to Wu Qian, the diuretic and diaphoretic mentioned in the text include the following prescriptions:

Diuretics: Decoction of *Yuebei* (Clause 14-23), Decoction of Greater *Qinglong* and Decoction of Lesser *Qinglong* (Clause 12-21).

Diaphoretics: *Wuling* Powder (Clause 12-29), Decoction of Polyporus Umbellatus (Clause 13-14).

CLAUSE 14-19

Master: Pulse on the wrist is slow and deep. Deep pulse signifies a syndrome of edema; slow pulse indicates prevalence of Cold. When Cold and Water (edema) conflict with each other, *Fuyang* pulse will become hidden, which is an indication of indigestion. Deficiency of the Spleen Vital Energy will result in watery stool like duck excrement. Deficiency of the Stomach Vital Energy will cause edema throughout the body.

Pulse of Lesser Yang (1) is deep and weak, and pulse of Lesser Yin (2) is slender. In male patients, this indicates dysuria, and in female patients, amenia. Menstruation is a physiological activity involving the Blood. A menstrual disorder can cause edema. This is called edema caused by a Blood disorder. (3)

NOTES

1. Pulse of Lesser Yang: Pulse in the Cubit of the right wrist. (05-588)
2. Pulse of Lesser Yin: Pulse in the Cubit of the left wrist. (05-588)
3. You Yi: Diagnosis is based on the pulses of *Fuyang* and the wrist. It is a case with prevailing Cold and Water and stagnation of the Stomach Yang Vital Energy. When the Stomach Yang Vital Energy is dulled and fails to circulate normally, indigestion results. Without good digestion, the Spleen and the

Stomach become weary. The Spleen controls the Interior, so when the Spleen Vital Energy is weak, watery stool occurs. The Stomach controls the Exterior, so when the Stomach Vital Energy is weary, edema throughout the body occurs. Pulse of Lesser Yang reflects vitality; whereas pulse of Lesser Yin reflects the pathological condition of the lower outlet. When the Spleen and the Stomach are weary, the vitality is hindered and the lower outlet obstructed. In male patients, dysuria results and in female patients, amenia results. Both of these syndromes are caused by the stagnation of the Yang Vital Energy and the Yin Vital Essence. (05-588)

CLAUSE 14-20

Question: Edema may be caused by a Blood disorder or by pathogenetic Water. How can they be differentiated?

Master: In female patients, if amenia appears before edema, it is a case of edema caused by Blood disorder and quite difficult to treat. If edema appears before amenia, case is one of edema caused by Water-evil and thus is easily treated. Why then? First disperse the stagnant Water; then menstruation will resume.

CLAUSE 14-21

Question: The patient suffers from a case of edema with the following symptoms and signs: Dropsy in the face, extremities, and throughout the body; and dysuria. When treated, the patient ignores edema but reports chest pains and an ascending gas rushing upward to the throat, as if he had a piece of roast meat stuck in his throat. Doctor says that the patient should have a slight coughing and wheezing. Doctor is correct. What will the pulse be in such a case?

Master: Pulse in the wrist should be deep and tense. Deep pulse signifies Water, tense pulse Cold. Cold and Water conflict with each other and then stagnate at the *Guanyuan* point (1). At first, the case is mild; when the patient reaches middle age, he does not experience it. When the patient reaches the age of Yang-evanescence (2), his Nutrient Essence and Vital Resistance will no longer be in harmony. Yang becomes weary and Yin rampant, the stagnated Cold will begin to move. This stimulates the Kidney Vital Energy to ascend upward to the throat, causing a suffocating and choking feeling in the throat. Acute pain appears in the costal regions. Doctor understands this as a case of Remaining *Tanyin* Fluid-retention (*Liu yin*). Strong purgative is adopted. But the ascending gas is not reversed and the patient's condition remains unchanged. Emetic is adopted next. This makes the Stomach deficient, and sets off a feeling of restlessness. Other symptoms include parched throat with thirst, dysuria, indigestion, dropsy in the face, eyelids and extremities. Doctor then prescribes Pills of Semen Lepidii seu Descurainiae (*Tingli Wan*, prescription is lost). After taking the medicine, syndrome subsides somewhat. The patient then eats more food than he can digest. A recurrence occurs, accompanied by dropsy as serious as before, as well as pains and discomfort in the chest and the costal regions, and an ascending gas rushing upward similar to that in a case of *Bentun* (3). With the exuberant Water-evil rushing upward, the patient coughs, wheezes, and experiences adverse ascending feeling (4). Syndrome of adverse ascending should be treated first (5). Once the adverse ascending gas settles, coughing should be treated. When coughing settles, wheezing will evanesce spontaneously. Principle of the treatment is that new and acute diseases (6) should be treated first; and chronic and obstinate diseases (7) should be treated next. (8)

NOTES

1. Guanyuan (RN 4). An acupoint three inches below the umbilicus. Here *Guanyuan* indicates the Lower Portion of Body Cavity. (01-152)

2. The age of Yang-evanescence (*Yang shuai*): For male patients, this is forty-eight (the sixth eight-year cycle; for details, see *Canon of Medicine of the Yellow Emperor*). For female patients, this is thirty-five (the fifth seven-year cycle). At these ages, men and women's health begins to deteriorate, and the Yang Vital Energy begins to evanesce. (02-131)

3. *Bentun*: see Chapter VIII.

4. The symptoms are caused by the invasion of pathogenetic Water in the Lung.

5. Treatment should include prescriptions such as Decoction of Poria, Ramulus Cinnamomi, Fructus Schisandrae and Radix Glycyrrhizae. (Prescription see Clause 12-34)

6. In this case, this refers to adverse ascending gas, wheezing and coughing.

7. In this case, this refers to edema.

8. This clause is a case study of edema in which the mechanism and improper treatment of the syndrome are discussed. (02-131)

CLAUSE 14-22

Wind-edema with symptoms and signs of floating pulse, heaviness of body movement, perspiration and aversion to cold can be treated with Decoction of Radix Stephaniae Tetrandrae and Radix Astragali Hedysari. In cases wherein abdominal pain is observed, add Radix Paeoniae.

Decoction of Radix Stephaniae Tetrandrae and
Radix Astragali Hedysari*
(*Fangji Huangqi Tang*):

Radix Stephaniae Tetrandrae	1 *liang*
Radix Astragali Hedysari	1 *liang* 1 *fen*
Rhizoma Atractylodis Macrocephalae	3 *fen*
Radix Glycyrrhizae Praeparata	0.5 *liang*

Chop up five *qianbi* of the drugs per dose. Stew the drugs in one and a half cups of water with four pieces of Rhizoma Zingiberis Recens and one piece of Fructus Ziziphi Jujubae until eight *fen* remain. Filter the decoction and serve warm. A second dose can be served after a long interval.

Explanation of the Prescription: See Clause 2-22.

*This prescription also appears in Clause 2-22.

CLAUSE 14-23

Wind-edema accompanied by symptoms and signs of aversion to cold, dropsy throughout the body, floating pulse, spontaneous perspiration with neither thirst nor high fever can be treated with Decoction of *Yuebei*.

Decoction of *Yuebei*
(*Yuebei Tang*):

Herba Ephedrae	6 *liang*
Gypsum Fibrosum	0.5 *jin*
Rhizoma Zingiberis Recens	3 *liang*

Radix Glycyrrhizae	2 *liang*
Fructus Ziziphi Jujubae	15 pcs.

Stew Herba Ephedrae briefly in six *sheng* of water. Skim off the foam and add remaining drugs. Stew it until three *sheng* remain. Serve the lukewarm decoction in three doses. If aversion to cold is present, add one piece of Radix Aconiti Praeparata. For Wind-edema syndrome, add four *liang* of Rhizoma Atractylodis Macrocephalae.

Explanation of the Prescription: This is a Water-expellent with functions of dispersing the pathogenetic Water, eliminating the Heat, tonifying the Interior and the Stomach. Herba Ephedrae is used to smooth the flow of the Yang Vital Energy and disperse the Exterior syndrome. Gypsum Fibrosum eliminates the Heat. Radix Glycyrrhizae, Rhizoma Zingiberis Recens and Fructus Ziziphi Jujubae harmonize the Interior and the Exterior. Aversion to cold is a sign of the weary and deficient state of the Yang Vital Energy. Radix Aconiti Praeparata is therefore required. Rhizoma Atractylodis Macrocephalae is added to strengthen its dispersal of the Humidity. (01-153)

CASES

Case 1 (65-406):

Mr. Yao, 26-year-old farmer, first treatment on October 6, 1976. A week earlier, the patient contracted a cold, with fever and chill, headache, pain over the body and joints, parched and aching throat, cough with spitting of white phlegm. Before completely recovered, the patient worked hard. He developed dropsy face, general fatigue, lumbago, dropsy on legs, dysuria, chill and fever, pain in joints, cough, anorexia, parched feeling in mouth, pale-red tongue covered with thin, white coating, floating-speedy pulse.

Diagnosis: Syndrome caused by pathogenetic Wind invading the Lung, and loss of Water circulation, causing dropsy.

Decoction of *Yuebei* was prescribed to ventilate the Lung and disperse the Wind, eliminate the Heat and smooth the urination:

Herba Ephedrae	6 grams
Gypsum Fibrosum	16 grams
Rhizoma Imperatae	16 grams
Fructus Forsythiae	9 grams

Rhizoma Alismatis	9 grams
Semen Plantaginis	9 grams
Cortex Mori Radicis	9 grams
Talcum	12 grams
Radix Glycyrrhizae	3 grams
Rhizoma Zingiberis Recens	3 slices
Fructus Ziziphi Jujubae	3 pcs.

Second treatment on October 10. Dropsy subsided significantly when three doses of the decoction were served. Another three doses were given.

Third treatment: Dropsy subsided and urination was smooth. Another two doses of the decoction were given, one dose every other day.

Fourth treatment: All symptoms were gone. Urine test was normal.

Case 2 (48-113): Nephritic Edema

A boy of eight had puffy lower eyelids after returning from an outing one spring day. Two days later edema spread all over the body. He had swollen scrotum, fever and cough. The boy was hospitalized and antibiotics was given. Condition remained as it was. His parents consulted a doctor of Chinese medicine.

Examination: Dropsy all over the body, moderate fever with perspiration, chill, thirst, dysuria, floating pulse, thin and white tongue coating.

Diagnosis: Syndrome of Wind-edema. Decoction of *Yuebei* with additions was prescribed:

Herba Ephedrae	6 grams
Gypsum Fibrosum	30 grams
Radix Glycyrrhizae	3 grams
Rhizoma Zingiberis Recens	2 slices
Fructus Ziziphi Jujubae	5 pcs.
Herba Spirodelae	9 grams
Rhizoma Imperatae Recens	30 grams
Herba Plantaginis Recens	30 grams

Two doses of the decoction brought down fever, and edema began to retreat. Another three doses were effective. The patient's urine test was normal, and he was sent home.

Case 3 (46-262): Case Recorded in *Dr. Ding Ganren's Case Studies*

Mr. Guan had edema with dyspnea, scanty urination, thirst, floating-slippery and speedy pulse. It was a syndrome caused by pathogenetic factors over the Lung, making Wind and Water cause trouble. Decoction of *Yuebei* with additions was prescribed:

Herba Ephedrae	0.4 *qian*
Gypsum Fibrosum Praeparata	3 *qian*
Rhizoma Atractylodis Macrocephalae	1.5 *qian*
Semen Armeniacae Amarum	3 *qian*
Rhizoma Anemarrhenae	1.5 *qian*
Poria peel	3 *qian*
Pericarpium Arecae	2 *qian*
Cortex Mori Radicis	2 *qian*
Semen Benincasae	3 *qian*
Pericarpium Benincasae	3 *qian*
Cortex Zingiberis	0.5 *qian*

Case 4 (02-125): Case Recorded in Journal of *Jiangsu Chinese Medicine*, 11:2, 1965

Mr. Liu, 40-year-old farmer, first treatment on June 1954.

Examination: The patient was wearing a padded coat on a hot day. Severe dropsy on face and body, aversion to wind, fever, no perspiration, thirst, scanty urination, anorexia, cough with sputum, and dyspnea made him impossible to lie flat were the symptions.

Diagnosis: Syndrome of Wind-edema. Decoction of *Yuebei* with additions was prescribed:

Herba Ephedrae	6 *qian*
Gypsum Fibrosum	5 *qian*
Radix Glycyrrhizae	2 *qian*
Talcum (given in two servings, blend into the decoction before service)	4 *qian*
Rhizoma Zingiberis Recens	4 slices
Fructus Ziziphi Jujubae	12 pcs.

After the decoction was given, the patient was covered with quilt to keep warm. He perspired after an hour or so. Urination returned normal. The patient could breathe smoothly now. Dropsy greatly reduced. More doses were given to complete the treatment.

CLAUSE 14-24

Skin-edema with the following symptoms and signs can be treated with Decoction of Radix Stephaniae Tetrandrae and Poria: edema in the extremities, edema under the skin and slight twitching in the extremities.

Decoction of Radix Stephaniae Tetrandrae and Poria (*Fangji Fuling Tang*):

Radix Stephaniae Tetrandrae	3 *liang*
Radix Astragali Hedysari	3 *liang*
Ramulus Cinnamomi	3 *liang*
Poria	6 *liang*
Radix Glycyrrhizae	2 *liang*

Stew the drugs in six *sheng* of water until two *sheng* remain. Serve the decoction lukewarm in three doses.

Explanation of the Prescription: This clause discusses the symptoms and treatment of Skin-edema. Since the Spleen dominates the extremities, Water will stagnate in the extremities when the Spleen is in a weakened condition. Edema in the extremities hampers the normal flow of Yang Vital Energy. Antagonism between the edema and the Vital Energy manifests itself as slight twitching. Decoction of Radix Stephaniae Tetrandrae and Poria aims to facilitate the flow of the Yang Vital Energy and disperse the Water-evil from both the Interior and the Exterior. Radix Stephaniae Tetrandrae and Radix Astragali Hedysari function at the Exterior to disperse the Humidity from the skin. Ramulus Cinnamomi and Poria dredge through the Yang Vital Energy and drain the Water via the urine. When Ramulus Cinnamomi and Radix Astragali Hedysari are used together, they perform the function of dredging through the Yang, removing the Obstruction and stimulating the Vital Resistance. Radix Glycyrrhizae harmonizes the other drugs and aids Radix Astragali Hedysari in tonifying the Spleen. Once the Spleen resumes normal functioning, Water is dispersed. At the same time, the Kidney Water-evil will be regulated,* as it may have ascended and caused injury while the Spleen was weak. (02-125)

*According to the Five Evolutive phases, the Spleen checks the Kidney. Thus when the Spleen is strong, it will exercise a stronger influence over the Kidney.

CASES

Case 1 (02-126): Case Recorded in *Dr. Chen Yaogeng's Case Studies*

A boy of six suffered from severe dropsy all over the body. It first appeared in the chest, then extended all over the body and face. Abdomen was distended with lustrous skin. Finger print remained when pressed. Scrotum was swollen with dripping of urine, pulse was floating-weak, there was shortness of breath.

Diagnosis: Syndrome caused by deficient Spleen and impaired Kidney. When exposed to Wind and Cold, the syndrome flared up.

Decoction of Radix Stephaniae Tetrandrae and Poria with additions was prescribed:

Radix Stephaniae Tetrandrae	1 *qian*
Poria	1 *qian*
Radix Astragali Hedysari	1 *qian*
Ramulus Cinnamomi	6 *fen*
Radix Glycyrrhizae Praeparata	4 *fen*
Pericarpium Citri Reticulatae	6 *fen*
Pericarpium Arecae	1 *qian*

The decoction worked effectively.

Case 2 (64-536): Ascites, Case Recorded in Journal of *Jiangxi Chinese Medicine and Pharmacology*, 4:42, 1981

A boy of three and a half, first treatment in August 1979. Abdominal distention with ascitic fluid was (++). Stool was watery, sometimes with undigested food. Dropsy appeared on face and abdomen. Tongue was red, covered with thin, yellow coating. Pulse was slender-speedy.

Diagnosis: Spleen deficient.

Decoction of Radix Stephaniae Tetrandrae and Poria with additions was given.

Radix Stephaniae Tetrandrae	10 grams
Radix Astragali Hedysari	20 grams
Poria	20 grams
Rhizoma Atractylodis Macrocephalae	10 grams
Rhizoma Alismatis	10 grams
Rhizoma Imperatae	15 grams

Twenty doses of the decoction with alterations were served. Dropsy and ascites subsided significantly.

Second treatment: The same decoction was given, with addition of Herba Epimedii and Radix Codonopsis Pilosulae. Forty doses were used before ascites was totally gone.

Case 3 (65-409): Hydramnios, Case Recorded in Journal of *New Chinese Medicine* 2:16, 1977

Xiong, 24-year-old female farmer, first treatment on March 17, 1967.

In the third month of pregnancy, the patient's abdomen was bigger than normal, and became as big as a matured pregnancy by the fourth month. The patient had dyspnea, abdominal distress and scanty urination. Fetal death occurred. This was third pregnancy to end this way. When the patient was two months into her fourth pregnancy, she consulted the doctor.

Examination: The patient had good health otherwise. The pregnancy caused vertigo, trance, nausea and anorexia. Pulse was deficient-slippery and speedy. Tongue was covered with thin, white and slippery coating.

Diagnosis: The patient's frequent pregnancies had consumed her Body Resistance causing deficient Spleen and Kidney function allowing Water to accumulate as amniotic fluid.

Decoction of Radix Stephaniae Tetrandrae and Poria with additions was given to replenish the Spleen and Kidney and facilitate Water circulation:

Radix Stephaniae Tetrandrae	9 grams
Poria	12 grams
Radix Astragali Hedysari	12 grams
Radix Angelicae Sinensis	9 grams
Rhizoma Atractylodis Macrocephalae	9 grams
Semen Zanthoxyli	6 grams
Ramulus Cinnamomi	4.5 grams
Rhizoma Ligustici Chuanxiong	4.5 grams
Rhizoma Alismatis	9 grams
Pericarpium Arecae	9 grams
Semen Cuscutae	9 grams
Radix Morindae Officinalis	9 grams
Fructus Amomi	4.5 grams

Four doses were served. More than forty doses were given before delivery, which guaranteed normal labor in October 1967.

In February 1972, the patient in another pregnancy had the same tragedy in the fourth month of pregnancy, because she didn't consult her doctor again.

In June 1974, the fifth pregnancy. The patient came to the doctor in her second month and was given the same decoction, which enabled her to have her second baby normally.

CLAUSE 14-25

Syndrome of Interior-edema (1) can be treated with Decoction of *Yuebei* adding Rhizoma Atractylodis Macrocephalae, or

Decoction of Radix Glycyrrhizae and Herba Ephedrae.

NOTES

1. Interior-edema (*Li shui*): Some annotators believe this should be "Skin-edema." Treatment of Skin-edema varies in accordance with the symptoms: Skin-edema with Deficiency in the Exterior and perspiration should be treated with Decoction of Radix Stephaniae Tetrandrae and Poria (see Clause 14-24). Skin-edema with fever and Excess in the Exterior without perspiration should be treated with Decoction of *Yuebei* adding Rhizoma Atractylodis Macrocephalae. Skin-edema with no fever but with Water-evil requiring a diaphoretic for dispersal should be treated with Decoction of Radix Glycyrrhizae and Herba Ephedrae. (01-154)

Decoction of *Yuebei* adding Rhizoma Atractylodis Macrocephalae (*Yuebei Jia Zhu Tang*):

Add four *liang* of Rhizoma Atractylodis Macrocephalae to Decoction of *Yuebei* (see Clause 14-23).

Explanation of the Prescription: See Clause 14-23.

Decoction of Radix Glycyrrhizae and Herba Ephedrae (*Gancao Mahuang Tang*):

Radix Glycyrrhizae	2 *liang*
Herba Ephedrae	4 *liang*

Stew Herba Ephedrae briefly in five *sheng* of water. Skim off the foam and add Radix Glycyrrhizae. Stew the decoction again until three *sheng* remain. Serve one *sheng* of lukewarm decoction per dose. Cover the patient to induce a perspiration. If there is no perspiration, serve another dose. Keep the patient away from cold and wind.

Explanation of the Prescription: Herba Ephedrae releases the inhibited Lung Vital Energy. As the Lung is the upper source of the Water (Body Fluid), when the Lung Vital Energy is released, urination will be normal, and edema will disappear. Radix Glycyrrhizae harmonizes the Interior and reduces the excessively warm and dry quality of Herba Ephedrae. (01-155)

CASES

Case 1 (64-412): Dropsy

Chen, 25, female, first treatment on September 13, 1970. The patient had dropsy all over the body for four months, with the area below waist more serious. When pressed, finger print would remain for a long time. Symptoms: lumbago, cold feeling at waist, little urination, constipation, coldness in extremities, pallid face, pale, fat tongue covered with white coating. Pulse was deep-slender with Cubit position weak.

Diagnosis: Syndrome of dropsy caused by impaired Yang Vital Energy.

Decoction of Radix Glycyrrhizae and Herba Ephedrae with addition was given to warm and tonify the Yang and facilitate Water circulation:

Herba Ephedrae	4.5 grams
Radix Glycyrrhizae	5 grams
Radix Aconiti Praeparata	9 grams
Semen Pharbitidis	30 grams
Semen Plantaginis	12 grams

Second treatment: Five doses were served. Stool was loose and urination was smooth, reducing the dropsy. The patient felt better. The doctor prescribed the same decoction, with Herba Ephedrae reduced to 3 grams, and Radix Aconiti Praeparata to 6 grams.

Three doses were given. Then Pills of Eight-ingredients (for prescription see Chapter V, Appendix) were given to complete the treatment.

Case 2 (46-264):

In one of the annotations of the *Synopsis of the Golden Chamber*, namely, *Jinkui Jinshi* (Modern Explanation of the *Jinkui*), a malpractice of adoption of Decoction of Radix Glycyrrhizae and Herba Ephedrae was recorded:

A young doctor, Mr. Fang, treated a syndrome of Skin-edema of a patient in his sixties. After consultation, the doctor prescribed Decoction of Radix Glycyrrhizae and Herba Ephedrae. The patient died the next morning after profuse perspiration and extreme restlessness. The drug (Herba Ephedrae) was too strong a diaphoretic for an old, weak patient. Caution must be used in giving strong drugs like Herba Ephedrae to the aged and the weak.

CLAUSE 14-26

Syndrome of edema with deep and slender pulse belongs to Lesser Yin syndrome (1). Floating pulse signifies the existence of pathogenetic Wind. Syndrome of distention of a deficient nature without edema is a case of stagnation of the Vital Energy.

Treatment of edema syndrome is to adopt a diaphoretic. Edema with deep pulse should be treated with Decoction of Herba Ephedrae and Radix Aconiti Praeparata. Edema with floating pulse can be treated with Decoction of Semen Armeniacae Amarum.

NOTES

1. Lesser Yin syndrome (*Shaoyin zheng*): See Chapter V of *Shanghan Lun*.

Decoction of Herba Ephedrae and Radix Aconiti Praeparata*
(*Mahuang Fuzi Tang*):

Herba Ephedrae	3 *liang*
Radix Glycyrrhizae	2 *liang*
Radix Aconiti Praeparata	1 pc.

Stew Herba Ephedrae briefly in seven *sheng* of water. Skim off the foam and add the remaining drugs. Stew again until two and a half *sheng* remain. Serve eight *fen* of the lukewarm decoction per dose three times a day.

*This prescription also appears in Clause 302 of *Shanghan Lun* under the name of Decoction of Herba Ephedrae, Radix Aconiti Praeparata and Radix Glycyrrhizae (*Mahuang Fuzi Gancao Tang*) with slightly different dosages.

Explanation of the Prescription: Herba Ephedrae is used to clear the obstructed Exterior so as to induce perspiration. Radix Aconiti Praeparata tonifies the Yang and dredges the Channels and Collaterals. Radix Glycyrrhizae harmonizes the Interior. This prescription treats edema with Yang Deficiency. (01-155)

Decoction of Semen Armeniacae Amarum
(*Xingzi Tang*):

Prescription is lost. It may be Decoction of Herba Ephedrae, Semen Armeniacae Amarum, Radix Glycyrrhizae and Gypsum Fibrosum.*

*The original annotation gives the above prescription. Wei Litong prescribes Decoction of Herba Ephedrae, Semen Armeniacae Amarum, Radix Glycyrrhizae and Gypsum Fibrosum for a case with symptoms of a Heat nature. If Heat symptoms are not observed. Decoction of *San' ao* can be adopted.

Decoction of *San' ao* (*San' ao Tang*): Radix Glycyrrhizae, Herba Ephedrae, Semen Armeniacae Amarum. (See *Formularies of the Bureau of the People's Welfare Pharmacies.*) (01-155)

Decoction of Herba Ephedrae, Semen Armeniacae Amarum, Radix Glycyrrhizae and Gypsum Fibrosum (*Mahuang Xingren Gancao Shigao Tang*):

Herba Ephedrae	4 *liang*
Semen Armeniacae Amarum	50 pcs.
Radix Glycyrrhizae Praeparata	2 *liang*
Gypsum Fibrosum (break into small pieces, and place in a silk pouch)	0.5 *jin*

Explanation of the Prescription: See Clause 63 of *Shanghan Lun*.

CLAUSE 14-27

Skin-edema with coldness in the extremities can be treated with Powder of Ash of Pollen Typhae. (1)

(For prescription, see Clause 13-12).

NOTES

1. Wei Litong: Coldness in the extremities is caused by the Deficiency of the Vital Resistance. While the Water-evil of Skin-edema is rampant, it flows throughout the extremities; the Vital Resistance comes to a standstill and fails to circulate around the body. Without the Yang Vital Resistance, coldness in the extremities occurs.

CLAUSE 14-28

Question: Yellow-sweat syndrome is accompanied by the following symptoms and signs: swelling throughout the body (1), fever, perspiration and thirst. Symptoms similar to that of Wind-edema are also present. Sweat as yellow as juice of Cortex Phellodendri permeates the patient's clothing. The pulse is deep. What is the mechanism of the disease explained?

Master: When the patient sweats all over, he may jump into the water for a bath, at which time water will invade the body through the pores. Decoction of Radix Astragali Hedysari, Radix Paeoniae, Ramulus Cinnamomi and Vinegar can be adopted. (2)

NOTES

1. According to another edition, this phrase should read "heaviness in physical movement."

2. You Yi: Yellow-sweat is a syndrome similar to Wind-edema. It is different in that the pulse in Wind-edema is floating whereas the pulse in Yellow-sweat is deep; Wind-edema is accompanied by aversion to cold whereas Yellow-sweat does not have this symptom. Sweat as yellow as the juice of Cortex Phellodendri (bright yellow) is a symptom unique to Yellow-sweat. Wind-edema is caused when Wind-evil intermingles in the Exterior with the Water-evil. In Yellow-sweat syndrome, presence of Water-evil (edema) in the Exterior hinders the release of pathogenetic Heat. Condensed Heat conflicts with Water, making the sweat yellow.

Decoction of Radix Astragali Hedysari, Radix Paeoniae, Ramulus Cinnamomi and Vinegar
(*Huangqi Shaoyao Guizhi Kujiu Tang*):

Radix Astragali Hedysari	5 *liang*
Radix Paeoniae	3 *liang*
Ramulus Cinnamomi	3 *liang*

Stew the drugs in seven *sheng* of water and one *sheng* of *Kujiu* (vinegar) until three *sheng* remain. Serve one *sheng* of lukewarm decoction per dose. The patient will feel restless. If this dosage is maintained for six or seven days, the syndrome will subside though restlessness will not cease. This is due to obstruction caused by the vinegar.*

Explanation of the Prescription: This prescription harmonizes the Nutrient Essence with the Vital Resistance and disperses the Humidity. Ramulus Cinnamomi and Radix Paeoniae harmonize the Nutrient Essence with the Vital Resistance. Aided by *Kujiu* (vinegar), they are effective in eliminating the condensed Heat in the Nutrient Essence. Radix Astragali Hedysari leads the Humidity out through the Exterior. Once the Nutrient Essence and Vital Resistance achieve a state of harmony, the Humidity is dispersed and the Blood and the Vital Energy resume their normal flow, Yellow-sweat will evanesce. (02-128)

*You Yi: Vinegar in the prescription obstructs (slows down) the action of the drugs. Curative power of the drugs accumulates until cure is effected. The syndrome will disappear on the sixth or seventh day.

CASES

Case 1 (64-545): Case Recorded in Journal of *Shandong Chinese Medicine*, 1:34, 1982

Zhang, 22, female, first treatment on August 23, 1978. One morning the patient working hard at home had a good sweat. She cleaned herself with a cold towel and went to the cinema. When she came home, she sweats on the upper part of the body, a yellow and greasy secretion. Her shirt was stained yellow. She had general fatigue, anorexia, slight fever and retching. Menstruation was normal, urine slightly brown, sweat greasy and yellow. Tongue was in normal condition. Pulse was slippery.

Diagnosis: Syndrome of Yellow-sweat.

Decoction of Radix Astragali Hedysari, Radix Paeoniae, Ramulus Cinnamomi and Vinegar was prescribed:

Radix Astragali Hedysari	18 grams
Radix Paeoniae Alba	12 grams
Ramulus Cinnamomi	9 grams
Fructus Gardeniae	9 grams
Cortex Phellodendri	9 grams

Second treatment on August 24. After taking one dose of the decoction, yellow-sweat reduced. Another dose was given.

Third treatment on August 25. Yellow-sweat subsided. In three years, yellow-sweat never occurred again.

Case 2 (64-546): Case Recorded in Journal of *Sichuan Chinese Medicine*, 5:33, 1983

Wu, 36, female, first treatment on August 6, 1980. The patient had a cold shower after working and sweating on a mid-July day. The following day, she felt a general fatigue and vertigo and consulted the doctor. When she felt no better, she went to our hospital for treatment.

Examination: General fatigue, distended feeling in extremities, insomnia, yellow-sweat staining her shirt, thirst, shortness of breath, anorexia, palpitation, scanty urine and stool, cold feeling on both legs in tibia. Face was yellow (sclera was not yellow though), tongue was red with thin coating of yellow-white. Pulse was deep-moderate.

Diagnosis: Syndrome of Yellow-sweat.

Decoction of Radix Astragali Hedysari, Ramulus Cinnamomi and Vinegar with additions was prescribed:

Radix Astragali Hedysari	15 grams
Radix Paeoniae Alba	12 grams
Ramulus Cinnamomi	6 grams
Rhizoma Atractylodis Macrocephalae	12 grams
Semen Coicis	15 grams
Herba Artemisiae Scopariae	15 grams
Radix Ledebouriellae	6 grams
Radix Scutellariae	12 grams
Poria	12 grams

Second treatment: Three doses of the decoction were served which worked effectively. The same decoction was given in three doses, with alternations:

Subtract: Radix Ledebouriellae.

Add: Semen Dolichoris Album, 15 grams.

Syndrome was gone after the decoctions were consumed. No recurrence was reported.

CLAUSE 14-29

Yellow-sweat is accompanied by coldness in both hips. If both hips are hot, then it is a case of acute arthritis (1). If after eating a meal, the patient perspires and experiences night sweat, the case is one of a consumptive disease (2). In a case when the patient has fever following perspiration, scaly skin will be present. Continuous fever will lead to malignant boils.

The patient experiences heaviness of movement. After perspiring he may feel somewhat relaxed. When the case lasts for a long time, he will experience body twitching (3) which will lead to a chest pain. Other symptoms and signs include sweating above the waist with no sweating below the waist, and pain and limpness in the waist and hipbones as if something were stuck under the skin. In acute cases, there will be anorexia, pain and heaviness throughout the body, restlessness, irritation and dysuria, all symptoms of Yellow-sweat. Decoction of Ramulus Cinnamomi adding Radix Astragali Hedysari can be adopted.

NOTES

1. Acute arthritis (*Li jie*), see Chapter V.

2. Consumptive disease (*Xu lao*), see Chapter VI.
3. Body twitching is caused by Yang Deficiency.

(01-157)

Decoction of Ramulus Cinnamomi adding Radix Astragali Hedysari (*Guizhi Jia Huangqi Tang*):

Ramulus Cinnamomi	3 *liang*
Radix Paeoniae	3 *liang*
Radix Glycyrrhizae	2 *liang*
Rhizoma Zingiberis Recens	3 *liang*
Fructus Ziziphi Jujubae	12 pcs.
Radix Astragali Hedysari	2 *liang*

Stew the drugs in eight *sheng* of water until three *sheng* remain. Serve one *sheng* of lukewarm decoction. After a while, serve one *sheng* or more of hot porridge to assist action of the drugs. Cover the patient warmly to induce a light sweat. If there is no sweat, give another dose.

Explanation of the Prescriptions: Both Decoction of Radix Astragali Hedysari, Radix Paeoniae, Ramulus Cinnamomi and Vinegar (Clause 14-28) and this prescription are effective in treating Yellow-sweat by ventilating the Yang Vital Energy and dispersing the Water and the Humidity. In Clause 14-28, Radix Astragali Hedysari is the principal drug in the prescription, since the Exterior has become deficient due to perspiration throughout the body. Radix Astragali Hedysari is used to stabilize the Exterior. Prescription in this clause treats cases with sweating above the waist, thus Decoction of Ramulus Cinnamomi is adopted to induce a thorough perspiration. Radix Astragali Hedysari is added to tonify the Vital Energy and prevent profuse perspiration. (02-129)

CASES

Case 1 (64-550): Case Recorded in Journal of *Beijing Chinese Medicine*, 4:7, 1983

Han, 41, female, had cirrhosis of liver, diagnosed by her husband, a physician of Western medicine. Accompanying symptoms: dark complexion, moving pain in chest and flanks, swelling over Liver and Spleen regions, soreness and heaviness in hips hampering normal movement. Tongue was covered with white and greasy coating, pulse was deep-slender. Icteric index and bilirubin assay were normal. Skin and sclera were not yellow-stained. At first, no doctor asked the patient if she perspired. She told the doctor of Chinese medicine she often had perspiration with aversion to wind, with yellow-sweat staining the collar of her shirt.

Diagnosis: Syndrome of Yellow-sweat, to be treated by harmonizing the Nutrient Essence and Body Resistance, reinforce Vital Energy to stabilize Exterior defence to stop the yellow-sweat. Decoction of Ramulus Cinnamomi adding Radix Astragali Hedysari was prescribed:

Ramulus Cinnamomi	10 grams
Radix Paeoniae Alba	10 grams
Radix Glycyrrhizae Praeparata	6 grams
Rhizoma Zingiberis Recens	10 grams
Fructus Ziziphi Jujubae	4 pcs.
Radix Astragali Hedysari	10 grams

The patient was instructed to take decoction warm, then hot porridge. After that, covered herself warmly to induce perspiration.

Three doses were served. Syndrome was reduced. After six doses the patient began to walk by herself. Then liver trouble was treated.

Case 2 (65-418):

Mr. Xie, 29, first treatment on May 15, 1979. The patient had sudden pain below his right rib. At first the syndrome attacked once a year, and in recent years, the attacks were frequent. Anorexia and bitterness in mouth occurred. Two years ago, yellow-sweat appeared. Areas under the armpits were the worst affected location. The syndrome was aggravated in summer. Liver function test was normal. Pulse was slender-tight. Tip of tongue was red covered with thin, yellow coating.

Diagnosis: As costal pain appeared first, this was a syndrome caused by accumulation of Humidity-Heat of Liver-Gall Bladder system. Treatment was to eliminate and dissolve the Humidity-Heat, smooth the Liver function and remove the blood stasis.

Prescription:

Radix Bupleuri	10 grams
Radix Scutellariae	9 grams
Rhizoma Anemarrhenae	9 grams
Herba Lysimachiae	30 grams
Herba Agastachis	9 grams
Cortex Magnoliae Officinalis	12 grams

Fructus Aurantii	9 grams
Radix Glycyrrhizae Praeparata	5 grams
Radix Salviae Miltiorrhizae	15 grams
Rhizoma Corydalis	9 grams
Fructus Evodiae	4 grams
Radix Curcumae	12 grams
Radix Paeoniae Alba	12 grams

Second treatment: Six doses of the decoction were served. Costal pain was reduced. Pulse was slender-tight and speedy. Tip of tongue was red, covered with thin and white coating. The original decoction was prescribed, with alterations:

Subtract: Fructus Evodiae and Herba Agastachis.

Add: Herba Artemisiae Scopariae 15 grams, Rhizoma Ligustici Chuanxiong 9 grams.

The decoction was served for two months and the patient could go back to work for four hours a day. He was instructed to take ten doses of the decoction every month to stabilize the condition. One year later, no recurrence was reported.

Case 3 (65-419): Case Recorded in *Journal of Shandong College of Chinese Medicine*, 2:55, 1980

Zhou, 48, female farmer, first treatment in June 1979. One day in late-autumn, after working in the field, she was jumped into the river to swim. When she got home, she was attacked by cold and had puffy skin of yellow color, pitting edema, flaccid extremities, coldness on lower legs, yellow-sweat above waist, lumbago, restlessness, low fever in afternoon and dysuria.

The following decoction was prescribed:

Radix Astragali Hedysari	30 grams
Ramulus Cinnamomi	18 grams
Radix Paeoniae Alba	18 grams
Vinegar	half a cup

Mixed and divided into two servings, to be taken one in the morning, one in the evening. Six doses were served, which worked effectively. Edema was gone and skin returned to normal condition.

CLAUSE 14-30

Master: Pulse in the wrist is slow and hesitant. Slow pulse signifies existence of Cold, whereas hesitant pulse indicates the insufficiency of the Blood. *Fuyang* pulse is feeble and slow. Feeble pulse indicates weary state of the Vital Energy; slow pulse reveals prevalence of Cold. Cold and insufficiency of the Vital Energy bring about coldness in the extremities, resulting in Nutrient Essence conflicting with the Vital Resistance, which will bring about abdominal distention and a running borborygmus (1). Pathogenetic Cold will then move into the Urinary Bladder (2). Both the Nutrient Essence and the Vital Resistance are exhausted. When the Yang Vital Energy fails to circulate normally, coldness prevails in the body. When the Yin Vital Essence fails to circulate normally, numbness occurs. Only when the Yin and Yang are in harmony, can their interflow be strong enough to disperse the Cold-evil. In cases of an excessive nature, there will be repeated flatus. In cases of a deficient nature, incontinence of urination will occur (3). Such a case is caused by disorder of the Vital Energy (4).

NOTES

1. Borborygmus is a reaction to pathogenetic Cold moving in the intestine. (01-158)

2. When the pathogenetic Cold moves into the Urinary Bladder, incontinence of urination and flatus begin. (01-158)

3. Incontinence of urination is caused when the deficient Vital Energy fails to exercise its control over the Urinary Bladder. (01-158)

4. Wu Qian: The following sentence should come at the end of the clause: "Decoction of Ramulus Cinnamomi subtracting Radix Paeoniae adding Herba Ephedrae, Herba Asari and Radix Aconiti Praeparata can be adopted." (See Clause 14-31) (05-589)

CLAUSE 14-31

Edema caused by a disorder of the Vital Energy has the symptom of a hardened mass in the epigastrium the size of a plate with a round edge. This is a case caused by Water-evil. Decoction of Ramulus Cinnamomi subtracting Radix Paeoniae adding Herba Ephedrae, Herba Asari and Radix Aconiti Praeparata can be prescribed. (1)

NOTES

1. According to *Jinjian*, this clause is redundant. The prescription belongs at the end of Clause 14-30. For the treatment of the case described herein, see Clause 14-32.

Decoction of Ramulus Cinnamomi subtracting
Radix Paeoniae adding Herba Ephedrae,
Herba Asari and Radix Aconiti Praeparata
(*Guizhi Qu Shaoyao Jia Ma Xin Fuzi Tang*):

Ramulus Cinnamomi	3 *liang*
Rhizoma Zingiberis Recens	3 *liang*
Radix Glycyrrhizae	2 *liang*
Fructus Ziziphi Jujubae	12 pcs.
Herba Ephedrae	2 *liang*
Herba Asari	2 *liang*
Radix Aconiti Praeparata	1 pc.

Stew Herba Ephedrae briefly in seven *sheng* of water. Skim off the foam and add the remaining drugs. Stew again until two *sheng* remain. Serve the lukewarm decoction in three doses. Recovery will follow when the patient perspires and feels as if worms were crawling under the skin.

Explanation of the Prescription: See that under Clause 14-32.

CASES

Case 1 (65-421): Nephrotic Syndrome

Zhang, 42, female worker, suffered from nephrotic syndrome for six years. In the last six months, syndrome was aggravated: edema all over the body, with pitting edema on extremities, chest distress, panting, aversion to wind, dysuria, no perspiration, coldness on hands and tibia. Pulse was deep-slender, tongue was pink and fat, covered with thin, white coating.

Diagnosis: Syndrome caused by the deficient Kidney Yang which failed to control Water, allowing it to accumulate as edema. Normal circulation of Yang Vital Energy was hampered.

Treatment: To reinforce the Yang and help circulate stagnated Water to disperse edema. Prescription recorded in Clause 14-31 was a good cure for this syndrome:

Ramulus Cinnamomi	9 grams
Rhizoma Zingiberis Recens	12 grams
Radix Glycyrrhizae Praeparata	6 grams
Fructus Ziziphi Jujubae	5 pcs.
Herba Ephedrae	6 grams

Radix Aconiti Praeparata	9 grams
Herba Asari	3 grams
Cortex Mori Radicis	12 grams
Pericarpium Benincasae	30 grams
Polyporus Umbellatus	15 grams
Semen Plantaginis	9 grams
Poria	12 grams

After the first dose, quantity of urine increased. Second dose induced perspiration. When the third dose was given, edema was greatly reduced. Pulse was still slender, with stronger pulsation. Pink tongue was covered with thin and white coating.

Second treatment: Six doses of the decoction were given.

Third treatment: Syndrome was almost gone. Pills of Eight-ingredients (prescription see Chapter V, Appendix) were given to complete the treatment. In two years, no edema appeared again.

Case 2 (64-555): Case Recorded in Journal of *Henan Chinese Medicine*, 5:32, 1983

Mr. Zhou, 72, was still working. Two months earlier, he developed dropsy on legs and flaccid extremities. Palpitation, chest distress, anorexia, nausea and vomit were present. The patient consulted the doctor of Chinese medicine in March 1971.

Examination: Dropsy on face and pitting edema on legs accompanied by swelling scrotum. Coldness on extremities, anorexia, chest distress (without tenderness), frequent urination at night, loose stool were diagnosed. Tongue was pale-red, covered with white, slippery coating.

Diagnosis: Edema caused by Yang Deficiency of Spleen and Kidney.

Treatment: To warm the Kidney and reinforce the Yang to disperse the edema.

Prescription:

Ramulus Cinnamomi	10 grams
Radix Glycyrrhizae	6 grams
Herba Ephedrae	5 grams
Herba Asari	3 grams
Radix Aconiti Praeparata (stewed earlier than other drugs)	15 grams
Rhizoma Zingiberis Recens	10 grams
Fructus Ziziphi Jujubae	4 pcs.

Second treatment: After two doses of the decoction, edema on legs and scrotum subsided. The patient's mood was improved. Pulse was deep-slow and mightier. In the second prescription, Radix Aconiti Praeparata was increased to thirty grams (stewed thirty minutes earlier than other drugs).

Third treatment: Two doses were served. Extremities became warm and edema subsided. Appetite was improved. The doctor instructed him to rest and have low-salt diet.

Case 3 (02-130): Case Recorded in *Collection of Case Studies and Commentaries of Doctors in Fujian Province*

Lu, 24, female, suffered from edema over the body, pale face, chills and cold extremities. Pulse was deep-slow, tongue was covered with white, greasy coating. The patient had thirst but could drink little.

Diagnosis: Syndrome caused by exuberant Yin and vanishing Yang, resulting accumulation of Water. She had always had a deficient Spleen and Kidney condition.

Treatment: Decoction in Clause 14-31 was prescribed:

Ramulus Cinnamomi	3 *qian*
Herba Ephedrae	2 *qian*
Radix Glycyrrhizae	2 *qian*
Herba Asari	1 *qian*
Radix Aconiti Praeparata	2 *qian*
Rhizoma Zingiberis Recens	2 *qian*
Fructus Ziziphi Jujubae	10 pcs.

Second treatment: Two doses were served. A light perspiration was resulted. Extremities returned to normal and chills subsided. Another dose was given.

Third treatment: Syndrome was further reduced. Another dose was given. Further treatment was adopted before full recovery.

CLAUSE 14-32

A hardened mass in the epigastrium the size of a plate with a round edge is observed. This is caused by Water-evil. Decoction of Fructus Aurantii Immaturus and Rhizoma Atractylodis Macrocephalae will provide a cure.

Decoction of Fructus Aurantii Immaturus and Rhizoma Atractylodis Macrocephalae (*Zhi Zhu Tang*):

Fructus Aurantii Immaturus	7 pcs.

Rhizoma Atractylodis Macrocephalae 2 *liang*

Stew the drugs in five *sheng* of water until three *sheng* remain. Serve the decoction warm in three doses. When the abdomen becomes soft again, pathogenetic factors will have dispersed.

Explanation of the Prescriptions: For cases when a hardened mass as big as a plate appears in the epigastrium, the Master offers two prescriptions. Decoction of Ramulus Cinnamomi subtracting Radix Paeoniae adding Herba Ephedrae, Herba Asari and Radix Aconiti Praeparata is effective in softening hardened masses caused by the congelation of Yin Vital Essence. Decoction of Fructus Aurantii Immaturus and Rhizoma Atractylodis Macrocephalae is suitable for removing hardened masses caused by the stagnation of Water-evil. Other symptoms and signs appearing in the former case may include coldness in the extremities or throughout the body, pain in the bones, aversion to cold, and numbness. (02-130)

CASES

Case 1 (64-556): Case Recorded in *Collection of Case Studies and Commentaries of Doctors in Fujian Province*

A general, Mr. Wang, suffered from chest distress for eight years. A doctor was consulted. Pulse in all positions was slow-uneven. The doctor asked: "Your Majesty, are you suffering from obstruction by phlegm?"

The general replied: "No. I seldom spit phlegm. I feel distress and obstruction in chest and epigastrium after eating."

The doctor said: "Your pulse is slow and hesitant with irregular intervals, which is a sign of phlegm accumulation."

Pills of Fructus Aurantii Immaturus and Rhizoma Atractylodis Macrocephalae were prescribed. Two doses of the pills cured the ailment.

Case 2 (64-557): Case Recorded in Journal of *Henan Chinese Medicine*, 1:43, 1982

Feng, 50, female, first treatment on April 10, 1973. The patient had distention in the epigastrium, which lasted ten years. When examined, the doctor found a protruding area as big as a plate in the abdomen. When pressed, there was a jumping feeling. The patient's complexion was good, menses were normal, pulse was deep-slippery. Deep pulse indicated an Interior syndrome. Slippery pulse was a sign of Fluid accumulation. Decoction of Fructus Aurantii Immaturus and Rhizoma Atractylodis Macrocephalae was prescribed to disperse accumulation, tonify the Spleen and eliminate Water:

Fructus Aurantii Immaturus Praeparata	12 grams
Rhizoma Atractylodis Macrocephalae	12 grams

Second treatment on April 14. Four doses were served. The patient felt relief in the epigastric region and the protrusion disappeared. Another four doses were given to complete the treatment.

Appendix:

Decoction of Radix Stephaniae Tetrandrae and Radix Astragali Hedysari as recorded in *Waitai* is effective in curing Wind-edema with floating pulse, which indicates that the pathogenetic factors are resting in the Exterior. The patient may perspire on the head but there will be no other Exterior syndromes. He also experiences tenesmus. There is no disease in the region above the waist. Below the waist, edema extends to the genitalia, causing the patient great difficulty in moving his body.

(For prescription, see Clause 2-22.)

Commentary: In *Waitai*, a note under the prescription states that prescription is from *Prescriptions by Shenshi*. But this can also be traced back to Zhang Zhongjing's treatise. In *Waitai*, this prescription is given as Decoction of Radix Stephaniae Tetrandrae (*Mufangji Tang*), and contains the following ingredients:

Rhizoma Zingiberis Recens	3 *liang*
Fructus Ziziphi Jujubae	12 pcs.
Rhizoma Atractylodis Macrocephalae	4 *liang*
Radix Stephaniae Tetrandrae	4 *liang*
Radix Glycyrrhizae Praeparata	2 *liang*
Radix Astragali Hedysari	5 *liang*

CHAPTER XV

ON PULSE, SYMPTOM COMPLEX AND TREATMENT OF JAUNDICE

CLAUSE 15-1

The pulse in the wrist is floating and moderate. Floating pulse indicates the existence of Wind, whereas moderate pulse signifies an Obstruction syndrome (1), which is not a case of febrile disease caused by Wind (2). Condensed Heat will turn the patient's skin a yellowish color, since the corresponding color of the Spleen is yellow (3). The patient also experiences malaise and discomfort in the extremities. (4)

NOTES

1. Obstruction syndrome (*Bizheng*): See Chapter IX.

2. Febrile disease caused by Wind (*Zhongfeng*): See Clause 2 of *Shanghan Lun*.

3. The corresponding color of the Spleen is yellow: According to the Five Elements theory (Five Evolutive Phases, *Wuxing*), each Viscus has its own particular manifestations. See the diagram in Clause 23 of *Shanghan Lun*. Colors and organs are related as follows:

Liver — Blue
Heart — Red
Spleen— Yellow
Lung — White
Kidney— Black

4. This clause discusses the mechanism of Jaundice. Appearance of floating and moderate pulse in febrile disease signifies Exterior syndrome of a deficient nature. In many common diseases,* floating pulse signifies Wind-evil. "Wind" here can be understood as "Heat." Moderate pulse generally indicates a syndrome caused by Humidity. When Humidity and Heat intermingle and accumulate in the Exterior, Jaundice will occur. "Obstruction" means an accumulation of Heat and Humidity in the Spleen. Although the pulse is floating and moderate— also the pulse of febrile disease caused by Wind— it is actually not a febrile disease.

As the Spleen dominates the extremities and the muscle, when the Spleen is affected by Heat and Humidity, the patient feels malaise and discomfort in the extremities. When the accumulated Heat and Humidity in the Spleen invade the Blood and circulate in the Exterior, Jaundice occurs. (02-134)

*Or miscellaneous diseases.

CLAUSE 15-2

Fuyang pulse is tense and speedy. Speedy pulse indicates prevalence of Heat (1), enabling the Stomach to perform digestive function well. Tense pulse indicates prevalence of Cold (2), which will lead to abdominal distention after meals. Floating pulse in the Cubit indicates state of weakness in the Kidney (3), whereas tense pulse in *Fuyang* signifies the weakness in the Spleen (4). When Wind and Cold intermingle and conflict with each other, the patient will feel dizziness the moment he finishes his meal (5). Queasiness in the Stomach is due to murkiness (6) caused by indigestion. While this murkiness flows downward, dysuria results. When the Yin (7) is affected by Cold and the Urinary Bladder by Heat, the body will turn yellow (8). This is called Jaundice due to improper diet (*Gudan*).

Complexion on the forehead turns dark (9), and a slight perspiration is observed. The palms and arches are warm. These symptoms will become acute at dusk. The patient also suffers contraction in the Urinary Bladder (abdomen), though urination is normal. This is a case of Jaundice due to sexual intemperance (*Nulaodan*). If the abdomen is distended as if it were full of water, the case will be difficult to treat (10).

The patient feels hot and restless in the chest with anorexia and repeated nausea. This is a case of Jaundice due to overdrinking (*Jiudan*) (11).

NOTES

1. Prevalence of Heat in the Stomach. (01-162)
2. Prevalence of Cold in the Spleen. (01-162)
3. Floating pulse in the Cubit appears in cases of Jaundice due to sexual intemperance when the Kidney is deficient and affected by pathogenetic Heat. (02-135)
4. Tense pulse appearing in *Fuyang* indicates prevalence of Cold and Hu-

midity in the Spleen. This is a case of Jaundice due to improper diet. (02-135)

5. Wind and Cold intermingle and conflict with each other: Here Wind and Cold indicate the pathogenetic factors in general, and can be understood as "Humidity and Heat." When Spleen and Stomach are affected by Humidity and Heat, food is not easily digested, and the patient feels uncomfortable after meals. When the pathogenetic factor ascends, dizziness is caused; when it descends, dysuria occurs. (02-135)

6. Murkiness: This indicates the pathogenetic Humidity and Heat resting in the Stomach. (02-135)

7. Yin here indicates the Yin Vital Essence of the Spleen. (01-162)

8. The Spleen is related to pathological changes of the Humidity factor. When it is affected by Cold, the Spleen ceases its normal control of Humidity. When Cold congeals for a period of time, it will turn into pathogenetic Heat, which will then flow into the Urinary Bladder. In such circumstances, pathogenetic Heat and Humidity cannot find escape, so they turn the skin yellow. This is the pathology of Jaundice due to improper diet (*Gudan*). (01-162)

9. A dark forehead is an indication of the original color of the Kidney. When the original color of any Viscus appears on the face or on any part of the body, this indicates that the corresponding Viscus is exhausting its Vital Energy. (02-135)

10. Jaundice due to sexual intemperance is characterized by dark forehead and normal urination. From this it can be inferred that the case is not caused by Water-evil (edema is always accompanied by dysuria). The case is caused by the Deficiency of the Kidney. When the case is aggravated to the point that the abdomen is distended as if it were full of water, this signifies the exhaustion of both the Kidney and the Spleen. Such a case is difficult to treat. (02-135)

11. Jaundice due to over-drinking (*Jiudan*) is caused by over indulgence in wine. When Humidity and Heat accumulate in the chest, they will ascend to affect the Heat, resulting in restlessness. While Heat and Humidity prevail in the Stomach, the Stomach's normal function of carrying the lucid upward and the turbid downward is hampered, resulting in anorexia and nausea. (02-135)

CLAUSE 15-3*

Greater Yang syndrome with slow pulse: The patient cannot eat large quantities of food. If he does, he will experience epigastric uneasiness, dizziness and dysuria. These symptoms indicate *Gudan* (Jaundice due to improper diet). Although purgative is given, abdominal distention is unaffected. The reason is that the pulse is slow (1).

NOTES

1. Diagnosis is based principally on "slow pulse." Other symptoms and signs include white and thin tongue coating, loose stool, emotional depression, coldness in extremities, fever, but no thirst. Skin complexion is dark yellowish. This is termed Yin Jaundice (*Yin Huang*) by later annotators. Cases of Yang Jaundice (*Yang Huang*) should be accompanied by the following symptoms and signs: Restlessness, thirst, speedy pulse, red tongue with white or yellow coating, fever, reddish urine, lustrous yellowish skin. One point deserves attention: The slow pulse mentioned above must be weak; if it is slow and mighty accompanied by abdominal distention and constipation, this is a case of Greater Yang syndrome with Interior Excess. (02-136)

* This clause also appears in *Shanghan Lun* (Clause 195).

CLAUSE 15-4

Jaundice due to over-drinking will have symptoms and signs of dysuria, hot feeling in the chest and warm feeling on the arches.

CLAUSE 15-5

Jaundice due to over-drinking is not accompanied by fever. The patient is generally quiet and relaxed but experiences abdominal distention, tends to vomit, and has a parched feeling in the nasal cavities. In such cases, emetic can be adopted at first when the pulse is floating. Purgative can be given first when the pulse is deep-tight. (1)

NOTES

1. The patient is quiet and relaxed. That is to say, he experiences no hot feeling in his chest. Abdominal distention is caused when Humidity and Heat accumulate in the Stomach and the Intestine. When the pathological condition ascends, the patient tends to vomit and feels parched in his nasal cavities. In general, emetic can be adopted when the patient vomits. If there is abdominal distention, purgative should be adopted. However when both abdominal distention and vomiting are observed, either an emetic or a purgative can be used. In such cases, pulse is an important basis for diagnosis. Floating pulse is an indication that the pathological condition is located in the upper part of the body cavity. An emetic should be adopted when the pulse is floating. Deep pulse indicates that the pathological condition is located in the Interior, and a purgative can be adopted. Nevertheless, before treating the syndrome, other symptoms and signs should also be taken into consideration together with the pulse. (02-136)

CLAUSE 15-6

Jaundice due to over-drinking with a hot feeling in the chest and nausea can be treated with a dose of emetic. (1)

NOTES

1. Clauses 15-4 to 15-6 discuss syndrome of Jaundice due to over-drinking. Reading them together offers an overall understanding of the symptoms and treatment of the disease. (02-136)

CLAUSE 15-7

Jaundice due to over-drinking treated by purgative may become Black Jaundice (1) after a period of time. Black Jaundice has the symptoms of bluish eyes, dark facial complexion, and an uncomfortable hot feeling in the chest, as if the patient has eaten too much garlic. The stool is black. The skin is numb, insensate to scratching. The pulse is floating-weak. Although the skin complexion is dark, there is a slight yellow tinge. This is evidence of the pathological changes (2).

NOTES

1. Black Jaundice is a complication resulting from improper use of purgative in treating Jaundice due to over-drinking. (02-137)

2. This is evidence of the pathological changes: From the complexion, it can be inferred that Black Jaundice is a result of the improper use of a purgative in treating Jaundice due to over-drinking. (01-163)

CLAUSE 15-8

Master: Jaundice accompanied by fever, restlessness, wheezing, fullness in the chest and a parched feeling in the mouth is treated with Fire therapy (1) to induce perspiration. Heat from the Fire therapy combines with the Heat in the Interior to make the case more serious. Jaundice originates in the Humidity factor (2). The whole body will then turn yellow and hot, with a hot feeling in the abdomen indicating the prevalence of Heat in the Interior. Purgative should be adopted to eliminate the Heat.

NOTES

1. Fire therapy: Therapies include acupuncture with moxa stick, hot-needle

acupuncture or fumigation to forcibly induce perspiration. (02-137)

2. Jaundice originates in the Humidity factor: The case is acute with excessive Interior Heat, but is nevertheless related to Humidity. Without Humidity, there would be no Jaundice. Humidity is aggravated by improper application of Fire therapy. Purgative should be adopted urgently to reduce the accumulated Heat. (02-137)

CLAUSE 15-9

Deep pulse with symptoms of thirst and dysuria foretells a syndrome of Jaundice (1).

NOTES

1. Wu Qian: Deep pulse indicates that pathological condition is located in the Interior. Thirst of water serves as evidence of condensed Heat. Dysuria will cause the Humidity to accumulate in the Interior. When Humidity and Heat intermingle and accumulate in the Interior, Jaundice will occur. (05-602)

CLAUSE 15-10

Symptoms and signs of abdominal distention, restlessness, irritation which prevent the patient from falling asleep and a dull yellow complexion all over the body indicate a syndrome of Jaundice. (1)

NOTES

1. Abdominal distention is an Interior syndrome. Observed together with the other symptoms and signs described in the clause, it can be seen that the accumulated Heat is moving outward. Jaundice will follow. (05-603)

CLAUSE 15-11

Eighteen days are the length of time of a cycle of Jaundice. After receiving treatment for ten or more days, the syndrome should subside. If syndrome does not subside but becomes aggravated, the case is difficult to treat (1).

NOTES

1. Gao Shishi: The last eighteen days of each season are periods during which the Spleen Vital Energy is strong.* Ten days are a set period relating to the Earth. As Jaundice originates from disorders of the Spleen (Earth), eighteen

days will be the proper length of a cycle of Jaundice. Nevertheless, treatment should be timely. It is estimated that within ten days or so, the disease can be cured. If the syndrome does not subside, this is evidence of the exhaustion of the Spleen (Earth) Vital Energy, and will be difficult to treat. (05-606)

*See Clause 1-1.

CLAUSE 15-12

Jaundice with thirst is difficult to treat; Jaundice without thirst is curable. Jaundice originating in Yin (the Interior) will be accompanied by nausea and vomiting; Jaundice originating in Yang (the Exterior) will be accompanied by aversion to cold with trembling and fever. (1)

NOTES

1. Wu Qian: Before the onset of Jaundice the patient experiences thirst and dysuria. After the onset, if the patient is still thirsty, it demonstrates that the pathogenetic Heat has not subsided but has become more rampant, making case difficult to deal with. If the patient is no longer in great thirst of water, it demonstrates that the Heat is subsiding. Therefore it is a curable case. When Jaundice originates in Yin (the Interior), nausea and vomiting will occur. This demonstrates that the pathological condition is located in the Interior. Jaundice originating in Yang (the Exterior) will be accompanied by aversion to cold with trembling and fever, all Exterior syndromes. This clause discusses prognosis of Jaundice in relation to thirst and the presence of the Interior and Exterior syndromes as seen in the relevant symptoms and signs. (05-602)

CLAUSE 15-13

The patient has fever and chills and is reluctant to eat. If he eats, he will experience vertigo and uneasiness in his chest. This condition will last for a period of time after which his skin will turn yellow. This is Jaundice due to improper diet (*Gudan*). Decoction of Herba Artemisiae Scopariae can be adopted. (1)

NOTES

1. This clause deals with the mechanism and treatment of Jaundice due to improper diet, with prevalence of Heat and Humidity. Such Jaundice may result from climatic pathogenetic factors or from an improper diet and indigestion which will hamper the normal transmitting function of the Spleen. Humidity and Heat will then accumulate and cause a case of Jaundice. At the initial stage, fe-

ver, chills and anorexia are observed. Fever and chills mentioned here are not part of an Exterior syndrome. The vaporization of Humidity and Heat obstructs the normal flow of the Nutrient Essence and the Vital Resistance, and fever and chills appear consequently. When Humidity and Heat accumulate, the physiological function of the Spleen and the Stomach will be affected resulting in anorexia. Though reluctant to eat, the patient forces himself to eat. This will lead to indigestion, which will in turn exacerbate Humidity-Heat. Humidity and Heat cannot find a path in which to flow downward (since Spleen's function of transmission is hampered), they will ascend abnormally and cause vertigo and uneasiness in the chest. As the activity of the Vital Energy is obstructed by Humidity-Heat, urination is blocked. Dysuria hinders the outflow of Humidity and Heat. The accumulated Humidity-Heat will turn into Jaundice if it is left untreated for a long time. (02-139)

Decoction of Herba Artemisiae Scopariae*
(*Yinchenhao Tang*):

Herba Artemisiae Scopariae	6 *liang*
Fructus Gardeniae	14 pcs.
Radix et Rhizoma Rhei	2 *liang*

Stew Herba Artemisiae Scopariae in one *dou* of water until six *sheng* remain. Add remaining drugs and stew until three *sheng* remain. Filter the decoction and serve lukewarm in three doses. After taking the decoction, the patient's urine should be as red as the juice of Fructus Gleditsiae Sinensis. Abdominal distention will be reduced during the night. Jaundice leaves the body with the urine.

*This prescription also appears in *Shanghan Lun*, Clause 163.

Explanation of the Prescription: Fever and chills of Jaundice due to an improper diet come from the Interior and are dispersed at the Exterior. Thus treatment should be to eliminate Interior Humidity and Heat. Herba Artemisiae Scopariae and Fructus Gardeniae eliminate the Heat, Humidity and Jaundice. Radix et Rhizoma Rhei purges the condensed Heat and indigestion. The combination of the three drugs has the effect of expelling Jaundice from the body via the urine and stool. (01-166)

CLAUSE 15-14

Patients affected by Jaundice have fever in the afternoon (1) and chills. This is a case of Jaundice due to sexual intemperance, with symptoms and signs of abdominal distention, strain in the Urinary Bladder, yellowish complexion all over the body, dark forehead, and warmth in the arches. This will gradually turn into Black Jaundice (2). The patient's abdomen is distended as if it were full of water. The stool is black and watery. Causa morbi is overexertion in sexual activity. It is not a case of edema. Jaundice accompanied by abdominal distention is generally difficult to treat. Powder of Nitrum and Alumen can be adopted. (3)

NOTES

1. *Ribusuo* is the original wording for "afternoon," and is a period from 3:00 to 5:00 p.m.

2. Black Jaundice (*Heidan*): See Clause 15-7.

3. This clause discusses mechanism and treatment of Jaundice due to sexual intemperance with complication of blood stasis. Most Jaundice syndromes are caused by condensation and vaporization of Humidity and Heat in the Greater Yang Channel. Fever in the afternoon without chills is one of the symptoms. But in this case, afternoon fever and chills are accompanied by symptoms of abdominal distention, strain in the Urinary Bladder, yellowish complexion all over the body, dark forehead, warmth in the arches of feet, all indications of Jaundice due to sexual intemperance with pathogenetic Heat in the deficient Kidney. When melena (black stool) and watery stool are observed, disease becomes Jaundice due to sexual intemperance with complication of blood stasis. (02-140)

Powder of Nitrum and Alumen
(*Xiaoshi Fanshi San*):

Nitrum
Alumen

Pound the substances in equal quantities into powder. Take one *fangcunbi* of the powder with thin barley porridge three doses a day. Jaundice will drain out of the body along with the urine and stool. Urine should be yellow and stool black.

Explanation of the Prescription: Nitrum, salty and cold, functions in the Blood to resolve the blood stasis and disperse the Heat. Alumen, sour and salty, eliminates the Heat in the Kidney. When used together, they can disperse the Humidity-Heat and drain them from the body along with urine and stool. Mineral drugs generally have an unfavorable influence on the Stomach, thus thin barley porridge is used to wash down the drug because it can protect the Stomach and Spleen Vital Energy. (01-167)

CASES

Case 1 (64-586): Case Recorded in *Records of Chinese and Western Medicine in Combination* by Zhang Xichun

Su, lady of sixty-six, contracted Jaundice in mid-spring. The disease started when she lost her temper and was exposed to cold weather.

Examination: Skin was yellow and pupils dark yellow. Symptoms: yellow urine, white and dry stool, a feeling of heat in the chest and thirst with anorexia. Pulse on the left wrist was tight-long and hard, on the right slightly floating and mighty. Tongue was dry, covered with thin, white coating.

Diagnosis: Liver invaded by excessive Heat, cold weather made it worse. Pills of Nitrum and Alumen were prescribed, also a decoction prepared.

Prescription No. 1 (pills):

Nitrum	1 *liang*
Alumen (flour of barley, or wheat)	1 *liang*

Made pills and served two *qian* in one serving. A decoction was prepared to wash them down.

Prescription No. 2 (decoction):

Rhizoma Dioscoreae	1 *liang*
Radix Paeoniae Alba	8 *qian*
Fructus Forsythiae	3 *qian*
Talcum	3 *qian*
Fructus Gardeniae	2 *qian*
Herba Artemisiae Scopariae	2 *qian*
Radix Glycyrrhizae	2 *qian*

After the pills and decoction, one aspirin was given to induce perspiration, to disperse Exterior syndrome.

Second treatment: Four doses were given. Aspirin induced perspiration. Hot feeling and thirst subsided. The patient could eat. Stool was black. Yellow in urine and skin faded.

Case 2 (64-587): Case Recorded in Journal of *Shanghai Chinese Medicine and Pharmacology*, 7:33, 1956

Mr. Huang, 57-year-old farmer, first treatment on August 15, 1955.

Examination: The patient had yellow sclera and skin, abdominal distention, edema over the body and mental distress. He had experienced epigastric and abdominal distention for six months. Jaundice started twenty days earlier. Stool was loose, urine red, pulse soft and slender. Tongue was dry, covered with white and greasy coating. There was pitting edema on both legs. Hepatomegaly was reported.

Treatment: Powder of Nitrum and Alumen was prescribed. Treatment lasted five months, from August 15, 1955 to January 16, 1956. By September 12, ascitic fluid and jaundice subsided.

Case 3 (65-446): Acute Infective Hepatitis, Case Recorded in Journal of *Shanxi Medicine and Pharmacology*, 4:47, 1978

A girl of five suffered from acute infectious hepatitis. First treatment in October 1977.

Examination: Fever, general lassitude, anorexia, emaciation, abdominal distention, yellow urine, tenderness at right rib.

Liver function test:

GPT: 520 unit
Icteric index: 6 unit
TTT: 18 unit
TFT: + + +

Diagnosis: Acute infective hepatitis. Powder of Nitrum and Alumen prescribed:

Alumen	10 unit
Rhizoma Dioscoreae	10 unit
Nitrum	3 unit

Pounded the above drugs into powder and made pills of 1.5 grams each with honey. Served two pills, three times a day.

Ten days of treatment worked effectively. Symptoms subsided.

Recheck of the liver function:

GPT: under 100 unit
Icteric index: 7 unit
TFT: (—)

CLAUSE 15-15

Jaundice due to over-drinking accompanied by symptoms of restlessness and irritation in the Heart or pain and hot feelings can be treated with Decoction of Fructus Gardeniae and Radix et Rhizoma Rhei. (1)

NOTES

1. This clause discusses syndrome and treatment of Jaundice due to overdrinking. Restlessness and irritation will appear in cases of Jaundice due to overdrinking. When such feelings become aggravated, the patient experiences pain and hot feelings, indicating rampant excessive Heat in the Stomach. Decoction of Fructus Gardeniae and Radix et Rhizoma Rhei is adopted to eliminate the excessive Heat. According to the ingredients in the prescription, it can be inferred that the following symptoms should be present: fever, restlessness preventing the patient from falling asleep, constipation, dysuria and skin as yellow as an orange. (02-141)

Decoction of Fructus Gardeniae and Radix et Rhizoma Rhei (*Zhizi Dahuang Tang*):

Fructus Gardeniae	14 pcs.
Radix et Rhizoma Rhei	1 *liang*
Fructus Aurantii Immaturus	5 pcs.
Semen Sojae Praeparatum	1 *sheng*

Stew the drugs in six *sheng* of water until two *sheng* remain. Serve the decoction lukewarm in three doses.

Explanation of the Prescription: This prescription treats Jaundice with a prevailing syndrome of a Heat and excessive nature. Its efficacy is similar to that of Decoction of Herba Artemisiae Scopariae, the prescriptions are not the same. Comparatively speaking, Decoction of Fructus Gardeniae has a stronger efficacy of harmonizing the Stomach to ease restlessness; whereas Decoction of Herba Artemisiae Scopariae has a stronger function of loosing the bowels and eliminating the Humidity. Pathological condition in the former case is located in the epigastrium (the Stomach), and the latter in the abdomen (Intestines). In Decoction of Fructus Gardeniae and Radix et Rhizoma Rhei, Fructus Gardeniae and Semen Sojae Praeparatum eliminate the accumulated Heat in the Heart (the Stomach). Radix et Rhizoma Rhei and Fructus Aurantii Immaturus are used to clear away the indigestion and turbidity in the Stomach and the Intestine. (02-141)

CASES

Case 1 (65-448): Case Recorded in *Collection of Classified Cases of Famous Doctors in China*

Mr. Wan, 64, an alcohol addict. One hot, humid, mid-summer day, the patient drank too much and Jaundice developed. Fever, dark-yellow complexion, thirst of water, dysuria and constipation followed. The patient was confined to bed, and the doctor was sent for.

Diagnosis: Pulse in all positions was deep-excessive and speedy. Tongue coating was yellow and dry. It was a Jaundice caused by excessive Humidity and Heat. The following decoction was prescribed:

Fructus Gardeniae	9 grams
Radix et Rhizoma Rhei	9 grams
Herba Artemisiae Scopariae	30 grams
Cortex Magnoliae Officinalis	4.5 grams
Caulis Akebiae	4.5 grams

Second treatment: Two doses were served. Stool and urination returned to normal. Jaundice was subsiding. Pulse was becoming moderate. The same decoction was prescribed, with alterations:

Subtract: Caulis Akebiae.

Add: Poria 9 grams, *Liu Yi San* (powder of Talcum and Radix Glycyrrhizae, ratioed 6:1) 12 grams.

Third treatment: Two doses were given. Jaundice reduced. As the patient was old, the following alterations were made to make the decoction milder:

Subtract: Radix et Rhizoma Rhei.

Add: Semen Coicis 12 grams.

CLAUSE 15-16

General therapy in all cases of Jaundice is the adoption of a diuretic. If pulse is floating, diaphoretic should be adopted. Decoction of Ramulus Cinnamomi adding Radix Astragali Hedysari will provide a cure. (1)

(For prescription, see Clause 14-29).

NOTES

1. This clause discusses the general principles of treating Jaundice at its onset. Generally speaking, dysuria is the causa morbi of Jaundice. This is due to the pathological changes which take place when the Vital Energy ceases its normal function of promoting the urination. When dysuria is present, the accumulated Humidity and Heat cannot escape and turn into Jaundice. Thus the

conventional treatment is to adopt a diuretic. But there are exceptions. At the onset of Jaundice, the patient experiences chills and fever with spontaneous perspiration and floating pulse; this is an Exterior syndrome unrelated to the Interior condensed Heat. The diaphoretic, Decoction of Ramulus Cinnamomi, should be adopted to harmonize the Nutrient Essence with the Vital Resistance and dispel the Exterior syndrome. Radix Astragali Hedysari is added to assist the Body Resistance in its efforts to disperse the pathological condition. (02-141)

CLAUSE 15-17

Decoction of Lard and Human Hair can be adopted in all cases of Jaundice. (1)

NOTES

1. This prescription is not effective for all cases of Jaundice. It is not applicable in cases of Jaundice caused by the condensation of Humidity and Heat. It is only effective for Jaundice caused by accumulation of Dryness. At first, Humidity-Heat condensation was the causa morbi but after a long period of time, they turn into Dryness. Other symptoms will include abdominal distention and constipation. (02-142)

Decoction of Lard and Human Hair
(*Zhugao Fa Jian*):

Lard	0.5 *jin*
Human hair*	3 egg-size balls

Place the human hair in the lard. Stew until hair dissolves. Serve the decoction in two doses. Pathogenetic factor will be excreted with the urine.

*Human hair, according to a case study as quoted on page 142 of *Jinkui S*, should be "ash of human hair" (Crinis Carbonisatus).

CASES

Case 1 (51-392):

Doctor Xu Zhongke recorded in his *Case Studies* the treatment of Jaundice with Decoction of Lard and Human Hair:

Mr. Luo suffered from jaundice with enlarged abdomen. He had tried many decoctions but got no relief. He consulted me. I prescribed:

Lard	4 *liang*
Crinis Carbonisatus	4 *liang*

One dose of the decoction worked.

CLAUSE 15-18

Powder of Herba Artemisiae Scopariae and *Wuling* can be adopted to treat the syndrome of Jaundice. (1)

NOTES

1. According to another edition, this clause reads, "Decoction of Herba Artemisiae Scopariae and *Wuling* Powder can be adopted to treat the syndrome of Jaundice."

Decoction of Herba Artemisiae Scopariae: See Clause 15-13.

Wuling Powder: See Clause 12-29.

Powder of Herba Artemisiae Scopariae and *Wuling*
(*Yinchen Wuling San*):

Powder of Herba Artemisiae Scopariae	10 *fen*
Wuling Powder	5 *fen*

Combine the powders and take one *fangcunbi* before meal per dose three times a day.

Explanation of the Prescription: This is a prescription for the initial stage of Jaundice accompanied by symptoms and signs of fever and chills, anorexia and dysuria. The prescription is designed to eliminate Heat and disperse the Water and Humidity. From the ingredients it can be inferred that this is a case of Jaundice with serious Humidity-evil and slight Interior Heat. (02-142)

CASES

Case 1 (51-393): Case Recorded in *Collection of Case Studies of Doctors in Hubei Province*

Mr. Hong's son, nine years old, first treatment in autumn 1951. The boy liked to sit on damp ground to play and had suffered indigestion for a long time. His skin turned yellow and his pupils bright yellow. He had dropsy appeared on feet and face, flaccid extremities, reluctance to move, anorexia, thirst, scanty and reddish urine, white and slippery tongue coating, moderate and weak pulse. This lasted twenty days before consultation with the doctor.

Diagnosis: Jaundice caused by excess Humidity and weak Spleen. Powder of Herba Artemisiae Scopariae and *Wuling* was prescribed:

Herba Artemisiae Scopariae	9 grams
Ramulus Cinnamomi	3 grams
Rhizoma Atractylodis Macrocephalae	3 grams
Poria	6 grams
Rhizoma Alismatis	6 grams
Polyporus Umbellatus	3 grams

The doctor instructed that one dose (in three servings) of drugs be served consecutively per day. After two doses, Jaundice began to retreat. The sixth dose cured the ailment.

Case 2 (64-594): Case Recorded in *Collection of Case Studies of Veteran Doctors in Hunan Province*

Mr. Jin, 54, suffered from diarrhea for a long time. Then he had indigestion, Jaundice on face and pupils and extremities. Other symptoms were: vertigo, epigastric distress, abdominal distention, puffy extremities, anorexia, scanty and yellow urine, soft and moderate pulse, tongue covered with thick and greasy coating.

Diagnosis: Syndrome caused by rampage of Humidity due to the impaired condition of Spleen and Stomach.

Treatment: To reinforce the Yang, to motivate Spleen function and disperse Jaundice.

Prescription:

Herba Artemisiae Scopariae	15 grams
Polyporus Umbellatus	10 grams
Rhizoma Alismatis	6 grams
Poria	10 grams
Rhizoma Atractylodis Macrocephalae	10 grams
Cortex Cinnamomi	3 grams

Second treatment: Ten doses of the decoction were served. Jaundice, abdominal distention and dropsy subsided. Another ten doses of the decoction with minor alterations were given, which worked effectively.

Third treatment: All symptoms subsided. There was slight abdominal distention and appetite not good. The following decoction was prescribed to tonify the Spleen and regulate the flow of the Vital Energy:

Radix Codonopsis Pilosulae	12 grams
Rhizoma Atractylodis Macrocephalae	10 grams
Rhizoma Zingiberis	6 grams
Fructus Aurantii Immaturus	6 grams
Herba Artemisiae Scopariae	12 grams
Radix Glycyrrhizae	3 grams
Fructus Ziziphi Jujubae	3 pcs.

The syndrome was gone after several doses.

CLAUSE 15-19

Syndrome of Jaundice accompanied by symptoms and signs of abdominal distention, dysuria with reddish urine, and spontaneous perspiration is a case with harmonious Exterior (1) and Excess in the Interior. A purgative should be adopted. Decoction of Radix et Rhizoma Rhei and Nitrum will provide a cure.

NOTES

1. Harmonious Exterior means there is no Exterior syndrome such as chills and fever, etc.

Decoction of Radix et Rhizoma Rhei and Nitrum
(*Dahuang Xiaoshi Tang*):

Radix et Rhizoma Rhei	4 *liang*
Cortex Phellodendri	4 *liang*
Fructus Gardeniae	15 pcs.
Nitrum	4 *liang*

Stew the first three herbs in six *sheng* of water until two *sheng* remain. Filter the decoction and add Nitrum. Stew again until one *sheng* remains. Serve the decoction in a single dose.

Explanation of the Prescription: Jaundice accompanied by abdominal distention and dysuria with reddish urine is caused by rampant Humidity and Heat in the Interior. Spontaneous perspiration indicates there are no exogenous pathogenetic factors in the Interior. Interior Excess caused by rampant Humidity and Heat should be treated with a purgative. Decoction of Radix et Rhizoma Rhei and Nitrum is effective in such cases. Radix et Rhizoma Rhei eliminates the Excess and fullness. Cortex Phellodendri and Fructus Gardeniae eliminate the Humidity and the Heat. Nitrum disperses the sensation of fullness and distention. (01-169)

CASES

Case 1 (02-143):

A gentleman suffering from Jaundice had received treatment by several doctors, but the disease was no better. The syndrome lasted a few months when the patient's skin was darker yellow, resembling the color of an orange. Pupils were yellow, urine scanty and yellow. The patient was restless and short of breath. When the doctor pressed the patient's ribcage, the color did not disperse. Syndrome was severe Jaundice. Combination of Decoction of Herba Artemisiae Scopariae, and Decoction of Radix et Rhizoma Rhei and Nitrum in large dosage was prescribed. The decoction was administered three to four times a day. Treatment lasted 30 days. Jaundice retreated and urination returned to normal.

Case 2 (64-598): Case Recorded in Journal of *Hubei Chinese Medicine*, 6:27, 1981

Mr. Guo, 48, suffered from Jaundice. Symptoms: Fever and chill (later fever and sweat on head), vertigo, nausea, restlessness, thirst, lower abdominal distention, tenderness on ribcage, no stool for four days, bright-yellow skin, scanty urine, slippery-speedy and mighty pulse.

Diagnosis: Jaundice caused by accumulation of Humidity and Heat.

Combination of Decoction of Radix et Rhizoma Rhei, Nitrum and Decoction of Herba Artemisiae Scopariae was prescribed:

Herba Artemisiae Scopariae	18 grams
Fructus Gardeniae	18 grams
Radix et Rhizoma Rhei	9 grams
Cortex Phellodendri	9 grams
Natrii Sulfas	9 grams
Poria	18 grams
Semen Dolichoris Album	18 grams

Second treatment: Five doses were administered. Stool and urine returned to normal. In the next treatment, the same decoction was prescribed, with alterations:

Subtract: Radix et Rhizoma Rhei and Natrii Sulfas.

Add: Radix Bupleuri 6 grams, Radix Gentianae 5 grams.

Eight doses were administered and in two weeks, the patient returned to work.

CLAUSE 15-20

Jaundice with urine of a normal color, abdominal distention, wheezing and a tendency to loose stool should not be treated with drugs in cold quality to eliminate the Heat. Adoption of drugs of a cold quality to eliminate the Heat will bring about nausea. Decoction of Lesser Rhizoma Pinelliae (see Clause 12-26) is a good cure for nausea. (1)

NOTES

1. Decoction of Lesser Rhizoma Pinelliae treats one of the complications resulting from improper treatment of Jaundice, and not the syndrome of Jaundice itself. When nausea appears with Jaundice as a result of improper treatment, Decoction of Lesser Rhizoma Pinelliae can be adopted. In treating serious cases, Radix Ginseng can be added to the prescription. (02-143)

CLAUSE 15-21

Syndrome of Jaundice with abdominal pain and nausea can be treated with Decoction of Radix Bupleuri. (This is very likely Decoction of Lesser Radix Bupleuri, see Clause 17-15.) (1)

NOTES

1. Wu Qian: Nausea and abdominal pain indicate the prevalence of excessive Heat in the Stomach. However, before adopting Decoction of Greater Radix Bupleuri (see Clause 10-12), tidal fever and constipation should be observed. If there is no tidal fever or constipation, Decoction of Lesser Radix Bupleuri subtracting Radix Scutellariae adding Radix Paeoniae can be adopted to act as a harmonizer. (05-611)

CLAUSE 15-22

In male patients, Jaundice with normal urination should be treated with Decoction of Lesser *Jianzhong* to tonify the Deficiency. (1)

(For prescription, see Clause 6-13.)

NOTES

1. This clause discusses the treatment of Jaundice due to Deficiency and consumptive disease. Patients who suffer from Jaundice generally have dysuria. But in this case, urination is normal, indicating the prevalence of Interior Deficiency. Such Jaundice is caused by the Deficiency of the Blood and the Stomach. Female patients may also have such Jaundice. Treatment should follow that given in consumptive diseases. See also Clause 6-13 and Clause 100 of *Shanghan Lun*. (02-144)

Appendix:

Decoction of Pedicellus Melo is effective in treating syndrome of Jaundice.

Prescription see Clause 2-27.

Decoction of Herba Ephedrae and Wine is effective in treating syndrome of Jaundice.

Decoction of Herba Ephedrae and Wine (from *Qianjin*)
(*Mahuang Chunjiu Tang*):

Herba Ephedrae 3 *liang*

Stew Herba Ephedrae in five *sheng* of rice wine until two and a half *sheng* remain. Serve the decoction in one dose. In winter, wine should be used. In spring, water can be used.

Explanation of the Prescription: This prescription is effective for Jaundice with accumulated Humidity-Heat at the Exterior as well as Exterior Cold. (01-170)

CHAPTER XVI

ON PULSE, SYMPTOM COMPLEX AND TREATMENT OF CONVULSIONS AND PALPITATION, HEMATEMESIS, EPISTAXIS, HEMATOCHEZIA, CHEST FULLNESS AND BLOOD STASIS

CLAUSE 16-1

Pulse in the wrist is moving and weak. Moving pulse indicates convulsions. Weak pulse indicates palpitations.

Remark: This chapter deals principally with syndromes and treatment of cases caused by Blood disorders. Only two clauses deal with convulsions and palpitation (Clauses 16-1 and 16-13). Chest fullness is a symptom that may occur in syndromes caused by Blood disorders. But since they are related to cases caused by Blood disorder or to the Heart (the Heart dominates the Blood), they are included in the same chapter. (01-172)

CLAUSE 16-2

Master: Pulse in the Cubit is floating. Eyeballs are yellowish with blurred vision. Epistaxis occurs occasionally. When yellowish color in the eyeballs fades and the vision returns to normal, epistaxis will cease. (1)

NOTES

1. You Yi: Floating pulse in the Cubit indicates the existence of pathogenetic Fire in the Kidney. Yellowish eyeballs reflects condensed Heat in the Liver. Epistaxis will not cease under such conditions. The Blood is of a Yin character. When it is forced out by the Heat-evil in the Kidney and the Liver, it ascends abnormally and will most likely cause epistaxis. When yellowish color fades and the vision returns to normal, this reflects the subsiding of the

pathogenetic Heat in both the Kidney and the Liver, and thus epistaxis will cease.

CLAUSE 16-3

The Master says: Epistaxis in spring and summer belong to the category of Initial Yang syndromes; epistaxis in autumn and winter belong to the category of Greater Yang syndromes. (1)

NOTES

1. Some annotators explain this clause as follows: Initial Yang syndromes are Exterior syndromes. During spring and summer, the Yang Vital Energy floats and rests in the Exterior. Epistaxis during this period results from a disorder of the Initial Yang Channel. The Greater Yang syndromes are Interior syndromes. During autumn and winter, Yang Vital Energy hides in the Interior. Epistaxis at this time must result from a disorder of the Greater Yang Channel. The Initial Yang syndromes generally include syndromes of the Exterior (described in Chapter I of *Shanghan Lun*). Etiology of the Greater Yang syndromes may include:

a) Diseases caused by exhaustion of the Body Fluid in the Viscera and the Bowels;

b) Diseases caused by scorching of the pathogenetic Heat in the Three Portions of Body Cavity, and

c) Diseases caused by excessive Heat in the Greater Yang Channel.

Nevertheless, in most cases of epistaxis, Heat is always the principal pathological condition. In treating specific cases, a thorough analysis should be carried out before making final diagnosis. (01-173)

CLAUSE 16-4*

Diaphoresis is not recommended for patients who suffer from frequent epistaxis. If it is adopted, the veins on the patient's forehead will be tense and protruding, his eyeballs will be motionless and he will suffer from insomnia (1).

NOTES

1. Patients with frequent epistaxis suffer loss of blood. Further loss of Nutrient Essence (Blood) through perspiration will obviously bring about syndromes stated in the clause. (04-52)

*This clause also appears in Clause 86 of *Shanghan Lun*.

CLAUSE 16-5

The patient's face is pale but he has no fever or chills. Epistaxis will occur when deep-tight pulse is diagnosed. In other cases, pulse is floating and weak (1). When pressed deeply, the pulse disappears, indicating a case of hematochezia. Restlessness and coughing indicate a case of hematemesis.

NOTES

1. Wu Qian: Pulses in these two sentences are out of order. It should read, "... Epistaxis will occur when *floating-tight* pulse is diagnosed. In other cases, the pulse is *deep and weak*." Thus, pulse and symptoms could agree. This must be a copying mistake. (05-551)

CLAUSE 16-6

Case is fatal when the patient has hematemesis with coughing, inspiratory dyspnea, fever, speedy pulse and restlessness that prevents him from lying quietly in bed. (1)

NOTES

1. This clause discusses the prognosis of hematemesis. Hematemesis not only consumes the Blood, but also exhausts the Vital Energy. Fever and speedy pulse in a patient suffering loss of blood (hematemesis) is an indication of a gravely deficient state of the Blood and the gradual loss of the Vital Energy. Coughing, inspiratory dyspnea and restlessness that prevents the patient from lying quietly are indications of the exhaustion of the Yin and evanescence of the Yang. Prognosis is extremely unfavorable. (02-148)

CLAUSE 16-7

Coughing in a patient who frequently drinks (wine) will lead to hematemesis, especially a patient drinks to excess and too often (1).

NOTES

1. A patient who drinks frequently will have excessive Heat in the Lung and the Stomach. Prolonged coughing will injure the tissues of the Lung. Hematemesis and spitting of blood will follow. (01-174)

CLAUSE 16-8*

The pulse is tight and huge. When pressed deeply, it is not as strong as a true tight pulse. Though huge, it is void within. Such pulse is called "void-tight." Tight pulse of reduced strength indicates prevalence of pathogenetic Cold. Void pulse reflects Interior Deficiency. When void-tight pulse occurs in female patients, this indicates premature delivery or mild, chronic bloody vaginal discharge. In male patients, it indicates loss of blood and sperm.

CLAUSE 16-9**

Diaphoresis is not recommended for those who suffer from frequent hemorrhaging. If it is adopted, there will be perspiration, trembling, shivering and chills. (1)

NOTES

1. Patients who suffer from hemorrhaging are deficient and weak in Yin Vital Essence. Even though Exterior syndromes are present, diaphoresis is prohibited. If diaphoresis is given, the Blood will be further exhausted. At the same time, the Yang Vital Energy will evanesce along with the Body Fluid and evanescence of the Yang will occur. When tendons and veins are no longer nourished and warmed by the Yang Vital Energy, trembling and shivering with chills will occur. (02-149)

*Text of this clause also appears in Clause 6-12.

**This clause also appears in Clause 87 of *Shanghan Lun*.

CLAUSE 16-10

The patient experiences a sense of fullness in the chest, withered lips, bluish tongue and parched mouth. He is thirsty but merely holds the water in his mouth with no intention of swallowing it. He has no fever or chills. He has no abdominal distention but claims to be suffering from this. His pulse is feeble, huge and slow (1). This is a case of blood stasis. (2)

NOTES

1. His pulse is feeble, huge and slow: Though appearing huge, this pulse lacks strength. It beats slowly and hesitantly. (02-149)

2. This clause discusses the pulse and symptoms of cases caused by blood

stasis. Blood stasis will obstruct the normal flow of Vital Energy resulting in fullness in the chest. Blood stasis in the Interior hampers supply of fresh blood to the lips and tongue, resulting in withered lips and bluish tongue. Flow of Body Fluid is also hampered, thus the patient's mouth is parched. As this is caused not by the exhaustion of the Body Fluid but by blood stasis, which blocks normal circulation of Body Fluid, the patient needs only to hold water in his mouth to moisten the dryness and does not need to swallow it. "No fever or chills" is evidence that the case is not caused by climatic pathogenetic factors. The patient has no abdominal distention but claims to have such a symptom. He feels a distention in his abdomen but this cannot be located. This distention is caused by the stagnation of Vital Energy resulting from blood stasis. It is neither caused by indigestion nor edema. (02-149)

CLAUSE 16-11

Symptoms and signs are similar to those in a case of a Heat nature, with restlessness, sensation of fullness, thirst and parched mouth. But the pulse does not suggest a case of a Heat nature (1). This is called "hidden Yin" (*Yin fu*), a case caused by blood stasis. A purgative which can remove the blood stasis should be adopted (2).

NOTES

1. Pulses of a Yang nature, such as floating, speedy, grand and excessive, generally suggest cases of a Yang (Heat) nature. Pulses of a Yin nature, such as slow, feeble, deficient and weak, generally reflect cases of a Yin (Cold) nature. The pulse mentioned in this clause must be of a Yin nature, which is contradictory to the symptoms.

2. The patient feels symptoms of a Heat nature, though the pulse reflects no Heat syndrome. It can then be inferred that the Heat is concealed in the Blood. The Vital Energy is not affected. Treatment should follow the principle of removing the blood stasis. Once the stasis is removed, the condensed Heat will also diminish. (02-149)

CLAUSE 16-12

Syndrome caused by Scorching therapy (1) can be treated with Decoction of Ramulus Cinnamomi *Jiuni*.

NOTES

1. Syndrome caused by Scorching therapy: Symptoms and signs are not given in this clause. Clause 112 of *Shanghan Lun* is a similar clause in which

symptoms and signs are recorded as follows:

"Febrile disease caused by Cold, floating pulse: Scorching therapy used as diaphoresis will cause loss of Yang (*Wang Yang*). Manic behavior, irritation and restlessness will occur. To cure this syndrome, Decoction of Ramulus Cinnamomi *Jiuni* can be adopted."

Decoction of Ramulus Cinnamomi *Jiuni*
(*Guizhi Jiuni Tang*):

Ramulus Cinnamomi	3 *liang*
Radix Glycyrrhizae Praeparata	2 *liang*
Rhizoma Zingiberis Recens	3 *liang*
Concha Ostreae	5 *liang*
Os Draconis	4 *liang*
Fructus Ziziphi Jujubae	12 pcs.
Ramulus et Folium Dichroae	3 *liang*

Stew Ramulus et Folium Dichroae in one *dou* and two *sheng* of water until one *dou* remains. Pound remaining drugs into powder and add to the decoction. Stew again until three *sheng* remain. Filter the decoction and serve one *sheng* of lukewarm decoction as a dose.

Explanation of the Prescription: This prescription treats convulsions caused by Scorching therapy. When the patient is scorched to induce a perspiration, the Heart Yang is injured. Palpitations, convulsions and irritation, manic behavior and restlessness that prevent the patient from lying quietly will occur. Decoction of Ramulus Cinnamomi (substract Radix Paeoniae, as it is of a softening and Yin nature) is used to assist the Heart Yang. Os Draconis and Concha Ostreae are added to reduce the convulsions and irritation. When Heart Yang is deficient, phlegm is likely to accumulate in the chest. Ramulus et Folium Dichroae clears the phlegm. As the prescription is applicable to cases with acute symptoms of convulsions and manic behavior, it is called *Jiuni* ("rescuing the adversity"). This prescription is applicable to all cases with the above-mentioned symptoms and signs, whether or not they are caused by Scorching therapy. (02-150)

CLAUSE 16-13

Palpitations can be treated with Pills of Rhizoma Pinelliae and Herba Ephedrae. (1)

NOTES

1. This clause discusses the treatment of palpitations due to Water-evil. When the Water stagnates in the Interior, it will ascend and invade the Heart, affecting the Yang Vital Energy in the Heart. Palpitations result. Pills of Rhizoma Pinelliae and Herba Ephedrae eliminate the Fluid-retention and reverse the adversity. But the strength of the drugs should be controlled to some extent to protect the Yang Vital Energy. Thus the drug is made in pill form to provide a slow and continuous delivery. (02-150)

Pills of Rhizoma Pinelliae and Herba Ephedrae
(*Banxia Mahuang Wan*):

Rhizoma Pinelliae
Herba Ephedrae

Pound the drugs in equal quantities into powder. Blend with honey and form pills the size of Semen Phaseoli. Take three pills per dose three times a day.

Explanation of the Prescription: This prescription is applicable to syndromes of palpitation caused by Fluid-retention stagnating in the epigastrium. Rhizoma Pinelliae disperses the Fluid-retention and reverses the adversity. Herba Ephedrae in pill form will not act as a diaphoretic, but will regulate the Heart Yang and assist Rhizoma Pinelliae in dispersing the Fluid. Once the Fluid is eliminated, palpitations will subside. (01-176)

CASES

Case 1 (46-306) Case Recorded in *Mr. Zhang Yiqing's Case Studies*:

Mr. Zhang had palpitation and an empty feeling in the chest. Pulse was slender and soft, but slippery at the right Bar position. This was a syndrome caused by stagnation of phlegm-Water in the chest and accumulation of Humidity in lower body cavity with the Heart Yang floating at the upper portion, resulting in palpitation.

Prescription:

Rhizoma Pinelliae Praeparata
Semen Armeniacae Amarum Praeparata
Poria
Pericarpium Citri Reticulatae
Bulbus Allii Aacrostemi
Juice of Rhizoma Zingiberis Recens

CLAUSE 16-14

Syndrom es with repeated hematemesis can be treated with Decoction of Cacumen Biotae.

Decoction of Cacumen Biotae
(*Boye Tang*):

Cacumen Biotae	3 *liang*
Rhizoma Zingiberis	3 *liang*
Folium Artemisiae Argyi	3 bundles

Add one *sheng* of liquid taken from horse faeces* to five *sheng* of water. Add drugs and stew until one *sheng* remains. Serve the lukewarm decoction in two doses.

*Liquid taken from horse faeces was used in ancient times to stop bleeding. In modern practice, children's urine (especially that of boys under the age of ten) is used as a replacement. In order to strengthen the action of hemostasis, the three drugs used in this prescription can be first processed by stir-frying. (02-150)
According to *Jinkui E*, "liquid of horse faeces" here is "horse urine." (p. 177)

Explanation of the Prescription: Xu Bin: "Repeated hematemesis" suggests that drugs of a cold quality with hemostatic qualities were adopted but did not succeed in curing the hematemesis. Hematemesis resulting from Yang Deficiency suggests that the blood is flowing outside of its normal channels. Loss of blood will also cause the Yin to become deficient. Thus Cacumen Biotae, one of the best Yin-tonifiers, is adopted as the principal ingredient in the prescription. Folium Artemisiae Argyi assists the principal drug and helps the blood return to its normal channels. Rhizoma Zingiberis warms the Stomach. Liquid from horse faeces compels the pathogenetic Fire to descend. Boy's urine can be used to replace liquid from horse faeces.

CASES

Case 1 (46-308):

Mr. Peng, 43, suffered from bronchiectasis with spitting of blood. The patient had a history of tuberculosis. Generally, such a syndrome is due to deficient Yin and Heat in the Blood, and should be treated by nourishing the Yin and clearing Heat in the Lung. In this case, the cough with spitting of thin phlegm and a chill were different. Tongue was covered with a thin, white coating. Pulse was deep-moderate. This was a syndrome caused by deficient and cold Lung Vital Energy which lost control of the Blood. Decoction of Cacumen Biotae was given to warm the Lung and control the loss of blood:

Cacumen Biotae	12 grams
Rhizoma Zingiberis (carbonated)	5 grams
Folium Artemisiae Argyi	3 grams
Boy's urine (blend into the decoction before service)	1 cup

Two doses were administered. Hematemesis stopped.

Second treatment: Decoction of *Liu Jun Zi* was prescribed, with additions:

Pericarpium Citri Reticulatae
Rhizoma Pinelliae
Poria
Radix Glycyrrhizae
Radix Ginseng
Rhizoma Atractylodis Macrocephalae
Rhizoma Zingiberis
Herba Asari
Fructus Schisandrae

Three doses were administered. Cough subsided and appetite improved. The syndrome was alleviated.

Case 2 (48-467):

Mr. Wang, 42, suffered from gastric ulcer for more than five years and had hematemesis three times. The night before cousultation, the patient vomited a cup of coffee-like blood with dregs of food. He had several hematemesis of small quantity. Black feces were found in the stool. He was pale and depressed. Tongue was pale red, with tooth prints on edge. Pulse was soft-slender and speedy. It was a syndrome caused by deficient Interior Vital Energy, which lost control of Blood. Decoction of Cacumen Biotae with additions was given:

Cacumen Biotae	12 grams
Rhizoma Zingiberis (carbonated)	4.5 grams
Folium Artemisiae Argyi (carbonated)	9 grams
Os Spiellae	12 grams
Bulbus Fritillariae Thunbergii	9 grams
Rhizoma Bletillae	9 grams
Lignum Dalbergiae Odoriferae	6 grams
Fructus Perillae	9 grams
Powder of Radix Notoginseng (blend into the decoction before service)	3 grams

After two doses of decoction, hematemesis stopped. Decoction of *Liu Jun Zi* was given as a harmonizer of the Interior conditions.

Case 3 (48-468): Case Recorded in Journal of *New Chinese Medicine*, Vol. 4, 1975

The journal reported case studies of successful treatment with Decoction of Cacumen Biotae of eight cases of hematemesis in pulmonary tuberculosis. One case described as follows:

Mr. Xie, 33, first treatment on June 19, 1972. The patient suffered from pulmonary tuberculosis for eight years. In the last eight months, he had bloody sputum. The morning of June 10, he had dyspnea and spat large quantity of blood sputum (more than 300 ml). Other symptoms: fever, shortness of breath, insomnia, pallid face with rosy cheeks, pain in chest and epigastrium, loose stool, tastelessness in mouth, pale-red and fat tongue covered with thin, yellow coating, weak, speedy pulse. Decoction of Cacumen Biotae was prescribed:

Cacumen Biotae	15 grams
Rhizoma Zingiberis	9 grams
Folium Artemisiae Argyi	9 grams
Boy's urine (blend into the decoction before service)	50 ml

Three doses were served. The patient felt better and bloody sputum was reduced in quantity. The morning of June 11, he had only 10 ml bloody sputum. Stool was in good shape.

Second treatment: Nine grams of Colla Corii Asini were blended into the decoction. Eight doses were consumed. Bloody sputum that had lasted eight months was gone. Ten days later the patient was sent home.

CLAUSE 16-15

In a case of hematochezia, blood is observed after the stool. This is called "Distant hematochezia" (*Yuan xue*). Decoction of Loess can be adopted.

Decoction of Loess
(*Huangtu Tang*):
Also effective in curing hematemesis and epistaxis.

Radix Glycyrrhizae	3 *liang*
Radix Rehmanniae	3 *liang*
Rhizoma Atractylodis Macrocephalae	3 *liang*
Radix Aconiti Praeparata	3 *liang*
Colla Corii Asini	3 *liang*
Radix Scutellariae	3 *liang*
Loess (taken from an earthen stove)	0.5 *jin*

Stew the drugs in eight *sheng* of water until three *sheng* remain. Serve the lukewarm decoction in two doses.

Explanation of the Prescription: This prescription is effective in curing hematochezia of a Cold and deficient nature. Blood after the stool comes from above the rectum and is called "Distant hematochezia" (distant from the anus). This is due to weakened Spleen when Vital Energy is damaged by Cold and Deficiency. The blood seeps into the intestine. (The Spleen controls Blood circulation). Decoction of Loess warms the Spleen and controls the Blood. Loess taken from an earthen stove has the function of warming the Interior, astringing the loose bowels and stopping the bleeding. Assisted by Radix Aconiti Praeparata and Rhizoma Atractylodis Macrocephalae, they have the function of warming the Yang and tonifying the Spleen. Radix Rehmanniae and Colla Corii Asini tonify the Blood and stop the bleeding. Radix Glycyrrhizae harmonizes the Interior. Radix Scutellariae, bitter and cold, is adopted to prevent the bleeding that may result from adopting drugs of a warm and dry quality. (02-151)

CASES

Case 1 (48-444):

Mr. Song, 43, had hematochezia after having a stool with dark purple blood. This lasted two years.

Examination: Pallid and puffy face, palpitation, trance, reluctance to speak, anorexia, edema in both legs and useless extremities. Abdomen was cold, inviting pressure. Tongue was pale covered with thin coating. Pulse was slender-weak and strengthless.

Decoction of Loess with alterations was given to warm the Spleen and control the Blood:

Radix Codonopsis Pilosulae	15 grams
Rhizoma Atractylodis Macrocephalae	12 grams
Radix Aconiti Praeparata	6 grams
Colla Corii Asini (blend into the decoction before service)	9 grams
Rhizoma Rehmanniae Praeparata	12 grams
Radix Glycyrrhizae	3 grams
Rhizoma Zingiberis Praeparata	6 grams
Loess	30 grams

Stewed Loess separately, filtered the decoction and the rest of drugs.

Decoction was served seven consecutive days. Hematochezia stopped and dropsy subsided. Drugs to harmonize the Spleen was given to stabilize the condition.

Case 2 (48-445):

Mr. Xu, 52, had a gastric ulcer and suffered from a vague epigastric pain and acid regurgitation. The night before consultation, melena occurred on two occasions. Test of occult blood was (+ + +). Other symptoms: pale face, vertigo, aversion to cold, general lassitude, tenderness in epigastrium, pale tongue with purple edge, covered with white, slippery coating, slender-weak pulse.

Warm drugs were needed to stop the bleeding. Decoction of Loess was prescribed:

Rhizoma Atractylodis Macrocephalae Praeparata	12 grams
Radix Aconiti Praeparata	6 grams
Halloysitum Rubrum	30 grams
Rhizoma Zingiberis Praeparata	6 grams
Colla Corii Asini (blend into the decoction before service)	9 grams
Os Spiellae Usta	30 grams

Radix Codonopsis Pilosulae	15 grams
Fructus Ziziphi Jujubae	4 pcs.

After five doses of the decoction, hematochezia subsided. Drugs to harmonize the Interior and tonify the Vital Energy were given to complete the treatment.

Case 3 (48-445):

Mr. Liang, 42, had suffered from hematemesis and epistaxis for a week. Nasal cavity was parched. The patient became restless, felt hot at night, had palpitation, shortness of breath and insomnia. Tongue was covered with white and slippery coating. Pulse was deep and weak.

Diagnosis: Syndrom caused by pathological condition of Spleen Deficiency and Stomach Excess. Treatment was to tonify the Spleen, reinforce the Vital Energy, eliminate the Fire in Stomach and moisten the Yin. The following decoction was prescribed:

Radix Rehmanniae	18 grams
Radix Scutellariae	9 grams
Rhizoma Atractylodis Macrocephalae	12 grams
Radix Glycyrrhizae	9 grams
Colla Corii Asini	9 grams
Halloysitum Rubrum	15 grams
Rhizoma Zingiberis (carbonated)	3 grams
Cacumen Biotae (carbonated)	12 grams
Rhizoma Imperatae	12 grams

Three doses were served. Symptoms subsided. Another three doses were given to stabilize condition.

CLAUSE 16-16

In cases of hematochezia, blood is observed before the stool. This is called "Near hematochezia" (*Jin xue*). Powder of Radix Angelicae Sinensis and Semen Phaseoli can be adopted. (1)

(Prescription see Clause 3-13.)

NOTES

1. Hematochezia in this clause is caused by Humidity-Heat-evil. Bleeding before stool is called "Near hematochezia" (near to the anus). Etiology is as follows: When Humidity-Heat accumulating in the large intestine prevails, it will force the blood to seep downward, causing "Near hematochezia." (02-152)

CLAUSE 16-17

Decoction of *Xiexin* is effective in syndromes with symptoms of restlessness (1), hematemesis and epistaxis.

NOTES

1. Restlessness: The original text is "Deficiency of the Heart Vital Energy" (*Xin Qi Bu Zu*). This may be a copying error. *Qianjin* gives it as "restlessness" (*Xin Qi Bu Ding*). (02-152)

Decoction of *Xiexin*
(*Xiexin Tang*):
Also effective in treating Cholera (*Huoluan*).*

Radix et Rhizoma Rhei	2 *liang*
Rhizoma Coptidis	1 *liang*
Radix Scutellariae	1 *liang*

Stew the drugs in three *sheng* of water until one *sheng* remains. Serve the decoction in a single draft.

Explanation of the Prescription: This prescription is applicable in cases of epistaxis and hematemesis due to a prevalence of excessive Heat. All three drugs are bitter and cold and can eliminate the exuberant Heat. Once the Heat descends, bleeding will cease. (02-152)

*According to some annotators, "also effective in treating Cholera (*Huoluan*)" should be deleted, as the prescription is not suitable in such cases.

CHAPTER XVII

ON PULSE, SYMPTOM COMPLEX AND TREATMENT OF NAUSEA AND VOMITING, RETCHING AND DIARRHEA

CLAUSE 17-1*

A patient constantly suffering from nausea and vomiting should not be treated with antiemetic if vomit includes purulent substances. Once the patient vomits up all of these substances, vomiting will stop. (1)

NOTES

1. Diagnosis should be made to discover cause of presence of purulent substance, and proper therapy should be adopted to eliminate the pus. (04-214)

* This clause also appears in *Shanghan Lun* (Clause 376).

CLAUSE 17-2

The patient first experiences nausea and vomiting followed by thirst. This indicates incipient self-cure (1). When the patient experiences thirst before nausea and vomiting, this indicates Fluid-retention in the epigastrium. This is a Fluid-retention syndrome (2). Under normal conditions, the patient experiencing nausea and vomiting should feel thirsty. When *Zhiyin* Fluid-retention (3) is located in the epigastrium, the patient will not feel thirsty. This is a *Zhiyin* Fluid-retention syndrome.

NOTES

1. The patient first experiences nausea and vomiting followed by thirst. This indicates that the Fluid-retention is rejected and the Stomach Yang Vital Energy restored. Thus self-cure is sure to follow. (02-155)

2. When the patient experiences thirst before nausea and vomiting, this in-

dicates Fluid-retention in the epigastrium, which hampers the normal circulation of Body Fluid in the mouth, resulting in thirst. To quench the thirst, the patient drinks a lot of water, which only aggravates Fluid-retention. Excessive Fluid-retention then ascends abnormally and causes nausea and vomiting. Because such nausea and vomiting are caused by Fluid-retention, the text states, "This is a Fluid-retention syndrome." (02-155)

3. *Zhiyin* Fluid-retention: See Chapter XII.

CLAUSE 17-3

Question: Speedy pulse indicates Interior Heat which normally promotes digestion and whets the appetite. But the patient experiences nausea and vomiting. Why does this happen?

Master: Diaphoresis has weakened the Yang Vital Energy and caused Deficiency in the diaphragm (1). A speedy pulse represents a "Guest Heat" (2) which cannot aid digestion. So cold and deficient Stomach causes nausea and vomiting (3). Tight pulse is diagnosed, which indicates a Deficiency. When the Stomach Vital Energy is exhausted, the patient will vomit the food eaten during the morning in the evening. This is called "Stomach Regurgitation" (*Wei fan*), resulting from the adoption of purgatives while pathogenetic Cold prevails in the upper part of the body (4). The pulse will turn tight. This is a case of Deficiency.

NOTES

1. Deficiency in the diaphragm (*Ge qi xu*) is a Deficiency of the Yang Vital Energy of the Heart and the Spleen. (04-75)

2. Guest Heat, or false Heat (*Ke re*): "Guest" is the opposite of "host," and generally indicates pathogenetic Heat caused by climatic factors (Exterior pathogens). Here the Guest Heat is of a deficient type. (04-75)

3. The above text also appears in Clause 122 of *Shanghan Lun*.

4. While pathogenetic Cold prevails in the upper part of the body, a purgative should not be adopted. It is an incorrect treatment. So the pulse becomes tight and deficient. (01-181)

CLAUSE 17-4

Pulse in the wrist is feeble and speedy. Feeble pulse demonstrates weary state of the Vital Resistance, which will cause the Nutrient Essence to become deficient. Deficient Nutrient Essence reflects insufficiency of the Blood, which will in turn give the patient a sensation of cold in the chest. (1)

NOTES

1. The Vital Energy is the dominant factor in the Nutrient Essence. When the Vital Energy is weak, the Nutrient Essence will be deficient. The Nutrient Essence is the source of the Blood. So deficient Nutrient Essence will bring about Blood insufficiency. Both the Vital Energy and Body Resistance are weakened; this is the cause of the cold feeling in the chest, which also reflects an insufficiency in the Yang Vital Energy of the Upper Portion of Body Cavity. Such a Deficiency also influences the Middle Portion, causing Stomach troubles and bringing with it cold and feeling of Deficiency, nausea and vomiting. The speedy pulse mentioned here is an indication of a false Heat. Feeble pulse is the principal manifestation in the diagnosis of the disease. (01-182)

CLAUSE 17-5

Fuyang pulse is floating and hesitant. Floating pulse indicates Deficiency (of the Stomach Vital Energy), whereas hesitant pulse signifies injured Spleen. When the Spleen is hurt, digestion is also hampered. So the patient vomits the food eaten during the morning in the evening, or vomits the food eaten at nigh the next morning. Indigestion prevails in the Stomach. This is a case of Stomach Regurgitation. When the pulse is tense-hesitant, the case will be difficult to treat. (1)

NOTES

1. When the pulse is tense-hesitant, the case will be difficult to treat: Tense pulse indicates prevalence of Cold and Yin in the Interior; hesitant pulse is evidence of the exhaustion of the Vital Energy, the Blood, the Body Fluid and the Spleen Yin. Therefore the case is difficult to treat. (01-182)

CLAUSE 17-6

No purgative should be adopted for patients who tend to vomit. (1)

NOTES

1. Treatment should be made in accordance with the specific conditions. When the patient tends to vomit, this shows that the pathological condition is located in the Upper Portion and is being dispersed by the Body Resistance. Treatment should follow the principle of easing the pathogenetic factor out from

the nearest channel (when pathogenetic factor is in the chest, vomiting is the easiest way out). When purgative is incorrectly adopted, it will not arrive at the location of the disease but lead the pathogenetic factors drain into the Interior, most likely causing complications. (02-156)

CLAUSE 17-7*

When nausea and abdominal distention are observed, diagnosis should be made by examining the front and the back (1). Therapy should facilitate the normal functioning. (2)

NOTES

1. The front and the back: urine and stool. (01-182)

2. Nausea in this clause is of an excessive nature. Either dysuria or constipation may be the cause of nausea and abdominal distention. (04-216)

* This clause also appears in *Shanghan Lun* (Clause 381).

CLAUSE 17-8

Decoction of Fructus Evodiae can be adopted for cases with nausea and fullness in the chest.

Decoction of Fructus Evodiae*
(*Zhuyu Tang*):

Fructus Evodiae	1 *sheng*
Radix Ginseng	3 *liang*
Rhizoma Zingiberis Recens	6 *liang*
Fructus Ziziphi Jujubae	12 pcs.

Stew the drugs in five *sheng* of water until three *sheng* remain. Serve seven *ge* of the lukewarm decoction per dose three times a day.

*This prescription also appears in Clause 243 of *Shanghan Lun*.

Explanation of the Prescription: Decoction of Fructus Evodiae treats Cold-evil congealed in the chest and the diaphragm. It has the function of relieving nausea caused by the prevalence of Cold-evil. When the Cold is dispersed, fullness will evanesce. Once, fullness evanesces, nausea diminishes. Fructus Evodiae disperses the Cold and reverses the adverse feeling. Rhizoma Zingiberis Recens warms the Interior. Radix Ginseng tonifies the Vital Energy. Fructus Ziziphi Jujubae tonifies the Spleen. (01-183)

CLAUSE 17-9*

Decoction of Fructus Evodiae is effective in curing nausea with saliva and headache. (1)

NOTES

1. Headache here is one of the symptoms of the Liver Channel syndrome of the Foot Greater Yin. It is located on the top of the head and on the forehead. Decoction of Fructus Evodiae warms and disperses the Cold and the Fluid-retention, as well as reverses the adverse feelings originating in the Liver. (01-183)

*This clause also appears in Clause 378 of *Shanghan Lun*.

CLAUSE 17-10

Decoction of Rhizoma Pinelliae *Xiexin* can be adopted for syndromes with the following symptoms and signs: Nausea and vomiting with borborygmus and Vital-energy Stagnation in the epigastrium.

Decoction of Rhizoma Pinelliae *Xiexin**
(*Banxia Xiexin Tang*):

Rhizoma Pinelliae	0.5 *sheng*
Radix Scutellariae	3 *liang*
Rhizoma Zingiberis	3 *liang*
Radix Ginseng	3 *liang*
Rhizoma Coptidis	1 *liang*
Fructus Ziziphi Jujubae	12 pcs.
Radix Glycyrrhizae Praeparata	3 *liang*

Stew the drugs in one *dou* of water until six *sheng* remain. Filter the decoction and stew again until three *sheng* remain. Serve one *sheng* of lukewarm decoction per dose three times a day.

*This prescription also appears in *Shanghan Lun*, Clause 149.

Explanation of the Prescription: This prescription treats nausea and vomiting caused by the intermingling of pathogenetic Cold and Heat. When pathogenetic factors sink into the Interior at a time while Deficiency prevails, Cold and Heat intermingle in the Stomach. This will cause the Middle Portion to become blocked. Vital-energy Stagnation will occur in the epigastrium. Normal ascending and descending functions are disturbed. When the Stomach Vital Energy ascends, nausea results. Borborygmus results when the Spleen ceases to exercise function of transmission. Decoction of Rhizoma Pinelliae *Xiexin* harmonizes the Interior and tonifies the Stomach. Radix Scutellariae and Rhizoma Coptidis eliminate the Heat. Rhizoma Pinelliae and Rhizoma Zingiberis reverse the adverse ascending and stop the nausea. Radix Ginseng, Radix Glycyrrhizae and Fructus Ziziphi Jujubae tonify the Interior Vital Energy. (02-160)

CLAUSE 17-11

Decoction of Radix Scutellariae adding Rhizoma Pinelliae and Rhizoma Zingiberis Recens can be adopted in cases with retching and diarrhea. (1)

NOTES

1. See Clause 172 of *Shanghan Lun*. The two clauses are closely linked.

Decoction of Radix Scutellariae adding Rhizoma Pinelliae and Rhizoma Zingiberis Recens (*Huangqin Jia Banxia Shengjiang Tang*):

Radix Scutellariae	3 *liang*
Radix Glycyrrhizae Praeparata	2 *liang*
Radix Paeoniae	2 *liang*
Rhizoma Pinelliae	0.5 *sheng*
Rhizoma Zingiberis Recens	3 *liang*
Fructus Ziziphi Jujubae	12 pcs.

Stew the drugs in one *dou* of water until three *sheng* remain.

Filter the decoction and serve one *sheng* of lukewarm decoction per dose, two doses during the day and one at night.

Explanation of the Prescription: This is a basic prescription for treating disorders of the Stomach. Retching is caused by ascending pathogenetic Heat whereas diarrhea results when Heat descends. This prescription eliminates the Heat and disperses the pathogenetic factors, eliminating the phlegm and sensation of fullness and harmonizing the Stomach to stop the nausea. Radix Scutellariae eliminates the Heat. Radix Paeoniae astringes the Yin. Radix Glycyrrhizae and Fructus Ziziphi Jujubae harmonize the Interior. Rhizoma Pinelliae eliminates the phlegm. Rhizoma Zingiberis Recens reverses the adverse feeling and stops the retching. (01-184)

You Yi: *Shanghan Lun* (Clause 172) analyses a case with retching and diarrhea caused by ascending and descending of pathogenetic Heat. In miscellaneous diseases, Fire originating in the Liver and the Stomach may also ascend and descend, causing retching and diarrhea. Rhizoma Pinelliae and Rhizoma Zingiberis Recens disperse the adversity in the Upper Portion. Radix Scutellariae and Radix Paeoniae eliminate the Heat in the Interior. When the Upper and the Lower Portions are affected at the same time, the Vital Energy in the Middle Portion will be in a disturbed condition. For this reason Radix Glycyrrhizae, Fructus Ziziphi Jujubae, assisted by Radix Paeoniae and Rhizoma Zingiberis Recens, are used to tranquilize the Interior and tonify the Body Resistance.

CLAUSE 17-12

The patient suffers nausea and vomiting. He cannot swallow what he has eaten. He should be given a dose of Decoction of Lesser Rhizoma Pinelliae to treat the syndrome. (1)

(For prescription, see Clause 12-26.)

NOTES

1. This clause discusses the treatment of nausea and vomiting caused by various pathological changes. Most cases of nausea and vomiting are caused by an abnormal ascending of the Stomach Vital Energy. The Stomach is an internal organ characterized by acceptance and digestion. Descending is its normal

movement. An ascent suggests a disorder of the Stomach Vital Energy. Nausea and vomiting that prevent the patient from swallowing what he has eaten will occur. Decoction of Lesser Rhizoma Pinelliae that has the function of reversing the adversity and stopping the nausea is therefore taken as a treat. (02-161)

CLAUSE 17-13

When the pathogenetic factors are located above the diaphragm, the patient suffers from nausea and vomiting. After vomiting, if the patient is thirsty, it is a sign of recovery and the patient should be served water immediately. If the patient is still thirsty after he is given water, Powder of Polyporus Umbellatus can be adopted.

Powder of Polyporus Umbellatus
(*Zhuling San*):

Polyporus Umbellatus
Poria
Rhizoma Atractylodis Macrocephalae

Pound the drugs in equal amounts into powder. Take one *fangcunbi* per dose three times a day.

Explanation of the Prescription: After repeated vomiting, the Stomach Vital Energy is seriously damaged and cannot resume normal functioning. In case too much water is given, Fluid-retention may occur. Powder of Polyporus Umbellatus is therefore adopted to tonify the Spleen and promote the normal distribution of Water. Polyporus Umbellatus is a Water-expellent. Poria tonifies the Spleen and facilitates Water circulation. Rhizoma Atractylodis Macrocephalae is added to tonify the Spleen. (01-185)

CASES

Case 1 (64-662): Case Recorded in *Collection of Case Studies of Veteran Doctors in Hunan Province*

Mr. Liu, 26, had an acute abdominal pain with severe distention, no stool and great thirst. When he drank a cup of tea, he would vomit a few moments later. After vomiting, he began to drink more tea, and vomited the water. Doctors of Western medicine diagnosed "intussusception," which required surgery. The patient was hesitant to have surgery. Syndrome was aggravated on the third day. A doctor of Chinese medicine was called.

Examination: Pulse was deep-tense and slippery.

Treatment: Powder of Polyporus Umbellatus (in decoction form) was prescribed:

Rhizoma Atractylodis Macrocephalae	5 *qian*
Poria	5 *qian*
Polyporus Umbellatus	5 *qian*

One dose of the decoction worked effectively in subduing the vomit and quenching the thirst. There was a smooth stool.

Second treatment: Decoction of Radix Aconiti Praeparata and Semen Oryzae Nonglutinosae (prescription see Clause 10-10) was prescribed. Abdominal pain and distention were gone.

CLAUSE 17-14*

Case will be difficult to treat if the following symptoms and signs are observed: Nausea and vomiting, weak pulse, normal urination, slight fever and coldness in the extremities. Decoction of *Sini* can be adopted to cure the case. (1)

NOTES

1. This is a case of nausea and vomiting caused by excessive Yin and deficient Yang. Excessive Essence Yin makes the pulse weak and urination normal. When it resists the Yang, nausea and vomiting with a slight fever results. Coldness in the extremities is caused by Deficiency of the Yang Vital Energy. Decoction of *Sini* is used to warm the Interior and rescue the Yang Vital Energy. (04-214)

Decoction of *Sini***
(*Sini Tang*):

Radix Aconiti	1 pc.
Rhizoma Zingiberis	1.5 *liang*
Radix Glycyrrhizae Praeparata	2 *liang*

*This clause also appears in *Shanghan Lun* (Clause 377).

**This prescription also appears in *Shanghan Lun* (Clause 29).

Second treatment on January 14. Vomit and cough were subsiding. Another four doses were given, which worked miraculously.

CLAUSE 17-17

Immediately after eating, food is vomited up. Such cases can be treated with Decoction of Radix et Rhizoma Rhei and Radix Glycyrrhizae (1).

NOTES

1. *Waitai* says this prescription is also effective for "vomiting water."

Decoction of Radix et Rhizoma Rhei and Radix Glycyrrhizae (*Dahuang Gancao Tang*):

Radix et Rhizoma Rhei	4 *liang*
Radix Glycyrrhizae	1 *liang*

Stew the drugs in three *sheng* of water until one *sheng* remains. Serve the decoction lukewarm in two doses.

Explanation of the Prescription: This prescription treats nausea and vomiting that occur immediately after the eating. Causa morbi is the prevalence of excessive Heat in the Stomach and the Intestine. Radix et Rhizoma Rhei eliminates the excessive Heat and clears the indigestion and turbid elements in the Stomach and the Intestine. Once the excessive Heat is eliminated and indigestion cleared away, nausea and vomiting, though not treated directly, will evanesce. This therapy treats the Lower Portion to heal the disease at the Upper Portion (*Shang Bing Xia Zhi*). (01-187)

CASES

Case 1 (62-398):

Mr. Li, 20, first treatment on November 10, 1971. The patient had repeated vomiting in the last fifteen days with epigastric pain, a hot feeling and constipation. Tongue was red and dry, covered with thin-yellow coating. Pulse was excessive and mighty as a whole but slippery at Bar position on the right wrist.

Diagnosis: Heat in the Lung transmitted to the Stomach, causing vomit. Drugs to clear the Heat and harmonize the Stomach were adopted.

Second treatment on November 12. The treatment did not work. After taking the decoction, the patient would vomit what he had eaten (this was new to the patient). Bad breath, pain, distention and a hot feeling in epigastrium, scanty, yellow urine were reported. There was no stool for three days. Tongue was slippery and mighty.

Diagnosis: Syndrome caused by accumulated Heat in the Stomach and obstruction of Vital Energy in the Bowel. Decoction of Radix et Rhizoma Rhei and Radix Glycyrrhizae was prescribed:

Radix et Rhizoma Rhei	12 grams
Radix Glycyrrhizae	3 grams

Third treatment: After one dose of the decoction, the patient no longer had vomiting, and stool was smooth. Another dose worked effectively. The syndrome was gone.

Case 2 (62-399):

Wang, female, 25-year-old farmer, first treatment on August 22, 1975. Two days earlier when the patient returned from the field after work on a hot summer day, she had vertigo and headache, epigastric pain and hot feeling, bitterness and parched mouth and bad breath, no fever. After eating, there was immediately a vomiting, (repeated after meals). Urine was scanty and yellow. Tongue was red and dry, covered with thin, yellow coating. Pulse was slippery and mighty.

Diagnosis: Syndrome caused by stagnation of Heat in Stomach which ascended, causing vomiting. Decoction of Radix et Rhizoma Rhei and Radix Glycyrrhizae was prescribed:

Radix et Rhizoma Rhei	12 grams
Radix Glycyrrhizae	3 grams

Second treatment on August 23. After taking the decoction, there was a smooth stool. Distention and hot feeling in epigastrium disappeared. The patient had two cups of porridge the same night and no vomit ensued. Vertigo and headache were also subsiding. There was still a parched feeling in mouth. Tongue was red and dry, free from coating. Pulse was slender-speedy. This showed stagnant Heat in the Stomach had been dispersed, but Stomach Yin was deficient.

Decoction of *Yiwei* (Radix Glehniae, Radix Ophiopogonis, Radix Rehmanniae, Rhizoma Polygonati Odorati, crystal sugar) was prescribed to moisten and tonify the Stomach.

On August 29, the doctor was told that after taking two doses of the decoction, the patient could go back to work.

Case 3 (62-399):

A boy of seventeen, first treatment on March 31, 1978. The patient had a cold with fever and was treated with diaphoretics. After perspiration, the fever went down, but vomiting occurred after each meal. The patient would then drink water (there was no vomit after drinking). Two days later he consulted the doctor.

Examination: There was a distended and hot feeling in epigastric region, no stool for two days. Urine was scanty and yellow. Tongue was red and dry, covered with thin and yellow coating. Pulse was tight-slippery and mighty.

Diagnosis: Syndrome with accumulation of pathogenetic Heat in the Stomach ascending, causing vomiting. Decoction of Radix et Rhizoma Rhei and Radix Glycyrrhizae was given:

Radix et Rhizoma Rhei	12 grams
Radix Glycyrrhizae	3 grams

Two doses were served, which stopped the vomiting.

CLAUSE 17-18

Stomach Regurgitation with vomiting and thirst can be eased with Decoction of Poria and Rhizoma Alismatis.

Decoction of Poria and Rhizoma Alismatis
(*Fuling Zexie Tang*):

Waitai states that this prescription is effective for *Xiaoke* (diabetes) with Stomach Regurgitation, vomiting of food which has just been eaten, and pulse that is barely palpable. In this case, one *sheng* of Fructus Tritici should be added to the prescription.

Poria	0.5 *jin*
Radix Glycyrrhizae	2 *liang*
Ramulus Cinnamomi	2 *liang*
Rhizoma Atractylodis Macrocephalae	3 *liang*
Rhizoma Zingiberis Recens	4 *liang*
Rhizoma Alismatis	4 *liang*

Stew the first five drugs in one *dou* of water until three *sheng* remain. Add Rhizoma Alismatis and stew again until two and a half *sheng* remain. Serve eight *ge* of the lukewarm decoction per dose three times a day.

Explanation of the Prescription: This prescription treats cases with nausea and thirst caused by Fluid-retention in the Stomach. When Stomach is affected by Fluid-retention, its normal function of descending is hampered, and Stomach gas ascends to cause nausea and vomiting. Fluid-retention also hampers the normal deployment of Body Fluid. This is the cause of thirst. With Fluid-retention in the Stomach, vomiting will not cease. After the vomiting, the patient is thirsty, but the water he drinks will only intensify the Fluid-retention and nausea and vomiting will occur again. Finally it turns into a case of Stomach Regurgitation with repeated vomiting and thirst. Decoction of Poria and Rhizoma Alismatis is adopted to disperse the Fluid-retention and facilitate Water circulation. Poria, Rhizoma Alismatis and Rhizoma Atractylodis Macrocephalae tonify the Spleen and help promote the Water circulation. Ramulus Cinnamomi, Radix Glycyrrhizae and Rhizoma Zingiberis Recens reinforce the Vital Energy and harmonize the Stomach. When the Vital Energy resumes its normal functioning and the Water resumes circulation, Fluid-retention will be dispersed and vomiting subsides. (02-162)

CASES

Case 1 (62-396):

Mr. Gou, 42, farmer, first treatment in August 1964. The patient had repeated vomiting for two years and could no longer work in the field. Diagnosis by a hospital was "chronic gastritis," but treatment did not seem to help.

Examination: He had one or two vomits every day. Vomitus was full of food and fluid, not smelly. The patient did not want water but his appetite was normal. Dropsy was all over the body, with pale face, and low spirit. Tongue lost its sense of taste, stool was loose, tongue was pale and moist, covered with thin, white coating. Pulse was moderate and slippery.

Diagnosis: Stomach Regurgitation caused by excessive Fluid-retention, while Spleen was deficient. Decoction of Poria and Rhizoma Alismatis was given to replenish the Spleen, smooth Water circulation to disperse retention:

Poria	15 grams
Rhizoma Alismatis	12 grams
Rhizoma Atractylodis Macrocephalae	12 grams
Ramulus Cinnamomi	9 grams

Rhizoma Zingiberis Recens	12 grams
Radix Glycyrrhizae	3 grams

Taboo: Cold and uncooked food was prohibited.

Second treatment (three days later): After two doses of the decoction, vomits stopped and appetite increased. Dropsy was dispersing, stool was loose, tongue was pale and moist, covered with thin and white coating. Pulse was deficient-moderate. Since the decoction worked, two to six doses were prescribed.

One year later, the patient reported that he took four doses of decoction and the syndrome was gone. After one month of rest and nursing care, he resumed work.

Case 2 (64-673): Case Recorded in Journal of *Jilin Chinese Medicine and Pharmacology*, 6:7, 1983

Mr. Zhou, 48, was accepted as an in-patient on March 9, 1983.

Examination: The patient suffered from gastric disease for ten years with repeated vomiting. Salivation per day could be as much as 2,000 ml. The patient was worn out, emaciated and depressed. A splashing sound could be heard in his stomach. Tongue coating was white; pulse was small-tight. Gastroscope examination showed a syndrome of chronic antral gastritis and pyloric hydrops.

Diagnosis: Syndrome caused by stagnation of Fluid-retention.

Treatment: To warm the Interior and harmonize the Stomach, smooth the Vital Energy flow and facilitate Water circulation. Combination of Decoction of Lesser Rhizoma Pinelliae (Clause 12-26) and Decoction of Poria and Rhizoma Alismatis were prescribed. After the decoction was prepared, Rhizoma Zingiberis Recens was chewed before taking the decoction

Two doses of the decoction reduced vomiting and another dose stopped it. The patient had good appetite and began to rebuild his health. One and a half months later, gastroscope examination showed improvement of pyloric hydrops.

Case 3 (51-437): Case Recorded in *Imperial Han Medicine*

A gentleman had Stomach Regurgitation and repeated vomiting with fluid and dregs of food. After the vomit, he was thirsty. He consulted several doctors and was treated many ways. None of the treatments worked. One doctor suggested a fast, which worked for a few days, but once the patient resumed his eating, vomit resumed. This condition had lasted five years.

Examination: The doctor palpated the abdomen and found it was full and distended from below the chest to the umbilicus.

Decoction of Poria and Rhizoma Alismatis was prescribed, which was effective. In a few days, the syndrome was gone.

CLAUSE 17-19

After the patient vomits, he is thirsty and drinks large quantities of water. Decoction of *Wenge* can be adopted to quench the thirst. This decoction is also effective in cases caused by a slight pathogenetic Wind with headache and tense pulse.

Decoction of *Wenge*
(*Wenge Tang*):

Wenge (Concha Meretricis seu Cyclinae or Galla Chinensis)	5 *liang*
Herba Ephedrae	3 *liang*
Radix Glycyrrhizae	3 *liang*
Rhizoma Zingiberis Recens	3 *liang*
Gypsum Fibrosum	5 *liang*
Semen Armeniacae Amarum	50 pcs.
Fructus Ziziphi Jujubae	12 pcs.

Stew the drugs in six *sheng* of water until two *sheng* remain. Serve one *sheng* of the lukewarm decoction per dose. When perspiration is induced the syndrome is subsiding.

Remark: Decoction of *Wenge* should be replaced by *Wenge* Powder described in Clause 141 of *Shanghan Lun*; *Wenge* Powder in that clause should be replaced by Decoction of *Wenge*. (01-188)

Wenge Powder
(*Wenge San*):

Wenge	5 *liang*

Pound the drug into powder. Take one *fangcunbi* of the powder with five *ge* of boiled water per dose.

CASES

Case 1 (64-675):

Mr. Li, 46, first treatment on March 5, 1980.

The patient had diabetes for three years. Symptoms: parched mouth and thirst, always hungry, frequent urination (sometimes turbid), black complexion, general lassitude, emaciation, red tongue with scanty coating, slender-speedy pulse. Middle of helix was withering.

Diagnosis: Syndrome caused by damaged and consumptive condition of Kidney.

Treatment: To moisten the Yin and stabilize the Kidney, clear the Heat and help produce Body Fluid. Decoction of *Wenge* was prescribed, with alterations:

Concha Meretricis seu Cyclinae	20 grams
Gypsum Fibrosum	60 grams
Herba Ephedrae	3 grams
Rhizoma Rehmanniae Praeparata	20 grams
Fructus Corni	15 grams
Rhizoma Dioscoreae	20 grams
Semen Cuscutae	10 grams
Plastrum Testudinis	30 grams

Twenty doses of the decoction were served consecutively. Drinking of water was ample and waste was under control. The patient put 6.5 kilograms on weight. Complexion was good, helix looked better. Tongue was red, covered with thin and white coating. Pulse was weak.

Second treatment: The above decoction was prescribed again, adding the followings:

Radix Pseudostellariae	20 grams
Rhizoma Atractylodis Macrocephalae	20 grams
Radix Astragali Hedysari	15 grams

Thirty doses were served before a full recovery was effected.

CLAUSE 17-20

Powder of Rhizoma Pinelliae and Rhizoma Zingiberis can be adopted in syndromes with nausea with copious salivation.

Powder of Rhizoma Pinelliae and Rhizoma Zingiberis
(*Banxia Ganjiang San*):

Rhizoma Pinelliae
Rhizoma Zingiberis

Pound the drugs in equal amounts into powder. Stew one *fangcunbi* of the powder in one and a half *sheng* of *jiangshui* water (see Clause 3-13) until seven *ge* remain. Serve the decoction in a single dose.

Explanation of the Prescription: The syndrome is caused by ascending of the Cold Fluid-retention which arouses nausea when the Interior Yang Vital Energy is deficient. Powder of Rhizoma Pinelliae and Rhizoma Zingiberis is adopted to disperse the Cold, warm the Interior and stop the nausea. *Jiangshui* water is used to strengthen drug's action in tonifying the Stomach and easing the nausea. (02-161)

CLAUSE 17-21

The patient feels a great discomfort in the chest, as if he were suffering from wheezing, nausea and vomiting. He is not actually suffering from these complaints, but feels extremely uncomfortable in his chest and is unable to quiet himself down. To tranquilize the patient, Decoction of Rhizoma Zingiberis Recens and Rhizoma Pinelliae can be adopted.

Decoction of Rhizoma Zingiberis Recens and Rhizoma Pinelliae (*Shengjiang Banxia Tang*):

Rhizoma Pinelliae	0.5 *sheng*
Juice of Rhizoma Zingiberis Recens	1 *liang*

Stew Rhizoma Pinelliae in three *sheng* of water until two *sheng* remain. Add in juice of Rhizoma Zingiberis Recens and stew again until one and a half *sheng* remain. Serve the decoction in four doses when it cools, three doses in the day and one dose at night. When the syndrome subsides, the rest of the decoction need not be taken.

Explanation of the Prescription: This prescription has the same ingredients as Decoction of Lesser Rhizoma Pinelliae (Clause 12-26), though here juice of Rhizoma Zingiberis Recens replaces Rhizoma Zingiberis Recens because it is more effective in dispersing the Fluid-retention. That hot-quality drugs are taken cool is in consideration of the resistance arising from the Cold Fluid-retention. When the decoction is taken hot, it may cause nausea and vomiting. Decoction is served in four doses to disperse the pathogenetic factors gradually. (01-189)

Summary of Treatments to Syndromes of Nausea and Vomit (64-682)

Pathology	*Principal symptoms and signs*	*Treatment (prescriptions)*
Deficiency and Cold	Vomit of saliva, chest fullness, headache	Decoction of Fructus Evodiae (Clause 17-8 and Clause 29 of *Shanghan Lun*)
	Nausea, slight fever, cold extremities, weak pulse	Decoction of *Sini* (Clause 17-14 and Clause 29 of *Shanghan Lun*)
	Vomit at dusk when food is taken in the morning	Decoction of Greater Rhizoma Pinelliae (Clause 17-16)
Excess and Heat	Nausea without vomit, diarrhea with hot feeling at anus	Decoction of Radix Scutellariae adding Rhizoma Pinelliae and Rhizoma Zingiberis Recens (Clause 17-11)
	Nausea and fever	Decoction of Radix Bupleuri (Clause 17-15 and Clause 37 of *Shanghan Lun*)
	Vomit right after food is taken, constipation	Decoction of Radix et Rhizoma Rhei and Radix Glycyrrhizae (Clause 17-17)
Intermingling of Heat & Cold	Nausea, borborygmus, fullness and distention in epigastrium	Decoction of Rhizoma Pinelliae *Xiexin* (Clause 17-10 and Clause 149 of *Shanghan Lun*)
Stagnation of Fluid-retention	Nausea, epigastric fullness, indigestion	Decoction of Lesser Rhizoma Pinelliae (Clause 17-12)

Summary of Treatments to Syndromes of Nausea and Vomit (64-682)

(Continued)

Pathology	*Principal symptoms and signs*	*Treatment (prescriptions)*
	Fluid-retention resting at above the diaphragm, thirst of water after vomit	Powder of Polyporus Umbellatus (Clause 17-13)
	Repeated vomit, thirst of water	Decoction of Poria and Rhizoma Alismatis (Clause 17-18)
	Cold Fluid-retention in Stomach, vomit of saliva	Powder of Rhizoma Pinelliae and Rhizoma Zingiberis (Clause 17-20)
	The patient seems suffering from wheezing, nausea, vomiting, feeling extremely uncomfortable in chest	Decoction of Rhizoma Zingiberis Recens and Rhizoma Pinelliae (Clause 17-21)

CLAUSE 17-22

Decoction of Pericarpium Citri Reticulatae can be adopted in syndromes with symptoms of nausea, retching and coldness in the extremities.

Decoction of Pericarpium Citri Reticulatae
(*Jupi Tang*):

Pericarpium Citri Reticulatae	4 *liang*
Rhizoma Zingiberis Recens	0.5 *jin*

Stew the drugs in seven *sheng* of water until three *sheng* remain. Serve one *sheng* of lukewarm decoction per dose. As soon as the decoction is taken, syndrome will subside.

Explanation of the Prescription: Coldness in the extremities is caused by Cold and Deficiency prevailing in the Stomach. Rhizoma Zingiberis Recens is used to disperse the Cold and stop the nausea.

Pericarpium Citri Reticulatae is used to smooth the flow of the Vital Energy and reverse the adverse ascending. (01-190)

CASES

Case 1 (02-163):

A gentleman had cholera in mid-summer. When vomit and diarrhea stopped, nausea and retching persisted. There was a coldness over the extremities. Pulse was extremely weak and slender. Drugs of warm and tonifying qualities had been used but did not help. The last doctor the patient consulted prescribed Decoction of Pericarpium Citri Reticulatae. The decoction was served little by little. Gradually it worked.

CLAUSE 17-23

Decoction of Pericarpium Citri Reticulatae and Caulis Bambusae in Taeniam can be adopted to ease nausea and retching.

Decoction of Pericarpium Citri Reticulatae and
Caulis Bambusae in Taeniam
(*Jupi Zhuru Tang*):

Pericarpium Citri Reticulatae	2 *sheng*
Caulis Bambusae in Taeniam	2 *sheng*
Fructus Ziziphi Jujubae	30 pcs.
Rhizoma Zingiberis Recens	0.5 *jin*
Radix Glycyrrhizae	5 *liang*
Radix Ginseng	1 *liang*

Stew the drugs in one *dou* of water until three *sheng* remain. Serve one *sheng* of lukewarm decoction per dose three times a day.

Explanation of the Prescription: Nausea and retching are generally caused by Cold and Deficiency in the Stomach. But in this case, Heat of a deficient nature intermingles with the Cold. Decoction of Pericarpium Citri Reticulatae and Caulis Bambusae in Taeniam is adopted to eliminate both symptoms. Pericarpium Citri Reticulatae is used to smooth the flow of the Vital Energy and harmonize the Stomach. Caulis Bambusae in Taeniam eliminates the Heat in the Stomach and reverses the adversity. Radix Glycyrrhizae and Fructus

Ziziphi Jujubae tonify the Interior. Radix Ginseng tonifies the Vital Energy. Rhizoma Zingiberis Recens warms the Stomach. Once the Stomach Vital Energy is restored, it will overcome the deficient Heat. This prescription is also effective for nausea and vomiting during early pregnancy, as well as acute and chronic gastritis. (01-190)

Li Wen: Nausea and retching may be caused by pathogenetic Cold or Heat in the Stomach. But this syndrome is caused by deficient Heat and adverse ascending in the Stomach. Radix Ginseng, Radix Glycyrrhizae and Fructus Ziziphi Jujubae are used to tonify the Deficiency. Pericarpium Citri Reticulatae and Rhizoma Zingiberis Recens disperse the adverse ascending. Caulis Bambusae in Taeniam, sweet and cold, is used as the principal ingredient to reverse the adversity and eliminate the Heat in the Stomach. (05-623)

CASES

Case 1 (02-164):

Mr. Lin, 34, had hiccup and retching for ten years. When the syndrome was aggravated, belching, nausea, salivation, insomnia, anorexia, constipation, scanty and red urine, thirst and epigastric pain appeared. Pulse was tight. Tongue was red, covered with yellow and greasy coating. The diagnosis of "nervous retching" was given by a hospital of Western medicine.

Diagnosis: A pathological condition of excessive Yang in the Liver and insufficient Yin in the Stomach with ascending Fire (Heat) from the Liver and Stomach.

Treatment: Decoction of Pericarpium Citri Reticulatae and Caulis Bambusae in Taeniam was prescribed to eliminate the Heat, nourish the Yin, harmonize the Stomach and bring down the adversity:

Pericarpium Citri Reticulatae	1.5 *qian*
Caulis Bambusae in Taeniam	3 *qian*
Rhizoma Polygonati Odorati	3 *qian*
Radix Ophiopogonis	2 *qian*
Radix Glycyrrhizae	1 *qian*
Herba Dendrobii	3 *qian*
Fructus Ziziphi Jujubae	3 pcs.
Rhizoma Zingiberis Recens	3 slices
Calyx Kaki	1 *qian*

Second treatment: Retching subsided and the patient could sleep well. There was a full and distended feeling in the chest. The same decoction was prescribed, with alterations:

Subtract: Fructus Ziziphi Jujubae and Calyx Kaki.

Add: Fructus Gardeniae, Semen Sojae Praeparatum, Semen Cardamomi Rotundi.

Third treatment: Retching stopped and other symptoms subsided. There was still a hot and uncomfortable feeling in chest. Pulse was moderate and tongue coating was slightly yellow. The following alterations made:

Add: Rhizoma Anemarrhenae.

Double the dosage of Herba Dendrobii.

Three doses were served. The syndrome was gone. No recurrence was reported in the following four months.

Case 2 (64-685):

Mr. Zhou, 22, had fever and headache for fifteen days, since he was hospitalized on May 21, 1980.

On the eighth day, he had repeated hiccups, which occurred 7-8 hours in the day and sometimes at night. Vomit, insomnia, anorexia, epigastric upset all ensued. Tongue proper was red. Pulse was slender and weak.

Diagnosis: A pathological condition of Stomach Deficiency complicated with pathogenetic Heat.

Decoction of Pericarpium Citri Reticulatae and Caulis Bambusae in Taeniam was prescribed:

Radix Codonopsis Pilosulae	15 grams
Caulis Bambusae in Taeniam	9 grams
Rhizoma Atractylodis Macrocephalae	12 grams
Poria	12 grams
Pericarpium Citri Reticulatae	9 grams
Rhizoma Zingiberis Recens	3 slices
Fructus Ziziphi Jujubae	4 pcs.
Fructus Hordei	9 grams
Radix Glycyrrhizae	2 grams

Three doses of the decoction cured the ailment.

Case 3 (65-513): Case Recorded in *Collection of Case Studies and Commentaries of Doctors in Fujian Province*

Mr. Zheng, in his thirties, suffered from febrile disease caused by summer-heat, with fever and chill, severe headache and loss of consciousness when fever was high. This lasted ten days after treatment of Chinese and Western medicines. Repeated hiccups occurred day and night, making it difficult for the patient to take medicine. He was irritable, and had flushed face, parched lips and mouth, and constipation. Tongue was covered with yellow-greasy and gray-turbid coating. Pulse was slippery-speedy and mighty at right Bar position.

Diagnosis: Febrile disease caused by summer-heat, maltreated by drugs of dry quality, resulted in accumulation of pathogenetic Heat in the Middle Portion.

Decoction of Pericarpium Citri Reticulatae and Caulis Bambusae in Taeniam adding Gypsum Fibrosum and Folium Bambusae was prescribed:

Pericarpium Citri Reticulatae	3 grams
Caulis Bambusae in Taeniam	24 grams
Radix Glehniae	12 grams
Radix Ophiopogonis	15 grams
Rhizoma Pinelliae	4.5 grams
Folium Eriobotryae	9 grams
Gypsum Fibrosum	90 grams
Folium Bambusae Recens	100 pcs.

After taking the decoction, fever subsided and hiccups occurred less frequently. Five doses of the following decoctions helped the patient recover from the ailment completely:

Radix Ophiopogonis	15 grams
Radix Scrophulariae	15 grams
Radix Rehmanniae	24 grams
Caulis Bambusae in Taeniam	24 grams
Rhizoma Phragmitis	30 grams
Gypsum Fibrosum	60 grams
Folium Eriobotryae	9 grams
Semen Oryzae Nonglutinosae	24 grams

Summary of Syndrome of Retching (64-686)

Pathology	*Symptoms*	*Principle of treatment*	*Prescription*
Excess and Heat	Hiccup and abdominal fullness, constipation	Purge the constipation	Decoction of *Tiaowei Chengqi* (Clause 29 of *Shanghan Lun*)
	Hiccup and abdominal fullness, dysuria	Smooth the urination	Decoction of Polyporus Umbellatus (Clause 13-14 and Clause 223 of *Shanghan Lun*)

Summary of Syndrome of Retching (64-686) (*Continued*)

Pathology	*Symptoms*	*Principle of treatment*	*Prescription*
Cold in Stomach and Stagnation of Vital Energy	Nausea, retching, coldness on extremities	Facilitate the flow of Yang Vital Energy, harmonize the Stomach	Decoction of Pericarpium Citri Reticulatae (Clause 17-22)
Stomach Deficiency complicated with Heat	Retching, irritation, shortness of breath, parched oral cavity	Eliminate Heat, tonify Deficiency, harmonize Stomach and bring down adversity	Decoction of Pericarpium Citri Reticulatae and Caulis Bambusae in Taeniam (Clause 17-23)

CLAUSE 17-24

When the Vital Energy of the Six Bowels evanesces and fails to reach the Exterior, the following symptoms and signs will appear: Coldness in the extremities, contraction of the feet and inspiratory dyspnea. When the Vital Energy of the Five Viscera evanesces in the Interior, continuous diarrhea will occur. An acute attack of diarrhea will cause numbness in the extremities. (1)

NOTES

1. This clause discusses the mechanism and prognosis of nausea and vomiting, retching and diarrhea, as well as the evanescence of the Vital Energy of the Five Viscera and the Six Bowels. The Six Bowels are Yang in nature, and control the Exterior. All the Six Bowels are dependent upon the condition of the Stomach. When the Stomach Vital Energy evanesces, the Vital Energy of the Six Bowels cannot reach and warm the extremities, thus coldness in the extremities result. The Six Bowels lose their normal function of acceptance as well as harmonization and descending, so nausea, vomiting and retching result. The Upper Portion receives no reinforcement from the Middle Portion, which is in a weary state, and the Vital Energy in the chest becomes deficient, bringing about inspiratory dyspnea. When Yang Vital Energy is weakened, it ceases providing nourishment to the tendons, and contraction of the feet occurs.

The Five Viscera are Yin in nature and control the Interior. All the Five Viscera are dependent on the condition of the Kidney. When Kidney Yang Vital Energy is deficient, the Vital Energy of all the Viscera cannot be deployed in the Interior and cause the hypofunctioning of the Vital Energy, resulting in uncontrollable diarrhea. Acute and chronic diarrhea will exhaust the Body Fluid, which will prevent nourishment and protection from reaching the extremities and tendons. This will result in the numbness in the extremities. (02-164)

CLAUSE 17-25*

Diarrhea with deep and tight pulse (1) will be accompanied by a descending feeling in the anus (tenesmus). Huge pulse (2) indicates that the syndrome is not coming to an end. When the pulse is feeble-weak and speedy (3), diarrhea will cease spontaneously. Although fever may be diagnosed, case will not be fatal.

NOTES

1. Pulse corresponds to the case. (04-209)
2. Huge pulse indicates prevalence of pathogenetic Heat. (04-209)
3. Feeble-weak and speedy pulse indicates diarrhea. But speedy pulse also indicates restoration of the Body Resistance. Thus syndrome will clear up. (04-209)

*This clause also appears in *Shanghan Lun* (Clause 365).

CLAUSE 17-26

Case will be fatal if the following symptoms and signs are observed: Diarrhea, coldness in hands and feet and barely palpable pulse. When moxibustion therapy can bring neither warmness to the extremities nor restoration of pulse, and if light dyspnea is present, case will be fatal (1). If pulse of Lesser Yin is weaker than *Fuyang* pulse, case is curable (2).

NOTES

1. Diarrhea, coldness in the extremities and barely palpable pulse indicate the extreme evanescence of Yang Vital Energy. Moxibustion therapy should be given immediately to save the patient. After moxibustion is adopted, if extremities do not become warm and pulse does not resume, and if light dyspnea is present, this case is one of complete dispersion of Yang Vital Energy, and will be fa-

tal. (04-208)

2. Pulse of Lesser Yin: *Taixi* pulse, reflecting Kidney Vital Energy. It is located at the foot Taixi point (KI 3). *Fuyang* pulse located at Chongyang point (ST 42) on the foot is where Stomach Vital Energy can be sensed.

When Kidney pulse (pulse of Lesser Yin, *Taixi* pulse) is weaker than Stomach pulse (*Fuyang* pulse), Stomach pulse (Yang in nature) will prevail. Thus when Yin syndrome has a Yang pulse, recovery is indicated. If Stomach Vital Energy still exists, possibility of recovery also exists. Thus the case can be cured. (04-208)

CLAUSE 17-27

In cases of diarrhea with light fever and thirst (1), self-cure will follow if the pulse is weak (2).

NOTES

1. "Light fever and thirst" signifies the restoration of Yang Vital Energy. (04-207)

2. "Weak pulse" indicates passing of the syndrome. (04-207)

Cheng Zhi: Restoration of the Yang Vital Energy and dispersion of pathogenetic factors are positive signs as far as diarrhea is concerned. Light fever with thirst indicates that the syndrome is becoming Yang. Weak pulse indicates passing of the syndrome, ensuring that self-cure will follow. If high fever and excessive pulse are observed in syndromes with diarrhea, case will be fatal. (05-270)

CLAUSE 17-28

Diarrhea will cease when speedy pulse, light fever and perspiration appear. When the pulse becomes tense (1), the syndrome is not healing.

NOTES

1. Tense pulse indicates prevalence of Cold. According to another edition "tense pulse" is "floating and tense pulse." (04-208)

Cheng Wuji: Diarrhea is a Yin syndrome. Speedy pulse is a Yang pulse. When Yang pulse appears in a Yin syndrome, it is a sign of recovery. Light fever with perspiration indicates the restoration of Yang Vital Energy, and diarrhea is sure to cease. Tense pulse always indicates syndromes of a Cold nature. When pulse is tense, Yin still prevails. Therefore the syndrome is not healing. (05-270)

CLAUSE 17-29*

Diarrhea with speedy pulse and thirst may lead to either self-cure or stool with bloody pus when pathogenetic Heat is excessive (1).

NOTES

1. Excessive restoration of Yang Vital Energy. (04-210)

*Clauses 17-26, 17-27, 17-28 and 17-29 also appear in *Shanghan Lun* (Clauses 360, 361, 362, and 367).

CLAUSE 17-30

Diarrhea accompanied by fever, perspiration and tight pulse will indicate a recovery. (1)

NOTES

1. Diarrhea is Yin in nature. But fever, perspiration and tight pulse all reflect the restoration of the Yang Vital Energy, and indicate a recovery. (01-192)

CLAUSE 17-31

Diuretic can be adopted in cases with diarrhea accompanied by flatus (1).

NOTES

1. Wei Litong: The lucid Vital Energy may leave the body via the urine, reflecting the physiological function of Yang. The turbid substance may leave the body via the stool, reflecting the physiological function of Yin. This is the normal state of a healthy person. When air (lucid Vital Energy) follows the stool in the form of flatus, it is evidence of the mingling of the lucid and the turbid, the Yin and the Yang. Therapy involves the adoption of a diuretic, enabling the lucid Vital Energy to return to its normal channels. Therefore, it is an excellent cure for diarrhea accompanied by flatus.

CLAUSE 17-32

Bloody pus will appear in diarrhea when the pulse under fore-finger is floating and speedy (1) and pulse under ring-finger is hesitant (2).

NOTES

1. Greater Yin syndrome has deep and slow pulse as it is of a deficient and Cold type. When floating and speedy pulse (pulse of excessive nature) appears in a Yin syndrome, it will indicate the restoration of the Yang Vital Energy. But if restoration of Yang is excessive, pathogenetic Heat will accumulate and damage the Yin and Blood. Diarrhea with bloody pus is the result. (04-209)

2. Wu Qian: Hesitant pulse under ring-finger: Exterior pathogenetic Heat will invade the Interior with diarrhea and damage the Yin. When pathogenetic Heat intermingles with Blood, bloody pus will result.

CLAUSE 17-33

Exterior syndromes should not be treated when diarrhea with undigested cereals is observed. After perspiration (through diaphoresis), abdominal distention will be present. (1)

NOTES

1. Diarrhea with undigested cereals indicates Deficiency and Coldness in the Spleen and Stomach. Diaphoresis will further weaken the Yang Vital Energy of the Spleen and the Stomach. When digestive system ceases its normal functioning, abdominal distention occurs. (04-209)

Remark: This clause is related to Clause 91 of *Shanghan Lun*.

CLAUSE 17-34

Syndrome will disappear following a period of vertigo and perspiration, preceded by the following symptoms and signs: Diarrhea with undigested cereals, deep and slow pulse, a slightly flushed face and fever. The patient will feel slight cold in extremities. This is caused by a Deficiency in the Lower Portion, which is evinced by the symptom of "Wearing Yang" (1) on the face.

NOTES

1. Wearing Yang (*Dai Yang*): See note of Clause 317 of *Shanghan Lun*.

CLAUSE 17-35

After diarrhea, the pulse disappears but coldness appears in hands and feet. Pulse resumes and extremities become warm again after one whole day. This indicates a favorable case. If pulse does not resume, case will be fatal. (1)

NOTES

1. Diarrhea is caused when Cold directly invades the Greater Yin Channel. Heavy loss of Body Fluid brings about a sudden dispersion of Yang Vital Energy. Some annotators suggest adoption of Decoction of *Baitong* (see Clause 314 of *Shanghan Lun*) and acupuncture at acupoints Guanyuan (RN 4) and Qihai (RN 6). (04-211)

CLAUSE 17-36*

When symptoms and signs of diarrhea, abdominal distention (1) and pain throughout the body (2) are observed, Interior coldness should be first treated with warm drugs after which the Exterior syndrome can be treated. Decoction of *Sini* can be used to warm the Interior and Decoction of Ramulus Cinnamomi can be used to disperse the Exterior syndrome. (3)

NOTES

1. Diarrhea and abdominal distention are symptoms of Interior Cold. (04-212)

2. Pain throughout the body is a symptom of an Exterior syndrome.

3. Treatment of cases with symptom complex in both the Interior and the Exterior cannot always be treated in the order "Exterior first followed by Interior," though this is a general law of treatment. Therapy should follow details of each case. Acute and urgent cases should be treated first. Diarrhea in this clause contains undigested cereal, an indication of acute Deficiency and Cold in the Interior. Thus the Interior syndrome is more acute than the Exterior syndrome and should be treated first.

*Clauses 17-32, 17-33, 17-34, 17-35 and 17-36 also appear in *Shanghan Lun* (Clauses 363, 364, 366, 368 and 372).

CLAUSE 17-37

Syndrome includes diarrhea with moderate pulse at the Inch, Bar and Cubit: When pressed, a hard mass is felt in the epigastrium. Purgative should be adopted urgently. Decoction of Greater *Chengqi* (for prescription see Clause 2-13 and Clause 208 of *Shanghan Lun*) will provide a cure (1).

NOTES

1. Li Wen: Diarrhea with moderate pulse at the Inch, Bar and Cubit with a hard mass in the epigastrium is a case of an excessive nature. If the pulse is feeble and weak, purgative should not be adopted. When moderate pulse in all three positions shows that the Interior is not deficient, thus purgative can be adopted urgently to stop the diarrhea. This treatment is based on a diagnosis of both the symptoms and the pulse. (05-627)

CLAUSE 17-38

Diarrhea with slow and slippery pulse is a case of an excessive nature (1). The purgative, Decoction of Greater *Chengqi*, should be given urgently. (2)

NOTES

1. Wu Qian: Slow pulse should not be slippery. The slow and slippery pulse mentioned in this clause exhibits slow pulsation when pressed lightly and slippery pulsation when pressed deeply. A slow pulse at the surface signifies a harmonious state in the Exterior. A slippery pulse in the depths indicates an Interior Excess. To stop the diarrhea caused by Interior Excess, a purgative should be adopted to eliminate the Excess. Once the Excess is eliminated, diarrhea will cease. (05-627)

2. You Yi: Slow pulse generally indicates a case of a Cold nature. When accompanied by a slippery pulse, it no longer signifies a case of a Cold nature but one of an excessive nature. This is because when pulsation is deterred by the Interior Excess, it will become slow. When Excess is the causa morbi of diarrhea, treatment of the diarrhea is achieved by eliminating the Interior Excess. That is why a purgative should be adopted urgently.

CLAUSE 17-39

When diarrhea is accompanied only by a slippery pulse, something is present in the Interior which must be eliminated. The purgative, Decoction of Greater *Chengqi*, should be adopted. (1)

NOTES

1. Zhao Liang: Diarrhea is generally a deficient case. But as a rule a slippery pulse reflects an excessive case. When pulse reflecting excessive case appears in a deficient case, something is blocking the Interior that needs to be cleared away. (05-628)

Cheng Lin: The medical canon says that a slippery pulse indicates indigestion. Thus a purgative should be adopted to disperse the indigestion, and the diarrhea will subside subsequently. (05-628)

CLAUSE 17-40

After the diarrhea subsides, it will recur on the same day and same month of each year (1), showing that the syndrome is not completely dispersed. The purgative, Decoction of Greater *Chengqi*, should be adopted to disperse the remaining pathological condition (2).

NOTES

1. Recur on the same day, and same month of each year: This means that the recurrence is related to the seasons, and not that the recurrence will occur at exactly the same date each year. (01-196)

2. Recurrence at the same time each year is due to the incomplete treatment of the syndrome at its onset or to the adoption of an astringent to stop the diarrhea. The pathogenetic factors will remain in the Intestine and the Stomach, and will stage a comeback either at the appropriate season or when induced by indigestion or improper diet. (02-166)

CLAUSE 17-41

Diarrhea with delirium indicates the existence of stercoroma. Decoction of Lesser *Chengqi* should be adopted. (1)

NOTES

1. Diarrhea in this clause refers to bad-smelling watery stool, different in nature from diarrhea with undigested cereals. Other symptoms and pulse of Interior Heat syndrome can also be diagnosed. (04-213)

Wang Hu: With diarrhea present, pathogenetic Heat should be dispersed. Thus how is it possible to diagnose delirium and stercoroma? This is a case with excessive pathogenetic Heat in the Greater Yang Channel syndrome. When indigestion cannot move downward because of static pathogenetic factors, some will congeal into a stercoroma and some will move downward in the form of watery stool. Thus stercoroma is the root of diarrhea. When stercoroma forces pathogenetic Heat upward to the Heart, delirium results. Diagnosis can be made by feeling the abdomen and the navel. It will be hard and painful if stercoroma is present. (05-172)

Decoction of Lesser *Chengqi**
(*Xiao Chengqi Tang*):

Radix et Rhizoma Rhei	4 *liang*
Cortex Magnoliae Officinalis Praeparata	3 *liang*
Fructus Aurantii Immaturus Praeparata	3 large pcs.

Stew the drugs in four *sheng* of water until one *sheng* and two *ge* remain. Filter the decoction and serve lukewarm in two doses. Stop taking decoction when loose stool is observed.

*This prescription also appears in Clause 208 of *Shanghan Lun*.

CLAUSE 17-42

Lesser Yin syndrome. Decoction of *Taohua* will cure diarrhea with sanious pus (bloody pus).

Decoction of *Taohua**
(*Taohua Tang*):

Halloysitum Rubrum	1 *jin***
Rhizoma Zingiberis	1 *liang*
Semen Oryzae Nonglutinosae	1 *sheng*

Stew the drugs in seven *sheng* of water until Semen Oryzae Nonglutinosae is well cooked. Filter the decoction and take seven *ge* of the decoction per dose mixed with one *fangcunbi* (two grams) powder of Halloysitum Rubrum three times a day. If one dose is efficacious, stop taking the decoction.

*This prescription also appears in Clause 306 of *Shanghan Lun*.
**0.5 *jin* in pieces, and 0.5 *jin* in powder.

Explanation of the Prescription: This decoction warms the Interior, and stops diarrhea. Halloysitum Rubrum stabilizes the Intestine and Stomach function. Rhizoma Zingiberis disperses the Interior Cold. Semen Oryzae Nonglutinosae tonifies the Body Resistance. (04-177)

Commentary: Decoction of *Taohua* is applicable to diarrhea of a Cold nature. If diarrhea is of a Heat nature, it will not be efficacious. Decoction of Radix Pulsatillae is the proper curative. See Clause 17-43.

CLAUSE 17-43

Decoction of Radix Pulsatillae will cure Hot Diarrhea (1) with a descending feeling in the anus.

NOTES

1. Hot Diarrhea: Diarrhea containing bloody pus caused by the descending Heat and Humidity. See Clause 363 of *Shanghan Lun*.

Decoction of Radix Pulsatillae
(*Baitouweng Tang*):

Radix Pulsatillae	2 *liang*
Rhizoma Coptidis	3 *liang*
Cortex Phellodendri	3 *liang*
Cortex Fraxini	3 *liang*

Stew the drugs in seven *sheng* of water until two *sheng* remain. Filter the decoction and take one *sheng* when lukewarm. If not effective, take a second dose.

Explanation of the Prescription: This is a basic prescription for treating Hot Diarrhea in the Greater Yin Channel. It has the function of eliminating Heat, drying Humidity and astringing diarrhea. (04-212)

CLAUSE 17-44*

After diarrhea, if restlessness appears again, and the epigastrium is soft when pressed, this will be restlessness of a deficient nature. Decoction of Fructus Gardeniae and Semen Sojae Praeparatum will provide a cure. (1)

NOTES:

1. Lin Lan: When diarrhea ceases, remaining pathogenetic Heat in the chest will cause restlessness. "Soft when pressed" indicates the case is not one of excessive pathogenetic Heat. So Decoction of Fructus Gardeniae and Semen Sojae Praeparatum is used to eliminate the pathogenetic Heat of a deficient nature. (05-76)

Decoction of Fructus Gardeniae and Semen Sojae Praeparatum** (*Zhizi Chi Tang*):

Fructus Gardeniae	14 pcs.
Semen Sojae Praeparatum (wrapped in silk)	4 *ge*

Stew Fructus Gardeniae in four *sheng* of water until two and a half *sheng* remain. Add Semen Sojae Praeparatum and stew until one and a half *sheng* remain. Filter the decoction and serve it in two doses. After the first dose, if emesis is observed, stop taking the decoction. (See Clause 76 of *Shanghan Lun*.)

*Clauses 17-41, 17-42, 17-43 and 17-44 also appear in *Shanghan Lun* (Clauses 306, 371, 374, and 375).

**This prescription also appears in Clause 76 of *Shanghan Lun*.

CLAUSE 17-45

The patient has diarrhea with undigested food as well as perspiration and coldness in the extremities. This is a case with Interior Cold and Exterior Heat (1). Decoction of *Tongmai Sini* will provide a cure.

NOTES

1. A case with Interior Cold and Exterior Heat: This is a case with real Cold in the Interior and false Heat in the Exterior. Interior Cold means the Cold that is prevailing in the Spleen and the Stomach, causing diarrhea and coldness in extremities. Exterior Heat is indicated by the symptoms of flushed face (or Wearing Yang, *Dai Yang*), light fever and perspiration. (01-198)

Decoction of *Tongmai Sini**
(*Tongmai Sini Tang*):

Radix Aconiti	1 large pc.
Rhizoma Zingiberis	3 *liang***
Radix Glycyrrhizae Praeparata	2 *liang*

Stew the drugs in three *sheng* of water until one *sheng* and two *ge* remain. Filter the decoction and serve lukewarm in two doses.

*This prescription also appears in Clause 317 of *Shanghan Lun*.
**Or 4 *liang* for a strong person.

Explanation of the Prescription: This prescription is applicable to cases of diarrhea caused by excessive Yin in the Interior and evanescent Yang in the Exterior. While the Interior and the Exterior are blocked, the Yin and Cold are active at the Interior, and the solitary Yang evanesces in the Exterior. Decoction with strong warm drugs should be urgently adopted to regulate the Yin and the Yang.

CLAUSE 17-46

Diarrhea with pain in the Lung can be treated with Decoction of *Zishen*. (1)

NOTES

1. Wu Qian: The meaning of this clause is obscure. Cheng Lin states that "pain in the lung" might be "pain in the abdomen." The original text cannot be traced.

Decoction of *Zishen*
(*Zishen Tang*):

*Zishen**	0.5 *jin*
Radix Glycyrrhizae	3 *liang*

Stew *Zishen* in five *sheng* of water until two *sheng* remain. Add Radix Glycyrrhizae and stew until one *sheng* and a half remain. Serve the lukewarm decoction in three doses. (It is doubtful that this is the prescription in the original text of Zhang Zhongjing.)

*See Clause 7-9.

Explanation of the Prescription: Diarrhea with pain in the lung is rarely seen in clinical practice. *Zishen* is also rarely used in prescriptions. This must be an instance of miscopying. (01-199)

CLAUSE 17-47

Diarrhea accompanied by flatus can be treated with Powder of Fructus Chebulae.

Powder of Fructus Chebulae
(*Kelile San*):

Fructus Chebulae Praeparata	10 pcs.

Pound the drug into powder and blend with porridge. Serve in a single draft. (It is doubtful that this is the prescription in the original text of Zhang Zhongjing.)

Explanation of the Prescription: Diarrhea accompanied by flatus is caused by descending Vital Energy into the bowels. The flatus mentioned here is not bad-smelling and the faeces are not sticky. Fructus Chebulae, warm and astringent, is effective in curing diarrhea accompanied by flatus. (01-199)

Summary of Syndrome of Diarrhea (64-714)

Disease	*Pathology*	*Principal symptoms*	*Treatment (prescriptions)*
Diarrhea	Deficiency and Cold	Diarrhea with undigested cereals, abdominal distention	*Decoction of *Sini* (Clause 17-14)
		Diarrhea with undigested cereals, perspiration and coldness on extremities, Interior Cold with Exterior Heat	Decoction of *Tongmai Sini* (Clause 17-45)

Summary of Syndrome of Diarrhea (64-714) (*Continued*)

Disease	*Pathology*	*Principal symptoms*	*Treatment (prescriptions)*
	Excess and Heat	Excessive pathogenetic factors resting in the Interior, diarrhea with greasy and foul stool	Decoction of Greater *Chengqi* (Clause 17-40), Decoction of Lesser *Chengqi* (Clause 17-41)
	Diarrhea with flatus	Diarrhea accompanied by flatus	Powder of Fructus Chebulae (Clause 17-47)
		Diarrhea with flatus, dominal fullness with borborygmus	Powder of *Wuling* (Clause 12-29)
Dysentery	Deficiency and Cold	Diarrhea with watery stool, abdominal pain which will reduce a little bit by pressure, tastelessness in mouth, no thirst, stool with sanious pus	Decoction of *Taohua* (Clause 17-42)
	Excess and Heat	Tenesmus, thirst of water, stool with sanious pus	Decoction of Radix Pulsatillae (Clause 17-43)
Complication	Deficient Heat	Restlessness after diarrhea, uneasy feeling in epigastrium	Decoction of Fructus Gardeniae and Semen Sojae Praeparatum

Appendix:

Decoction of Lesser *Chengqi* recorded in *A Supplement to the Prescriptions Worth a Thousand Gold* is effective in treating constipation with retching and delirium.

Decoction of Lesser *Chengqi*
(*Xiao Chengqi Tang*):

(Prescription see Clause 17-41.)

Decoction of Radix Scutellariae recorded in *Waitai* is effective in curing diarrhea with nausea and retching.

Decoction of Radix Scutellariae
(*Huangqin Tang*):

Radix Scutellariae	3 *liang*
Radix Ginseng	3 *liang*
Rhizoma Zingiberis	3 *liang*
Ramulus Cinnamomi	1 *liang*
Fructus Ziziphi Jujubae	12 pcs.
Rhizoma Pinelliae	0.5 *sheng*

Stew the drugs in seven *sheng* of water until three *sheng* remain. Serve the lukewarm decoction in three doses.

CHAPTER XVIII

ON PULSE, SYMPTOM COMPLEX AND TREATMENT OF ULCEROUS DISEASES OF SKIN, ACUTE APPENDICITIS AND *JINYIN* (ACUTE ECZEMA)*

CLAUSE 18-1

Floating and speedy pulse usually indicates a case of fever. But here the patient has chills. In case local pain is present, this may be due to carbuncles. (1)

NOTES

1. According to *Treatise on Febrile Diseases Caused by Cold with Annotations by Cheng Wuji*, the text should read:

Floating and speedy pulse indicates a case of fever. The patient has chills with normal intake of food. If there is local pain, the case is one of carbuncles caused by the accumulation of pathogenetic factors.

Cheng Wuji is correct in his explication of the clause.

This clause discusses the pulse, symptoms and mechanism of carbuncles at their first stage. Floating pulse indicates an Exterior syndrome, whereas speedy pulse indicates prevalence of pathogenetic Heat. The corresponding symptoms should include fever and chills with fever as the main symptom. But in this case, when the patient has chills, pulse and symptoms are contradictory. Formation of carbuncle is possible in such cases, especially when local pain is diagnosed. (02-172)

*According to *The Pulse Classic*, the title should read: On Pulse, Symptom Complex and Treatment of Carbuncles, Acute Appendicitis, Trauma and *Jinyin* (Acute Eczema).

CLAUSE 18-2

Master: In a case of carbuncles and swelling, diagnosis of pus can be made by feeling the focus. When focus is hot, pus must be present. If there is no hot feeling, there will be no pus (1).

NOTES

1. This is an original diagnosis of pus. Later scholars and doctors developed the following technique: To decide whether pus is present, softness and hardness, shape, painfulness and color should be all taken into consideration. (02-172)

CLAUSE 18-3

Cases of acute appendicitis may have the following symptoms and signs: Scaly skin, strained abdomen, and a mass in the abdomen that is soft when pressed. No hard mass can be felt. There is no fever, and the pulse is speedy. This is a case of carbuncles and pus in the intestine. Powder of Semen Coicis, Radix Aconiti Praeparata and Herba Patriniae can be adopted.

Powder of Semen Coicis, Radix Aconiti Praeparata and Herba Patriniae
(*Yiyi Fuzi Baijiang San*):

Semen Coicis	10 *fen*
Radix Aconiti Praeparata	2 *fen*
Herba Patriniae	5 *fen*

Pound the drugs into powder. Stew one *fangcunbi* of the powder in two *sheng* of water until one *sheng* remains. Take the medicine in a single draft. The patient will pass urine.*

Explanation of the Prescription: Semen Coicis eliminates the carbuncles and disperses the pus. Radix Aconiti Praeparata is used in small doses to stimulate the stagnant Vital Energy. Herba Patriniae, salty and cold, eliminates the accumulated Heat and disperses the bloody pus. After taking the medicine, pus will be defecated along with the stool. (01-202)

*The patient will pass urine: This may be incorrect. It should read: "A defecation will exhaust the carbuncles and pus." (02-174)

CASES

Case 1 (55-147):

Hu, 60, female, had suffered from chronic appendicitis for five to six years. There was pain over the lower abdomen on the right. When the patient was exposed to cold weather, worked too hard, or ate improperly, the symptoms were aggravated. Streptomycin and penicillin had been adopted, but the syndrome did not subside. Surgery was proposed, but the patient thought she was too old. She preferred to try Chinese medicine.

Examination: The patient was depressed and emaciated, and liked warm places. Coldness on extremities was present. There was tenderness at McBurney's point. Tongue was pale, covered with white coating. Pulse was deep-weak.

Powder of Semen Coicis, Radix Aconiti Praeparata and Herba Patriniae was prescribed (in decoction form):

Radix Aconiti Praeparata	15 grams
Semen Coicis	15 grams
Herba Patriniae Recens (the whole herb)	15 pcs.

Six doses of the decoction was served. Abdominal pain subsided totally. Within the following two years, it did not recur.

Case 2 (55-148):

Zhang, 39, female, had suffered from abdominal pain on the right for more than a year. There was tenderness, continuous pain. Menses lasted three months with scanty discharge, and resumed after ten days. This was diagnosed as "functional vaginal bleeding (endometrorrhagia)" by doctor of Western medicine.

Powder of Semen Coicis, Radix Aconiti Praeparata and Herba Patriniae was prescribed (in decoction form):

Semen Coicis	60 grams
Radix Aconiti Praeparata	12 grams
Herba Patriniae	30 grams
Cortex Moutan Radicis	12 grams

After taking the decoction, blood clots were found in the discharge. Abdominal pain and metrorrhagia subsided.

Case 3 (64-723):

A boy of ten had acute appendicitis.

Examination: The boy had a pale face and depressed look. Skin was dry and peeling. Tongue was moist, covered with yellow and white coating. Pulse was deep-slender, slippery and became strengthless when pressed deeply. There was lower abdominal pain and tenderness. A palpable mass as big as an egg could be felt in the lower abdomen.

First treatment: Decoction of Semen Coicis, Radix Aconiti Praeparata and Herba Patriniae was prescribed as follows:

Radix Aconiti Praeparata	30 grams
Semen Coicis	30 grams
Herba Patriniae	24 grams

Second treatment: Two doses were served. Abdominal pain reduced and mass disappeared. There was still tenderness. Tongue was moist, and yellow-white coating was found at root of tongue. Pulse was deep-slender and moderate. Another five doses of the decoction were served within five days. In the following year, no recurrence was reported.

CLAUSE 18-4

A case of acute appendicitis may be accompanied by the following symptoms and signs: Swelling mass in the abdomen as painful as gonorrhea when pressed; normal urination and sporadic fever with spontaneous perspiration and chills. When the pulse is slow-tense, this indicates that pus is not forming. Decoction of Radix et Rhizoma Rhei and Cortex Moutan Radicis can be adopted. After taking the decoction, bloody stool will be observed. If pulse is grand-speedy, this indicates the formation of pus and no purgative should be adopted.

Decoction of Radix et Rhizoma Rhei and Cortex Moutan Radicis (*Dahuang Mudan Tang*):

Radix et Rhizoma Rhei	4 *liang*
Cortex Moutan Radicis	1 *liang*
Semen Persicae	50 pcs.
Semen Melo	0.5 *sheng*
Natrii Sulfas	3 *ge*

Stew the first five drugs in six *sheng* of water until one *sheng* remains. Filter the decoction. Add Natrii Sulfas and stew until it boils. Serve the decoction in a single draft. If there is pus, it will be defecated with the stool. If there is no pus, bloody stool will be observed.

Explanation of the Prescription: Radix et Rhizoma Rhei and Natrii Sulfas disperse the accumulated pathogenetic Humidity and Heat in the intestines. Semen Persicae and Cortex Moutan Radicis unblock the blood stasis and remove the pus. Cortex Moutan Radicis also has the efficacy of cooling the Heat in the Blood. Semen Melo moistens the intestines and disperses the bloody pus. Thus this prescription is effective in eliminating Heat and dispersing the accumulated stasis and swelling. (01-203)

Commentary: Decoction of Radix et Rhizoma Rhei and Cortex Moutan Radicis, and Powder of Semen Coicis, Radix Aconiti Praeparata and Herba Patriniae have different effectiveness. The former is suitable to cases of acute appendicitis caused by excessive Interior Heat without pus formation; the latter is suitable for patients with weak constitutions suffering from chronic appendicitis with pus but without ulceration, and from Interior Deficiency and mild Interior Heat.

The text states, "Grand-speedy pulse indicates pus formation. No purgative should be adopted." This is a case of acute appendicitis with gangrenous pus. An operation is urgently needed in such cases. (02-174)

CASES

Case 1 (64-727): Case Recorded in *Collection of Case Studies and Commentaries of Doctors in Fujian Province*

Cheng, 24, female, had a stabbing pain at lower abdomen on the right, accompanied by fever and chill. Doctors of Western medicine diagnosed "appendiceal abscess" and treated the patient accordingly in the previous five days. The trouble was still there. She came to consult a doctor of Chinese medicine.

Examination: Pulse was grand and floating, tongue was covered with yellow and greasy coating, there was no stool in three days and urine was red accompanied by a hot feeling during urination. Syndrome caused by accumulation of pathogenetic Heat in the intestine.

First treatment: Decoction of Radix et Rhizoma Rhei and Cortex Moutan Radicis was prescribed to clear the Heat and dissolve the accumulation of evil factors:

Radix et Rhizoma Rhei	5 *qian*
Semen Persicae	1.5 *qian*
Flos Carthami	1.5 *qian*
Cortex Moutan Radicis	2 *qian*
Radix Aristolochiae	2 *qian*
Rhizoma Coptidis	2 *qian*
Rhizoma Corydalis	2 *qian*
Natrii Sulfas	2 *qian*

Second treatment: Two doses were served. There was a smooth stool and pain subsided. Another two doses were given, which cured the ailment. After a few days' care and nursing, the patient was sent home.

Case 2 (640-727): Case Recorded in Journal of *Zhejiang Chinese Medicine*, 4:172, 1983

Feng, 19, female, had in the last three days abdominal pain with nausea and vomit. Pain concentrated in the lower abdomen on the right with persistent and paroxysmal attacks and tenderness. Constipation and reddish urine, chill and fever were also diagnosed. Tongue was red, covered with yellow and greasy coating. Pulse was slippery-speedy. Diagnosis by doctors of Western medicine was "acute purulent appendicitis." Pathological condition resulted from accumulation of pathogenetic Heat. Decoction of Radix et Rhizoma Rhei and Cortex Moutan Radicis was prescribed:

Radix et Rhizoma Rhei	24 grams
Natrii Sulfas Exsiccatus	15 grams
Cortex Moutan Radicis	10 grams
Semen Persicae	30 grams
Semen Benincasae	30 grams
Caulis Sargentodoxae	30 grams
Herba Patriniae	30 grams
Herba Taraxaci	30 grams

Consuming of decoction was followed by a smooth stool, which reduced the pain. Several doses given cured the pain completely by the seventh day of the treatment.

Case 3 (48-449): Cases Recorded in Journal of *Bare-foot Doctors*, Vol. 9, 1976

The journal carried a report on the use of Decoction of Radix et Rhizoma Rhei and Cortex Moutan Radicis in treatment of local infection due to vasoligation.

Prescription:

Radix et Rhizoma Rhei	9 grams
Natrii Sulfas	9 grams
Cortex Moutan Radicis	12 grams
Semen Persicae	9 grams
Rhizoma Atractylodis	9 grams
Semen Coicis	18 grams
Semen Benincasae	30 grams
Radix Glycyrrhizae	3 grams

Indication: Swelling of epididymis, nodules of spermatic cord, with dragging pain to lower abdomen and waist, vertigo, anorexia, red urine and constipation.

Therapeutic effect: Seventy-four cases were cured, averagely within two days for less serious cases, and eight days, for more serious cases. Here is one case:

Mr. Fu, 37, suffered from local infection due to vasoligation. The second day after surgery, there was local swelling and pain on epididymis, nodules of spermatic cord and dragging pain to lower abdomen and lumbar region. Urine was yellow with urodynia, vertigo and constipation. Terramycin was given but did not help. The third day after the operation, the patient was given the decoction with alterations:

Radix et Rhizoma Rhei	18 grams
Natrii Sulfas	18 grams
Cortex Moutan Radicis	12 grams
Semen Persicae	9 grams
Rhizoma Atractylodis	9 grams
Semen Coicis	18 grams.
Semen Benincasae	30 grams
Radix Glycyrrhizae	3 grams
Resina Olibani	9 grams
Resina Commiphorae Myrrhae	9 grams

After taking two doses of the decoction, all the symptoms subsided. Stool was smooth. In the second treatment, the following alterations was made:

Subtract Resina Olibani and Resina Commiphorae Mýrrhae.

Change Radix et Rhizoma Rhei into Radix et Rhizoma Rhei Praeparata.

Two doses worked effectively.

CLAUSE 18-5

Question: Floating-feeble and hesitant pulse (1) in the wrist generally indicates a case with loss of blood or perspiration. In case there is no perspiration, how should it be diagnosed?

Master: This must be a case of trauma causing loss of blood. (2)

NOTES

1. According to *The Pulse Classic*, the pulse is "feeble and weak."

2. Li Wen: Profuse perspiration will cause the Yang to evanesce and the pulse will become feeble. Loss of blood injures the Yin, which will make the pulse hesitant. Both feeble and hesitant pulses are Yin in nature, and are caused by either profuse perspiration or by loss of blood. In any case, this pulse reflects the exhaustion and evanescence of the Nutrient Essence and the Vital Resistance. (05-634)

CLAUSE 18-6

Powder of Semen Vaccariae can be adopted in cases of trauma.

Powder of Semen Vaccariae
(*Wangbuliuxing San*):

Semen Vaccariae (collected on the eighth day of the eighth month)	10 *fen*
Folium Sambucus Chinensis (collected on the seventh day of the seventh month)	10 *fen*
Cortex Mori Radicis (southeast portion, collected on the third day of the third month)	10 *fen*
Radix Glycyrrhizae	18 *fen*
Pericarpium Zanthoxyli Praeparata	3 *fen*
Radix Scutellariae	2 *fen*
Rhizoma Zingiberis	2 *fen*
Radix Paeoniae	2 *fen*
Cortex Magnoliae Officinalis	2 *fen*

Roast Semen Vaccariae, Folium Sambucus Chinensis and Cortex Mori Radicis over a slow charcoal fire until the exterior is charred and the interior browned (this is called "charring"). Do not allow the drugs to burn exteriorly. Pound all the drugs separately into powder and mix together. Take one *fangcunbi* per dose. In case of a minor carbuncle, the powder can be applied locally to the affected part. In acute cases, the powder can be taken orally. After childbirth, woman can also take it when necessary. On windy and cold days, Cortex Mori Radicis should be subtracted from the prescription.

Dry the first three drugs (Semen Vaccariae, Folium Sambucus Chinensis and Cortex Mori Radicis) in a shady place for one hundred days before using them.

Explanation of the Prescription: This prescription aims at stopping bleeding and preventing the invasion of pathogenetic climatic factors. (05-634)

Powder of Pus-dispersion
(*Pai Nong San*):

Fructus Aurantii Immaturus	16 pcs.
Radix Paeoniae	6 *fen*
Radix Platycodi	2 *fen*

Pound the drugs into powder and blend with an egg yolk. The powder should weigh about the same as the yolk. Take the medicine with water once a day.

Decoction of Pus-dispersion
(*Pai Nong Tang*):

Radix Glycyrrhizae	2 *liang*
Radix Platycodi	3 *liang*
Rhizoma Zingiberis Recens	1 *liang*
Fructus Ziziphi Jujubae	10 pcs.

Stew the drugs in three *sheng* of water until one *sheng* remains. Serve five *ge* of the lukewarm decoction per dose twice during the day.

Commentary: These two prescriptions are applicable to many ulcerous diseases of skin and carbuncles, and are widely used in practice. (01-205)

CLAUSE 18-7

Jinyinchuang (1), a form of skin sore, will be curable when it develops from the mouth to the extremities. When it spreads from extremities towards the mouth, case will be fatal. (2)

NOTES

1. *Jinyinchuang*, a form of skin sore, spreads from one part of the body throughout the rest of the body. At first, it resembles scabies and is accompanied by repeated itching. Later it may develop and begin to secrete yellowish fluid. (01-205)
2. This clause also appears in Clause 1-12.

CLAUSE 18-8

Powder of Rhizoma Coptidis can be applied to *Jinyinchuang*.

Powder of Rhizoma Coptidis
(*Huanglian Fen*):

(Prescription has been lost.)

CASES

Case 1 (64-732): Case Recorded in *Dr. Ran Xuefeng' s Case Studies*

Mr. Jiang was traveling on a passenger ship on the Yangtze River in the 1940s. Dr. Ran was on the same carrier. When Mr. Jiang heard that Mr. Ran, a famous doctor at the time, was aboard, he consulted him.

Examination: The patient was apparently suffering from *Jinyinchuang*. Skin sores appeared first on chest, then spread to the rest of the body and extremities. There was a secretion of yellow fluid from the sores. *Jinyinchuang* that spread from extremities to the chest was an uncurable case. But this was a case with skin sores spreading from chest to extremities, it was curable. Drugs to eliminate the Heat and detoxicate the poisonous factors were used. The following decoction was prescribed:

Flos Lonicerae	3 *qian*
Fructus Forsythiae	3 *qian*
Fructus Gardeniae	2.5 *qian*
Cortex Phellodendri	3 *qian*
Cortex Moutan Radicis	3 *qian*

Herba Taraxaci	4 *qian*
Rhizoma Smilacis Glabrae	6 *qian*
Radix Inulae Helenii	3 *qian*
Radix Achyranthis Bidentatae	3 *qian*
Radix et Rhizoma Rhei	1 *qian*

One dose of the decoction was served per day. After three doses, secretion of yellow fluid stopped and scabs were formed. Another three doses were given. Scabs fell off gradually. In the ten days of voyage, the patient was rid of the ailment and well when he left the ship.

CHAPTER XIX

ON PULSE, SYMPTOM COMPLEX AND TREATMENT OF DISEASES ON EXTREMITIES, HERNIA AND ASCARIASIS

CLAUSE 19-1

Master: *Fujue* is a disease caused by contraction on the dorsal side of the foot. The patient can walk forward comfortably but feels pain when walking backward. This is due to injury of the Initial Yang Channel. Puncture the calf for a length of two inches.

CLAUSE 19-2

The patient has swollen fingers and arms and twitching of the body. Decoction of Veratrum Nigrum and Radix Glycyrrhizae can be adopted. (1)

NOTES

1. The disease is caused by stagnant phlegm in the chest and the diaphragm. Decoction of Veratrum Nigrum is an emetic which can induce vomiting up of the pathogenetic factors. (01-207)

Decoction of Veratrum Nigrum and Radix Glycyrrhizae
(*Lilu Gancao Tang*):

(Prescription has been lost.)

CLAUSE 19-3

Zhuanjin (spasm) is a syndrome with stiff arms and legs and slightly tight pulse which moves to and fro in a straight line. When the spasm invades the abdomen, Powder of Chicken Excrement can be adopted.

Powder of Chicken Excrement
(*Jishibai San*):

White of chicken excrement

Pound the drug into powder and blend with six *ge* of water. Take when lukewarm in one dose.

CLAUSE 19-4

Yinhushan (hernia) (1) that causes swelling in the scrotum on one side and shrinking on the other with ascending and descending feelings can be treated with Powder of Spider.

NOTES

1. *Yinhushan*, literally "Yin fox-hernia," indicates that the hernia is as uncertain as a fox. (02-177)

Powder of Spider
(*Zhizhu San*):

Spiders (prepared)	14 pcs.
Ramulus Cinnamomi	0.5 *liang*

Pound the drugs into powder. Take eight *fen* per dose with water twice a day. Pills can also be made with honey.

Explanation of the Prescription: Powder of Spider has the function of dispersing the stagnation and regulating the physiological activities. When assisted by Ramulus Cinnamomi, pungent and warm, it can disperse the pathogenetic Cold in the Liver Channel of the Greater Yin. But spiders are poisonous and caution is advised. In such cases, later scholars prefer the following drugs, all which regulate the Liver and smooth the flow of Vital Energy: Fructus Meliae Toosendan, Rhizoma Corydalis, Radix Aucklandiae, Fructus Foeniculi, Rhizoma Cyperi and Radix Linderae. (02-177)

CASES

Case 1 (64-739): Case Recorded in Journal of *Henan Chinese Medicine*, 1:41, 1984

I had treated all hernias with Powder of Spider for sixty years, about one thousand cases. None of the patient had been poisoned.

Prescription:

Spiders (baked them in a new tile over fire)	14 pcs.
Cortex Cinnamomi	5 *qian* (15 grams)

Pound the drugs into powder. Serve two times a day, three grams per serving.

A boy of seven had a hernia since he was a baby. When he was only a few months old, the mother could see the scrotum enlarge when he cried. This made him cry even harder. When examined at seven, the doctor could identify a hernia on the right side, with the intestines descending into the scrotum. When the boy was lying down the intestines could be pushed back into place and the scrotum became smaller. As soon as he stood up the intestines descended again. Powder of Spider was served. Within a week, the syndrome was gone. There was no recurrence in the following ten years.

CLAUSE 19-5

Question: Describe the pulse in a case of abdominal pain caused by ascarides.

Master: Pulse should be deep or tight. If it is grand-huge, it indicates a case of ascariasis.

CLAUSE 19-6

Ascariasis will cause the patient to vomit saliva and experience paroxysmal pains in the epigastrium and the abdomen. Toxic drugs that dispel the ascarides have been adopted, but they are not effective. Decoction of Radix Glycyrrhizae, Rice Powder and Honey can be adopted.

Decoction of Radix Glycyrrhizae, Rice Powder and Honey (*Gancao Fen Mi Tang*):

Radix Glycyrrhizae	2 *liang*
Rice powder*	1 *liang*

Honey (Mel) 4 *liang*

Stew Radix Glycyrrhizae in three *sheng* of water until two *sheng* remain. Filter the decoction. Add rice powder and honey and stew again until it resembles thin porridge. Serve one *sheng* of lukewarm decoction per dose. Stop taking when the syndrome subsides.

*Some annotators believe this is lead powder (*Qian fen*) which can kill the ascarides. Because it is poisonous, caution is advised.

Explanation of the Prescription: Lead powder kills the ascarides. Based on clinical practice, dosage should be as follows:

Lead powder	3 grams
Radix Glycyrrhizae (can be used in a larger amount than given in original prescription)	
Honey (Mel) (minimum)	30 grams

When syndrome subsides, stop taking the medicine. This is a precaution designed to protect the Body Resistance. (02-178)

CLAUSE 19-7*

If coldness in extremities is caused by ascarides, the patient should vomit ascarides. When the patient is quiet and feels occasionally restless, it is a case of coldness in the Viscera (1). When ascarides appear above the diaphragm, restlessness results but ceases shortly. The patient will be nauseous and vomit after eating, after which he will become restless. When ascarides smell food and crawl upward, the patient will vomit ascarides. Pills of Fructus Mume can cure coldness in the extremities caused by ascariasis.

NOTES

1. Coldness in the Viscera: Weakness and evanescence of the Stomach and Intestine function. (04-197)

Wu Qian's remark: "It is a case of coldness in the Viscera" makes no sense. It should read "It is *not* a case of coldness in the Viscera." (05-256)

*This clause also appears in *Shanghan Lun* (Clause 338).

Pills of Fructus Mume
(*Wumei Wan*):

Fructus Mume	300 pcs.
Herba Asari	6 *liang*
Rhizoma Zingiberis	10 *liang*
Rhizoma Coptidis	16 *liang*
Radix Angelicae Sinensis	4 *liang*
Radix Aconiti Praeparata	6 *liang*
Pericarpium Zanthoxyli	4 *liang*
Ramulus Cinnamomi	6 *liang*
Radix Ginseng	6 *liang*
Cortex Phellodendri	6 *liang*

Pound the drugs separately into powder and mix together. Soak Fructus Mume in vinegar overnight. Remove the kernels of Fructus Mume and steam in a pot under five *dou* of rice. When rice is well-cooked, pound it with Fructus Mume until creamy. Continue this with the powdered drugs and pound two thousand times with honey. Form pills the size of Chinese parasol seeds. Take ten pills before meals, three times a day. Dosage can be increased to twenty pills. Avoid eating cold dishes, hard-to-digest food and strongly spiced food.

Explanation of the Prescription: Rhizoma Coptidis and Cortex Phellodendri eliminate the Heat at the Upper Portion. Rhizoma Zingiberis, Radix Aconiti Praeparata, Herba Asari and Pericarpium Zanthoxyli warm the coldness at the Lower Portion. Fructus Mume, sour in taste, stimulates the function of the Liver and relieves the Stomach (kills ascarides). Radix Angelicae Sinensis tonifies the Liver Blood. Ramulus Cinnamomi harmonizes the Vital Energy of the Liver. Radix Ginseng regulates the Interior Vital Energy, since warm and cold drugs are used simultaneously. This prescription is suitable in cases of "upper Heat and lower Cold." (Clause 338 of *Shanghan Lun* should be consulted.) (04-197)

CHAPTER XX

ON PULSE, SYMPTOM COMPLEX AND TREATMENT OF GYNOPATHY DURING PREGNANCY

CLAUSE 20-1

Master: The pulse of a woman patient is moderate, but the pulse at the Cubit is slender and weak (1). She is also thirsty and has no appetite. No fever or chill is observed. This indicates a pregnancy. Decoction of Ramulus Cinnamomi can be adopted (see Clause 17-36). This syndrome generally appears on the sixtieth day of pregnancy. In case of improper treatment, syndrome will appear with complications of vomiting and diarrhea at the end of the first month of pregnancy. At this point, Decoction of Ramulus Cinnamomi is no longer suited to the case (2).

NOTES

1. The pulse during pregnancy is generally slippery and slightly speedy. (01-211)

2. The syndrome is aggravated due to incorrect treatment, and vomiting and diarrhea are observed. At this point, Decoction of Ramulus Cinnamomi is no longer recommended for the case. Instead of taking medicine, the patient should follow a proper diet. If syndrome still does not subside, treatment should be adopted according to case. (02-180)

CASES

Case 1 (65-564): Case Recorded in *The Great Wall Medical News*, 1:20, 1982

Zhang, 25, first treatment on January 25, 1980. The patient told doctor she had menolipsis for two and a half months with headache, nausea and vomit and had not eaten for three days.

Examination: The patient had normal constitution, but showed signs of malnutrition: pale face, pale tongue covered with thin and white coating, no fever and chill. Pulse was slippery and speedy.

Diagnosis: The patient had a weak Spleen and Stomach. Being pregnant, she had severe nausea and vomit. This was morning sickness due to deficient Spleen and Stomach. The decoction was prescribed as follows:

Ramulus Cinnamomi	9 grams
Radix Paeoniae Alba	12 grams
Rhizoma Zingiberis Recens	7 grams
Fructus Ziziphi Jujubae	5 pcs.
Radix Glycyrrhizae	7 grams
Fructus Amomi	10 grams
Poria	9 grams
Rhizoma Atractylodis Macrocephalae	15 grams
Radix Codonopsis Pilosulae	12 grams

Two doses of the decoction cured the ailment.

Case 2 (65-564): Case Recorded in Journal of *Zhejiang Chinese Medicine*, 1:26, 1965

Liu, 24, first treatment on December 6, 1963. Menstruation had ceased for three months. General lassitude, nausea and vomit, thirsty but could not take water, tastelessness in mouth, anorexia, vertigo, sleepiness, chill and fever were diagnosed. Pulse was slippery and slender, tongue coating was pale and white.

Diagnosis: Pregnancy. Decoction of Ramulus Cinnamomi (Ramulus Cinnamomi, Radix Paeoniae, Radix Glycyrrhizae, Rhizoma Zingiberis Recens and Fructus Ziziphi Jujubae) was prescribed.

Second treatment on December 10. All symptoms subsided. Pulse was slippery and weak, tongue was pink. Decoction of Ramulus Cinnamomi *Xinjia* (Ramulus Cinnamomi, Radix Paeoniae, Radix Glycyrrhizae, Radix Ginseng, Fructus Ziziphi Jujubae, and Rhizoma Zingiberis Recens, also see Clause 62 of *Shanghan Lun*) was given. Two doses were effective in curing morning sickness. The patient had her baby in July the following year.

CLAUSE 20-2

A woman patient who originally suffered from *Zheng* disease (1) ceases menstruating for a period of less than three months, but continues to suffer from mild chronic bloody vaginal discharges. She also feels a quickening in the abdomen above the navel, which is caused by *Zheng* disease. If menstruation is normal for three months prior to conception and if the patient feels the quickening during the sixth month after conception, fetus will be normal. In case menstruation ceases for three months and is followed by mild chronic bloody vaginal discharge, blood stasis will result. Bloody discharge does not cease because *Zheng* has not yet subsided. Stasis should be removed with Pills of Ramulus Cinnamomi and Poria.

NOTES

1. *Zheng*: A disease with a mass or blood stasis in the abdomen. (01-212)

Pills of Ramulus Cinnamomi and Poria
(*Guizhi Fuling Wan*):

Ramulus Cinnamomi
Poria
Cortex Moutan Radicis
Semen Persicae
Radix Paeoniae

Pound the drugs in equal amounts into powder. Blend with honey and form pills the size of rabbit feces. Take one pill before every meal. If not effective increase dosage to three pills.

Explanation of the Prescription: Ramulus Cinnamomi, warm in quality, dredges through the blood channels, Cortex Moutan Radicis and Semen Persicae remove the stasis. Poria is used to facilitate the normal flow of Water and Blood. Radix Paeoniae is added to protect the Blood, harmonize the Nutrient Essence and nourish the Liver. (01-212)

CASES

Case 1 (65-567): Case Recorded in *Journal* of *Zhejiang College of Chinese Medicine*, 3:2, 1979

Xu, 32, first treatment on July 1965. The patient had not been pregnant in ten years of married life. In the past six months she had irregular menstral periods sometimes lasting 15 days. The discharge was bright red, large in quantity, mixed with purple clots. After bed rest a moving mass could be palpated in the lower abdomen on the left. There was tenderness and contracture in the lower abdomen.

Diagnosis by Western docters was "hysteromyoma". Because the patient wanted to have a child she was reluctant to have surgery and went to a Chinese doctor for treatment.

Examination: The patient had a pale face, but no other symptoms that suggested any other disease.

Diagnosis: Syndrome of blood disorder to be treated by regulating the blood and removing the stasis.

Decoction of Ramulus Cinnamomi and Poria was prescribed:

Ramulus Cinnamomi	3 grams
Radix Angelicae Sinensis	4.5 grams
Semen Persicae	6 grams
Cortex Moutan Radicis	6 grams
Rhizoma Cyperi	6 grams
Poria	9 grams
Radix Paeoniae Alba	9 grams
Radix Salviae Miltiorrhizae	9 grams
Faeces Trogopterorum	9 grams

Two doses a day were served at first. Mass in abdomen reduced, then one dose per day. Five months later, gynecological examination showed the subsidence of tumor. Menstruation returned normal consequently.

Case 2 (48-453): Pelvic Inflammation, Cases Recorded in Journal of *New Chinese Medicine*, Vol. 6, 1975

A report from a hospital of Huiyang County, Guangdong Province said that Decoction of Ramulus Cinnamomi and Poria was used to treat 200 cases of pelvic inflammation. Study of fifty cases showed the following:

Chronic pelvic inflammation: 35 cases
- 27 cases were cured;
- 8 cases did not show much improvement.

Subacute pelvic inflammation: 10 cases
- 8 cases were cured;
- 2 cases did not show much improvement.

Acute pelvic inflammation: 5 cases
- 4 cases were cured;
- 1 case did not show much improvement.

Number of days on average for symptoms to subside: 6.8-18.9 days.

Prescription:

Ramulus Cinnamomi	6 grams
Poria	12 grams
Semen Persicae	6 grams
Radix Paeoniae Alba	12 grams
Cortex Moutan Radicis	9 grams
Rhizoma Cyperi Praeparata	9 grams

Radix Angelicae Sinensis	9 grams
Rhizoma Corydalis	6 grams

Preparation 1: Stew the above drugs to make decoction. Serve the decoction before a meal and have the patient rest half an hour.

Preparation 2: Make pills, six grams each with honey. Serve one pill, two times a day.

Case 3 (48-453): Sterility, Case Recorded from *Dr. Yue Meizhong's Clinical Experience*

Yan, in her thirties, had not been pregnant in ten years of married life. One year earlier, she suffered from endometritis and had an operation. After that, menstruation stopped. Every other month, there occurred an epistaxis and hematemesis. Bloody vesicles with purulent secretion appeared in the skin. In the last three months epistaxis attacked more frequently. The vagina was dry and rough.

Treatment: Combination of Decoction of Ramulus Cinnamomi and Poria and Powder of Radix Angelicae Sinensis and Radix Paeoniae (see Clause 20-5) with additions was prescribed:

Ramulus Cinnamomi
Poria
Cortex Moutan Radicis
Semen Persicae
Radix Paeoniae
Radix Angelicae Sinensis
Rhizoma Atractylodis Macrocephalae
Rhizoma Alismatis
Rhizoma Ligustici Chuanxiong
Radix et Rhizoma Rhei
Flos Carthami

Acupuncture on Sanyinjiao (SP 6), Hegu (LI 4) and Guanyuan (RN 4) was practiced.

Twenty doses cured the ailment and helped resume the menstruation. A month later the patient was pregnant and had a baby boy.

Case 4 (48-454): Dysmenorrhea, Case Recorded in Journal of *Shanghai Chinese Medicine and Pharmacology*

Dai, 18, unmarried, had suffered from dysmenorrhea for three years. Before the menstruation period, she had severe abdominal pain, accompanied by acid regurgitation, anorexia, nausea, epigastric distress, insomnia and general lassitude. Pulse was tight-slender, tongue was covered with thin and greasy coating. There was tenderness at lower abdomen.

Prescription:

Ramulus Cinnamomi	3 grams
Poria	9 grams
Cortex Moutan Radicis	9 grams
Semen Persicae	9 grams
Radix Paeoniae Rubra	4.5 grams
Radix Paeoniae Alba	4.5 grams
Radix Angelicae Sinensis	15 grams
Herba Lycopi	9 grams
Rhizoma Pinelliae (prepared with ginger)	6 grams
Pericarpium Citri Reticulatae	4.5 grams

After two doses of the decoction, abdominal pain subsided. The patient no longer had nausea and acid regurgitation. Discharge in the menses was black blood.

Second treatment: The same prescription (subtracting Rhizoma Pinelliae) was given again. The decoctions worked. The doctor told her as soon as she felt the menses coming to take one dose every day till the second day of menses. The patient followed instructions for three months (three menstrual cycles), the drugs worked as anticipated.

CLAUSE 20-3

During the sixth and seventh month of pregnancy, the patient has fever and pulse is tight. Abdomen is distended, and this becomes aggravated. She had abdominal pains and a feeling of cold, as if the abdomen were being fanned. This indicates the opening of the uterus. Decoction of Radix Aconiti Praeparata should be adopted to warm the uterus.

(Prescription is missing.)*

*Though prescription is lost, Decoction of Radix Aconiti Praeparata is considered to be Decoction of Radix Aconiti Praeparata as recorded in the Lesser Yin Chapter of *Shanghan Lun*. The prescription appears in Clause 304 as follows:

Radix Aconiti Praeparata	2 pcs.
Poria	3 *liang*
Radix Paeoniae	3 *liang*
Rhizoma Atractylodis Macrocephalae	4 *liang*
Radix Ginseng	2 *liang*

Radix Aconiti Praeparata has the function of aborting the fetus, and is thus not suitable to pregnant patients. But since it is a case with severe Deficiency of the Yang Vital Energy, Radix Aconiti Praeparata must be used. It has the added efficacy of tranquilizing the fetus. (02-183)

CLAUSE 20-4

Master: Decoction of Colla Corii Asini and Folium Artemisiae Argyi can be prescribed in the following cases: mild chronic bloody vaginal discharge; mild chronic bloody vaginal discharge after miscarriage, and mild chronic bloody vaginal discharge with abdominal pain resulting from retarded growth of fetus.

Decoction of Colla Corii Asini and Folium Artemisiae Argyi*
(*Xiong Gui Jiao Ai Tang*):

Rhizoma Ligustici Chuanxiong	2 *liang*
Radix Glycyrrhizae	2 *liang*
Folium Artemisiae Argyi	3 *liang*
Radix Angelicae Sinensis	3 *liang*
Radix Paeoniae	4 *liang*
Radix Rehmanniae	6 *liang*
Colla Corii Asini	2 *liang*

Stew the first six drugs in five *sheng* of water and three *sheng* of rice wine until three *sheng* remain. Filter the decoction. Add Colla Corii Asini and allow it to dissolve thoroughly. Serve one *sheng* of lukewarm decoction per dose three times a day. If not effective, additional doses should be served.

*According to another edition, one *liang* of Rhizoma Zingiberis should be added to the prescription. Hu Qia (in fifth century A.D.) stated in *Hu Qia's Prescriptions* that this prescription is effective in stopping the movement of the fetus. Rhizoma Zingiberis is not included.

Explanation of the Prescription: Radix Angelicae Sinensis, Rhizoma Ligustici Chuanxiong, Radix Paeoniae and Radix Rehmanniae tonify the Blood and remove stasis. Colla Corii Asini and Folium Artemisiae Argyi nourish the Blood Cavity and warm the uterus. Radix Glycyrrhizae harmonizes the Yin and the Yang and regulates Blood circulation. This is a prescription with a tonifying and stabilizing effect applicable to most of the cases involving bloody discharge in female patients. (01-214)

CASES

Case 1 (48-475): Cases Recorded in Journal of *Zhejiang Chinese Medicine*, Vol. 7, 1959

Decoction of Colla Corii Asini and Folium Artemisiae Argyi was used to treat incomplete abortion. Of the forty-one cases treated, thirty-six were cured; five cases had some improvement. On average, 4.6 doses were needed to effect a treatment.

Indication: After abortion, if tissues were found at ostium of uterus and in uterine cavity, they should be taken out and Decoction of Colla Corii Asini and Folium Artemisiae Argyi with additions was taken, one dose per day till the subsidence of bleeding and closing of ostium of uterus.

The decoction promotes uterine contraction, exhausting the rudimentaries, removing stasis and suppressing pain, promoting metabolism and whetting appetite.

Prescription:

Radix Angelicae Sinensis (prepared with salt water)	9 grams
Rhizoma Zingiberis (carbonated)	4.5 grams
Radix Rehmanniae (carbonated)	12 grams
Radix Paeoniae Alba Praeparata	4.5 grams
Radix Glycyrrhizae Praeparata	2.4 grams
Folium Artemisiae Argyi (carbonated)	4.5 grams
Rhizoma Ligustici Chuanxiong (carbonated)	4.5 grams
Os Spiellae Praeparata	9 grams
Colla Corii Asini	12 grams

Case 2 (48-475): Threatened Abortion, Cases Recorded in Journal of *Chinese Medicine*, Vol. 3, 1967

Decoction of Colla Corii Asini and Folium Artemisiae Argyi adding Rhizoma Atractylodis Macrocephalae and Ramulus Loranthi was used to treat nineteen cases of threatened abortion. Two to five doses were used in varied cases. All were cured effectively.

Case 3 (48-476): Functional Endometrorrhagia (Uterine Bleeding), Cases Recorded in Journal of *Chinese Obstetrics and Gynecology*, May, 1959

The journal reported the using of Decoction of Colla Corii Asini and Folium Artemisiae Argyi in treating twenty-five cases of functional uterine bleeding. Among them, sixty-eight percent were cured effectively and thirty-two percent had marked progress. But the decoction was not effective in treating uterine bleeding. It was not effective in cases of hypermenorrhea or bleeding resulting from organic pathological changes.

Case 4 (64-759): Case Recorded in *Collection of Case Studies and Commentaries of Chinese Medical Doctors*

Yang, 31, first treatment on August 5, 1976. The patient was pregnant four months and had bloody discharge. The discharge was unexpected and not in large quantity. She suffered no abdominal pain. Pulse was slippery but weak.

Diagosis: Syndrome caused by overexertion, and damaged Spleen, which affected the Liver. Deficiency in both of the Viscera caused the leaking. The prescription was given to nourish the blood and soothe the fetus:

Colla Corii Asini (blend into the already stewed decoction before service)	9 grams
Folium Artemisiae Argyi	9 grams
Radix Rehmanniae	15 grams
Radix Paeoniae Alba	9 grams
Radix Angelicae Sinensis	9 grams
Rhizoma Ligustici Chuanxiong	3 grams
Radix Dipsaci	9 grams
Cortex Eucommiae Praeparata	9 grams
Radix Ginseng	9 grams
Radix Scutellariae	6 grams
Radix Glycyrrhizae	6 grams

Second treatment on August 9. Bleeding reduced. Another five doses were given, which worked as anticipated.

CLAUSE 20-5

Powder of Radix Angelicae Sinensis and Radix Paeoniae can be prescribed for pregnant women with chronic abdominal pain and contractions.

Powder of Radix Angelicae Sinensis and Radix Paeoniae (*Danggui Shaoyao San*):

Radix Angelicae Sinensis	3 *liang*
Radix Paeoniae	1 *jin*
Poria	4 *liang*
Rhizoma Atractylodis Macrocephalae	4 *liang*
Rhizoma Alismatis	0.5 *jin*

Rhizoma Ligustici Chuanxiong	0.5 *jin**

Pound the drugs into powder. Take one *fangcunbi* of the powder with wine per dose three times a day.

*According to another edition, 3 *liang*.

Explanation of the Prescription: Radix Angelicae Sinensis and Rhizoma Ligustici Chuanxiong tonify the Blood and ease pain. Radix Paeoniae is heavily dosed to moisten the Liver and dredge through the stagnation. Rhizoma Atractylodis Macrocephalae, Poria and Rhizoma Alismatis tonify the Spleen and drain the Humidity. This prescription eases pain and tranquilizes the fetus. For patients of weak build, dosage of Rhizoma Ligustici Chuanxiong should be reduced. (01-215)

CASES

Case 1 (48-457):

Shen, 38, had menses every two weeks. Menses were accompanied by abdominal pain and distention, dysuria, vertigo, anorexia, general lassitude, puffy face and eyelids. Tongue was pale, covered with thin coating. Pulse was tight. It was a syndrome caused by conflicting Spleen and Liver Vital Energies. Powder of Radix Angelicae Sinensis and Radix Paeoniae (in decoction form) was prescribed:

Radix Angelicae Sinensis	9 grams
Rhizoma Ligustici Chuanxiong	6 grams
Radix Paeoniae Alba	15 grams
Rhizoma Atractylodis Macrocephalae	12 grams
Poria	12 grams
Rhizoma Alismatis	12 grams

Decoction was given one dose per day for a week. Symptoms subsided. Treatment continued for another two weeks. Abdominal pain subsided and menstruation returned to normal.

Case 2 (48-458):

Once Doctor Yue Meizhong treated two girls who had abdominal pain due to gynecological troubles.

Miss Shao: She had abdominal pain accompanied by profuse leukorrhea and vertigo. A hospital of Western medicine diagnosed chronic pelvic inflammation. Powder of Radix Angelicae Sinensis and Radix Paeoniae was prescribed:

Radix Angelicae Sinensis	9 grams
Radix Paeoniae Alba	18 grams
Rhizoma Ligustici Chuanxiong	6 grams
Rhizoma Atractylodis Macrocephalae	9 grams
Poria	9 grams
Rhizoma Alismatis	12 grams

After several doses of the decoction, abdominal pain and vertigo subsided and leukorrhea was reduced.

Miss Gui: She had abdominal pain with a descending feeling accompanied by profuse leukorrhea and vertigo. Powder of Radix Angelicae Sinensis and Radix Paeoniae worked effectively. In follow-up treatment to clear away leukorrhea, Decoction for Removing Blood Stasis in Lower Abdomen (*Shao Fu Zhu Yu Tang*) was prescribed:

Fructus Foeniculi
Rhizoma Zingiberis
Rhizoma Corydalis
Resina Commiphorae Myrrhae
Radix Angelicae Sinensis
Rhizoma Ligustici Chuanxiong
Cortex Cinnamomi
Radix Paeoniae Rubra
Pollen Typhae
Faeces Trogopterorum

Case 3 (65-573):

Li, 24, was three months' pregnant. She had lower abdominal pain which reduced when palpated. The patient had a cyan and yellow complexion, with vertigo, blurred vision, irritation, anorexia, sporadic nausea and puffy legs. Tongue was pale fringed with red edge and covered with white-thin and greasy coating. Pulse was tight-slender, slippery and speedy.

This syndrome reflected a deficient condition of the Liver and Blood and Humidity-impaired Spleen that had lost control of Water circulation.

Powder of Radix Angelicae Sinensis and Radix Paeoniae with additions was prescribed, prepared in decoction form:

Radix Angelicae Sinensis	9 grams
Radix Paeoniae Alba	20 grams
Rhizoma Ligustici Chuanxiong	6 grams
Rhizoma Atractylodis Macrocephalae	10 grams

Poria	12 grams
Rhizoma Alismatis	12 grams
Pericarpium Citri Reticulatae	9 grams
Radix Scutellariae	9 grams
Ramulus Loranthi	9 grams
Radix Glycyrrhizae	6 grams
Terra Flava Usta	9 grams

Three doses cured the ailment.

CLAUSE 20-6

A pregnant woman is suffering from repeated nausea and vomiting. Pills of Rhizoma Zingiberis, Radix Ginseng and Rhizoma Pinelliae can be adopted.

Pills of Rhizoma Zingiberis, Radix Ginseng and Rhizoma Pinelliae (*Ganjiang Renshen Banxia Wan*):

Rhizoma Zingiberis	1 *liang*
Radix Ginseng	1 *liang*
Rhizoma Pinelliae	2 *liang*

Pound the drugs into powder and blend with juice of fresh ginger (Rhizoma Zingiberis Recens). Form pills the size of Chinese parasol seeds. Take ten pills per dose three times a day.

Explanation of the Prescription: Wu Qian: This is a case of nausea and vomiting during early pregnancy (*E zu*). The patient has suffered Cold Fluid-retention which has hampered fetal growth, making it difficult for the patient to eat. Rhizoma Zingiberis is used to eliminate the Cold. Rhizoma Pinelliae stops the nausea. As the repeated vomiting damages the Stomach Vital Energy, Radix Ginseng is added to protect the Vital Energy. (05-642)

Lou Quanshan: I have repeatedly used Rhizoma Pinelliae in the treatment of nausea and vomiting in female patients during early pregnancy. In no case has the fetus been hurt in any way. (It is commonly believed that Rhizoma Pinelliae is poisonous and should not be given to female patients during pregnancy.) (05-643)

Chen Xiuyuan: When Rhizoma Pinelliae is used together with Radix Ginseng, it will no longer be harmful to the fetus. (02-185)

CASES

Case 1 (64-763): Case Recorded in *Dr. Qian Boxuan's Case Studies of Gynecology*

Mrs. Guo, first treatment on June 18, 1959. The patient was forty-five days' pregnant. Nausea and vomit occurred ten days ago and was aggravated in the last four days. The patient could no longer eat or drink, and vomited yellow fluid. Vertigo and constipation were reported. Tongue was covered with thin and greasy coating. Pulse was slender-tight and speedy on the left and slippery-speedy on the right.

Diagnosis: Accumulation of phlegm and Humidity hampering the normal function of the Stomach, which should be warmed and tonified to dissolve the phlegm and drain the turbidity

Pills of Rhizoma Zingiberis, Radix Ginseng and Rhizoma Pinelliae were prescribed:

Radix Codonopsis Pilosulae	3 grams
Rhizoma Zingiberis	3 grams
Rhizoma Pinelliae	3 grams

Mixed and pounded the drugs into powder. Served 1.5 grams per dose with four drops of fresh ginger juice. The drug worked effectively.

Case 2 (64-764): Case Recorded in Journal of *Jiangxi Chinese Medicine and Pharmacology*, 1:61, 1981

Liao, 22-year-old nurse, had no menses for more than fifty days. She was vomiting clear fluid and saliva and could eat little food. When food was taken, she would vomit. The patient was chilly and preferred warmth.

Examination: The patient had a pale face, thin constitution, normal stool, clear and ample urination. Tongue was pink, covered with white-thick and slippery coating. Pulse was slow-slender and slippery.

Diagnosis: Syndrome caused by ascending phlegm and Fluid-retention due to cold and deficient Spleen and Stomach.

Treatment: Pills of Rhizoma Zingiberis, Radix Ginseng and Rhizoma Pinelliae were given to warm the Interior and bring down the adverse ascending:

Rhizoma Zingiberis	6 grams
Radix Codonopsis Pilosulae	12 grams
Rhizoma Pinelliae	6 grams
Rhizoma Zingiberis Recens	6 grams
Fructus Amomi	5 grams

Pericarpium Citri Reticulatae	6 grams

Stewed the drugs in a larger quantity of water than normal until a thick decoction was made. Served the decoction little by little.

After two doses, nausea and vomit reduced and the patient was less chilly. She began to eat a small amount.

Second treatment: The following prescription was given:

Radix Codonopsis Pilosulae	12 grams
Rhizoma Atractylodis Macrocephalae Praeparata	9 grams
Rhizoma Zingiberis	4 grams
Rhizoma Pinelliae	4 grams
Fructus Evodiae	3 grams
Pericarpium Citri Reticulatae	6 grams
Fructus Amomi	5 grams
Rhizoma Zingiberis Recens	4 grams

The decoction was prepared and served the same way as the first. The patient felt better. A baby girl was born in due course.

CLAUSE 20-7

A pregnant woman is eating normally but is suffering dysuria. Pills of Radix Angelicae Sinensis, Bulbus Fritillariae Thunbergii and Radix Sophorae Flavescentis can be adopted (1).

NOTES

1. A pregnant woman who eats normally but who suffers from dysuria is normal in the Upper and Middle Portions of Body Cavity but is suffering from Humidity-Heat in the Lower Portion. While Humidity-Heat prevails in the Lower Portion, the action of the Vital Energy of the Urinary Bladder is hampered, which in turn hampers the normal circulation of water, resulting in dysuria. (01-215)

Pills of Radix Angelicae Sinensis, Bulbus Fritillariae Thunbergii and Radix Sophorae Flavescentis
(*Danggui Beimu Kushen Wan*):
For male patients, half *liang* of Talcum should be added.*

Radix Angelicae Sinensis	4 *liang*
Bulbus Fritillariae Thunbergii	4 *liang*
Radix Sophorae Flavescentis	4 *liang*

Pound the drugs into powder. Blend with honey and form pills the size of Semen Phaseoli. Take three pills per dose. Dosage can be increased to ten pills.

*Later annotators generally delete this sentence.

Explanation of the Prescription: This prescription is effective in curing dysuria by dredging through the stagnation and eliminating the Humidity-Heat. Radix Angelicae Sinensis harmonizes the Blood and moistens the Dryness. Radix Sophorae Flavescentis eliminates the Heat and facilitates Water circulation. Bulbus Fritillariae Thunbergii unblocks the stagnation, normalizes the Vital Energy and disperses the Humidity-Heat. Some annotators think this prescription is for cases of constipation in pregnant women. (01-216)

CASES

Case 1 (65- 577): Case Recorded in Journal of *Zhejiang Chinese Medicine*, 11:506, 1981

Chen, 24, first treatment on June 15, 1976. The patient was three months' pregnant with her second child. In the last eight days she had dysuria and urinated only a few drops at a time. There was distention and a bearing down feeling, worse during urination. The patient could eat little and dared not drink, though she was thirsty. Pulse was deep-slender on the left, tight and slippery on the right. Tongue was red, covered with thin-white and slightly greasy coating.

Diagnosis: Syndrome caused by accumulated Heat when Blood was deficient. To nourish the Blood and moisten the dryness, eliminate Heat and disperse stagnation was the treatment.

Pills of Radix Angelicae Sinensis, Bulbus Fritillariae Thunbergii and Radix Sophorae Flavescentis with additions were prescribed:

Radix Angelicae Sinensis	12 grams
Bulbus Fritillariae Thunbergii	12 grams
Radix Sophorae Flavescentis	12 grams
Radix Bupleuri	12 grams
Radix Scutellariae	12 grams
Radix Paeoniae Alba	12 grams
Radix Adenophorae	12 grams
Radix Ophiopogonis	12 grams
Rhizoma Pinelliae	10 grams

Rhizoma Alismatis	10 grams
Fructus Ziziphi Jujubae	10 grams
Rhizoma Zingiberis Recens	6 grams
Fructus Meliae Toosendan	6 grams
Radix Glycyrrhizae	3 grams

One dose smoothed the urination.

Case 2 (65-577):

Doctor Qin Bowei explained the prescription of Clause 20-7 in his *Simplified Explanation of Synopsis of the Golden Chamber* as follows:

I just got a letter from Doctor Shen Jieye of Jinhua, Zhejiang Province, pointing out that Clause 20-7 was treatment for constipation rather than dysuria in pregnant women. This, according to Shen, is his grandfather's and his own clinical experience. The prescription is good for habitual constipation occurring in pregnant women or constipation accompanied by a dry cough.

Prescription:

Radix Angelicae Sinensis	4 unit
Bulbus Fritillariae Thunbergii	3 unit
Radix Sophorae Flavescentis	3 unit

Make pills with honey. After taking the pills, stool should be smooth and normal (once a day). Dry cough should subside. In our family tradition, when we saw cases of constipation in pregnant women who were too weak for a purgative, this prescription worked.

CLAUSE 20-8

A pregnant woman is suffering Fluid-retention syndrome with symptoms and signs of heaviness of movement, dysuria, aversion to cold and vertigo which is aggravated when the patient stands up. In such cases, Powder of Semen Malvae Verticillatae and Poria can be prescribed.

Powder of Semen Malvae Verticillatae and Poria
(*Kuizi Fuling San*):

Semen Malvae Verticillatae	1 *jin*
Poria	3 *liang*

Pound the drugs into powder. Take one *fangcunbi* per dose three times a day. When urination returns to normal, the syndrome disappears.

Explanation of the Prescription: Wu Qian: A pregnant woman is suffering Fluid-retention syndrome which causes edema and aversion to cold. When the Water is excessive in the Exterior, heaviness of movement results. When the Water is exuberant in the Interior, dysuria results. The active pathogenetic Water hampers the normal ascending of Yang Vital Energy to the head which brings about vertigo. Powder of Semen Malvae Verticillatae and Poria is used to clear the orifices to let out the pathogenetic factors and disperse the Fluid-retention. (05-643)

CLAUSE 20-9

Powder of Radix Angelicae Sinensis can be frequently prescribed as a tonic for women during pregnancy (1).

NOTES

1. Wu Qian: Women during pregnancy need not any medicine if no disease is present. When the patient is emaciated and has a fever, Powder of Radix Angelicae Sinensis should be taken frequently, as the patient's Blood may become exhausted and the fetus harmed by the prevalence of Heat. (05-644)

Powder of Radix Angelicae Sinensis
(*Danggui San*):

Radix Angelicae Sinensis	1 *jin*
Radix Scutellariae	1 *jin*
Radix Paeoniae	1 *jin*
Rhizoma Ligustici Chuanxiong	1 *jin*
Rhizoma Atractylodis Macrocephalae	0.5 *jin*

Pound the drugs into powder. Take one *fangcunbi* with wine per dose twice a day. If drug is taken frequently, delivery will be easy and the fetus will be born in healthy condition. This prescription is also effective for various postpartum diseases.

Explanation of the Prescription: You Yi: Pathogenetic Heat can be of great harm to pregnant women. That is why Radix Scutellariae is added to eliminate the Heat along with the other ingredients which tonify the Blood (Radix Angelicae Sinensis, Radix Paeoniae and Rhizoma Ligustici Chuanxiong). Rhizoma Atractylodis Macrocephalae is used to harmonize the Stomach Vital Energy. Zhu Zhenheng (1281-1358) believed that Radix Scutellariae and Rhizoma Atractylodis Macrocephalae were the best fetus-soothing drugs. This is not to say that the two drugs directly soothe the fetus, but that they can disperse Humidity-Heat, the principal factor affecting the fetus. Once Humidity-Heat is dispersed, fetus will be safe. (05-644)

CASES

Case 1 (65-580): Habitual Abortion

Mrs. Yuan had been pregnant five times all aborting during the second and third months. Now, pregnant again, she consulted Doctor Du Yumao.

Examination: The patient was thin, but did not seem to suffer other diseases. She was in normal spiritual condition and good appetite. There was no abdominal pain or lumbago. Pulse was slender and slippery. The doctor told her that he had treated many cases like hers and could help her protect the fetus this time. Pills of Radix Angelicae Sinensis with additions (in decoction form) were prescribed:

Radix Angelicae Sinensis	9 grams
Rhizoma Ligustici Chuanxiong	6 grams
Radix Scutellariae	6 grams
Rhizoma Atractylodis Macrocephalae	9 grams
Rhizoma Rehmanniae Praeparata	12 grams
Radix Dipsaci	12 grams
Ramulus Loranthi	12 grams
Herba Schizonepetae Praeparata	6 grams
Cortex Eucommiae Praeparata	12 grams

Three doses of the decoction were served. There was no unfavorable reaction. The decoction was given till the fifth month. A baby was born in due course.

Case 2 (65-581): Case Recorded in *Commentaries on Ancient and Modern Case Reports*

Dr. Zhu Danxi once treated a pregnant woman of thirty years, who had

had habitual abortions. The patient was irritable and apt to lose temper. Her complexion was dark with symptoms of excessive nature.

Diagnosis: Excessive Fire was hampering the formation of fetus, and should be eliminated.

Prescription:

Radix Scutellariae
Rhizoma Atractylodis Macrocephalae
Radix Angelicae Sinensis
Radix Glycyrrhizae

The decoction was served during the second month of pregnancy until the end of the third month. There was no abortion.

CLAUSE 20-10

Powder of Rhizoma Atractylodis Macrocephalae can be adopted as a tonic to protect the fetus.

Powder of Rhizoma Atractylodis Macrocephalae
(*Baizhu San**):

Rhizoma Atractylodis Macrocephalae	3 *fen*
Rhizoma Ligustici Chuanxiong	3 *fen*
Pericarpium Zanthoxyli	3 *fen*
Concha Ostreae**	

Pound the drugs into powder. Take one *qianbi* with wine three times in the day and once at night.

When the patient feels pain (in the abdomen), add Radix Paeoniae;

When the patient has acute pain in the epigastrium, double the dosage of Rhizoma Ligustici Chuanxiong;

If the patient has restlessness, nausea, vomiting, pain and anorexia, add one *liang* of Herba Asari and twenty large pieces of Rhizoma Pinelliae. After taking the medicine, if the patient still vomits, serve *cujiang* water. If still not efficacious, serve wheat juice (Fructus Tritici). The patient will become thirsty. Feed the patient barley porridge. When the syndrome subsides, continue serving barley porridge as a tonic.

*A prescription from *Waitai*.

**Dosage is lost. According to *Jinkui S*, the prescription includes:

Rhizoma Atractylodis Macrocephalae	4 *fen*
Rhizoma Ligustici Chuanxiong	4 *fen*
Pericarpium Zanthoxyli	3 *fen*
Concha Ostreae	2 *fen*

Explanation of the Prescription: This prescription treats cases of potential miscarriage (threatened abortion) caused by prevalence of Cold-Humidity in the deficient Spleen. Powder of Rhizoma Atractylodis Macrocephalae is adopted to tonify the Spleen and warm the Middle Portion and disperse the Cold-Humidity so as to soothe the fetus. The text states that Powder of Rhizoma Atractylodis Macrocephalae can be adopted as a tonic to protect the fetus. But this does not mean that this prescription is applicable to all cases irrespective of their symptoms and specific nature. (02-187)

CASES

Case 1 (65-582):

Dr. Xu Zhongke treated a pregnant woman for a persistant cough. Before conception she had been coughing up blood. When she consulted the doctor she was emaciated and had abdominal pain. Powder of Rhizoma Atractylodis Macrocephalae adding Radix Paeoniae Alba was given. Two doses cured the troubles.

CLAUSE 20-11

The patient is in the seventh month of pregnancy when she catches a febrile disease caused by Cold, which causes abdominal distention and dysuria. She also feels heaviness in the region below the waist, similar to the feeling experienced in Fluid-retention syndrome. In the seventh month of pregnancy, the Initial Yin Channel should be nourishing the fetus, but it fails to do so. The Heart Vital Energy is in an excessive state. Treatment should be applying needle to acupoints Laogong (PC 8) and Guanyuan (RN 4). When urination begins to return normal, the syndrome will disappear (1).

NOTES

1. **Wu Qian**: Applying needle at Laogong (PC 8) and Guanyuan (CV 4) will induce a miscarriage. This appears incorrect. There are errors and omissions in the clause. (05-645)

Eupolyphaga seu Steleophaga	6 grams
Radix Achyranthis Bidentatae	15 grams
Radix Ginseng	15 grams
Radix Glycyrrhizae	3 grams

Three doses worked effectively. In the vaginal discharge, black clots and white mucous were found. Follow-up treatment was given to harmonize the Interior.

CLAUSE 21-6

On the seventh or eighth day after delivery, the patient does not suffer Initial Yang syndrome (see Chapter I of *Shanghan Lun*) but suffers abdominal distention and pain. This is a case of profuse lochia. Decoction of Greater *Chengqi* (see Clause 2-13) can be adopted when the following symptoms and signs are observed: constipation; fever with restlessness and irritability; and slightly excessive pulse; fever aggravated in the afternoon; poor appetite. If food is taken, delirium will occur but the patient will quiet down at night. This is a case with accumulated pathogenetic Heat in the Urinary Bladder. (1)

NOTES

1. This clause discusses the symptom complex of blood stasis and Greater Yang syndrome of Interior Excess. On the seventh or eighth day after delivery, presence of abdominal distention and pain reflect a case of profuse lochia with blood stasis in the uterus. Constipation, fever with restlessness and irritability which becomes aggravated in the afternoon and excessive pulse indicate prevalence of pathogenetic Heat in the Stomach and the Intestine. Anorexia is caused by Stomach Excess. Intake of food will aggravate the Heat and bring on a state of delirium. At night the Yin Vital Essence is restored, and thus delirium will be reduced. Decoction of Greater *Chengqi* is adopted to purge the Heat and ease defecation. Once the bowels are evacuated, blood stasis is also removed. If abdominal pain is still present after the adoption of the decoction, Decoction for Removing Blood Stasis can be adopted to remove the stasis. "Urinary Bladder" here indicates the Lower Portion of Body Cavity. (02-192)

Syndromes of Postpartum Abdominal Pain (64-787)

Pathology	*Symptoms and signs*	*Principle of treatment*	*Prescription*
Blood Deficiency and Cold	Vague abdominal pain that relieves a bit when warmed or pressed	Tonify the Blood, disperse the Cold, warm the Interior and ease the pain	Decoction of Radix Angelicae Sinensis, Rhizoma Zingiberis Recens and Mutton (Clauses 10-18, 21-3)
Stagnation of Blood and Vital Energy	Abdominal pain and distention, restlessness and chest distress, unable to sleep	Promote circulation of Vital Energy and remove blood stasis	Powder of Fructus Aurantii Immaturus and Radix Paeoniae (Clause 21-4)
Remaining of blood stasis	Stabbing pain in abdomen and/or with hard mass, urination was normal	Remove blood stasis	Decoction for Removing Blood Stasis (Clause 21-5)

CLAUSE 21-7

Postpartum disease caused by Wind (1) lasts for several dozen days. Symptoms and signs include slight headache, aversion to cold, sporadic fever, fullness in the chest, perspiration, nausea and retching. Although the syndrome lasts for a long time, it is still classified as a *Yangdan* syndrome (2). Decoction of *Yangdan* can be adopted. (Decoction of *Yangdan* is just Decoction of Ramulus Cinnamomi. Prescription see Clause 17-36.) (3)

NOTES

1. Postpartum disease caused by Wind (*Chan hou feng*) is febrile disease caused by Wind occurring after delivery. See Clauses 2 and 12 of *Shanghan Lun* for the symptoms and treatment of febrile disease caused by Wind (*Zhong feng*). (01-223)

Tonic Decoction of Radix Angelicae Sinensis from *Qianjin* is effective in treating postpartum weakness and Deficiency accompanied by acute pain in the abdomen and dyspnea, dragging pain in the waist and back, and anorexia. In the first month after delivery, four or five doses will help restore the patient's health.

Tonic Decoction of Radix Angelicae Sinensis
(*Neibu Danggui Jianzhong Tang*):

Radix Angelicae Sinensis	4 *liang*
Ramulus Cinnamomi	3 *liang*
Radix Paeoniae	6 *liang*
Rhizoma Zingiberis Recens	3 *liang*
Radix Glycyrrhizae	2 *liang*
Fructus Ziziphi Jujubae	12 pcs.

Stew the drugs in one *dou* of water until three *sheng* remain. Serve the decoction lukewarm in three doses on a single day. If the patient is extremely weak, add six *liang* of malt sugar and stew until it melts.

If the patient has suffered a great loss of blood, add six *liang* of Radix Rehmanniae and two *liang* of Colla Corii Asini, the latter being added when the decoction is prepared.

If Radix Angelicae Sinensis is not available, Rhizoma Ligustici Chuanxiong can be used, and Rhizoma Zingiberis Recens can be replaced by Rhizoma Zingiberis.

CHAPTER XXII

ON PULSE, SYMPTOM COMPLEX AND TREATMENT OF MISCELLANEOUS GYNECOLOGICAL DISEASES

CLAUSE 22-1

Febrile disease caused by Wind in women: The patient has tidal fever and chills during the seventh or eighth day after last day of menstruation period. This is a case of invasion of Heat in the Blood Cavity (1). Congelation of blood causes tidal chill and fever resembling malaria. Decoction of Lesser Radix Bupleuri can be adopted to cure the disease. (For prescription, see Clause 17-15.)

NOTES

1. Blood Cavity: See Note 1 of Clause 22-3.

CLAUSE 22-2

Febrile disease caused by Cold in women: At the onset of menstruation, the patient has fever and delirium with insanity at night but returns to normal during the day (1). These are symptoms of Heat invading the Blood Cavity. Be careful not to disturb Stomach Vital Energy and the Upper and Middle Portions of Body Cavity (2), a self-healing (3) will follow.

NOTES

1. The statement "delirium with insanity at night but returns to normal during the day" proves that this is a case of invasion of Heat into the Blood Cavity caused by a disease of the Blood rather than of the Vital Energy. As the Vital Energy is Yang in nature, the patient returns to normal in the day (day is Yang, night is Yin); Blood is Yin in nature, so she will suffer from delirium and insanity at night. (04-91)

2. A purgative will hurt the Upper Portion of Body Cavity and an emetic or purgative will hurt the Spleen and the Stomach in the Middle Portion of

Body Cavity. Some annotators suggest acupuncture therapy at Qimen (LR 14) and adoption of Decoction of Lesser Radix Bupleuri with additions and subtractions. (04-91)

3. Fang Youzhi: "Self-healing": During menstruation, pathogenetic Heat will follow the blood and drain out of the body. This is similar to "self-healing" after epistaxis (see Clauses 46 and 47 of *Shanghan Lun*). Zhang Zhongjing's intention here is to warn physicians not to prescribe acute remedies to disperse pathogenetic factors to avoid possible complications. (05-202)

CLAUSE 22-3

Febrile disease caused by Wind in women: The patient has fever and chill during menstruation. After seven or eight days, when fever disappears, her skin cools and pulse becomes slow. She experiences fullness below the costal margin similar to a Blocked-up Chest syndrome, as well as delirium, both of which are symptoms of Heat invading the Blood Cavity (1). Needle therapy at Qimen (LR 14) will release the pathogenetic Heat. (2)

NOTES

1. Blood Cavity (*Xue shi*) may refer to the following:

a) Liver, as the Liver stores blood;

b) *Chongmai*, the Conception Channel, as it is like a sea of blood; or

c) Womb, as menstruation flows from there.

2. Wu Qian: Qimen (LR14) is an acupoint of the Liver. As the Liver stores blood, acupuncture is practiced on Qimen to release the pathogenetic Heat when Heat invades the Blood Cavity. (05-201)

CLAUSE 22-4*

Greater Yang syndrome with delirium and excretion of blood indicates that pathogenetic Heat has invaded the Blood Cavity (1). When sweat appears on the head only, puncture at acupoint Qimen (LR 14) will release the Excess. Following this, heavy perspiration will lead to recovery.

NOTES

1. Wu Qian: Female patients will experience the syndrome of Heat invading the Blood Cavity during menstruation. Male patients will also experience the syndrome of Heat invading the Blood Cavity, which is manifested by delirium and gastrointestinal bleeding (stercorrhagia). (05-155)

*Clauses 22-1, 22-2, 22-3 and 22-4 also appear in *Shanghan Lun* (Clauses 143, 144, 145 and 216).

CLAUSE 22-5

The patient is suffocating as if there were a piece of roast meat stuck in her throat. Decoction of Rhizoma Pinelliae and Cortex Magnoliae Officinalis can provide a cure. (1)

NOTES

1. This case is caused by an accumulation of phlegm and by stagnation of the Vital Energy. Spiritual depression is one of the causes of the disease. When phlegm and Vital Energy stagnate, they may ascend and invade the throat, resulting in this syndrome. Symptoms and signs may include difficulty in swallowing and a feeling of a foreign body lodged in the throat which cannot be spat out or swallowed. But this does not affect normal food intake. Later scholars call this "*Meiheqi*" (globus hystericus). (02-198)

Decoction of Rhizoma Pinelliae and Cortex Magnoliae Officinalis (*Banxia Houpo Tang*):

Rhizoma Pinelliae	1 *sheng*
Cortex Magnoliae Officinalis	3 *liang*
Poria	4 *liang*
Rhizoma Zingiberis Recens	5 *liang*
Folium Perillae	2 *liang*

Stew the drugs in seven *sheng* of water until four *sheng* remain. Serve the decoction in four doses (three in the day and one at night).

Explanation of the Prescription: This prescription unblocks the stagnation, eliminates the phlegm and reverses the adversity. Rhizoma Pinelliae, Cortex Magnoliae Officinalis and Rhizoma Zingiberis Recens, pungent and bitter in taste, disperse the accumulation and reverse the adversity. Poria eliminates the Fluid-retention to eliminate the phlegm. Folium Perillae, fragrant in odor, facilitates the flow of Vital Energy and helps dissipate the stagnation. When the Vital Energy resumes its normal functioning and the phlegm is dispersed, the feeling of a foreign body lodged in the throat will disappear.

Meiheqi (globus hystericus) is not a disease exclusive to women. In clinical situations, drugs which regulate the Vital Energy, such as Rhizoma Cyperi and Pericarpium Citri Reticulatae, can be added to strengthen the action of the prescription. An expectorant, such as Fructus Trichosanthis and Semen Armeniacae Amarum can also be added. (02-198)

CASES

Case 1 (64-815):

Zhang, 52, first treatment on April 10, 1963. The patient felt something stuck in the throat which was diagnosed globus hystericus. She had abdominal distention and a feeling of gas rushing to the throat, and constipation. Passing flatus made the patient feel better. Tongue was covered with thin and greasy coating. Pulse was deep and tight.

Diagnosis: Syndrome caused by obstructed circulation of the Vital Energy and accumulation of phlegm.

Treatment: To dissolve the phlegm and unblock the stagnation of Vital Energy.

Prescription:

Rhizoma Pinelliae (prepared with ginger)	9 grams
Fructus Aurantii Immaturus Praeparata	9 grams
Caulis Bambusae in Taeniam (prepared with ginger)	9 grams
Semen Raphani Praeparata	9 grams
Fructus Trichosanthis	12 grams
Fructus Perillae	4.5 grams
Poria	9 grams
Cortex Magnoliae Officinalis	3 grams
Radix Glycyrrhizae	1.5 grams

Two doses of the decoction were served. After two more calls on April 12 and 15, the patient recovered completely.

Case 2 (64-816): Case Recorded in *Collection of Case Studies of Veteran Doctors in Hunan Province*

Zheng, 48, felt chest distress and suffocating feeling in throat. She could not vomit or swallow the obstructing object. One hospital diagnosed "hysteria." But the treatment that followed did not help.

Examination: Pulse was tight and moderate. Tongue was covered with thin, white coating. The syndrome was aggravated by overexertion. Mental depression resulted.

Diagnosis: Syndrome caused by accumulation and intermingling of phlegm and Vital Energy. Decoction of Rhizoma Pinelliae and Cortex Magnoliae Officinalis with additions was prescribed:

Rhizoma Pinelliae Praeparata	10 grams
Cortex Magnoliae Officinalis	6 grams
Poria	10 grams
Fructus Perillae	3 grams
Fructus Aurantii	6 grams
Fructus Trichosanthis	9 grams
Radix Curcumae	5 grams
Rhizoma Belamcandae	9 grams
Pericarpium Citri Reticulatae	5 grams
Fructus Eriobotryae	5 grams

Seven doses of the decoction reduced the symptoms. Later, drugs to relieve Liver strain were served, which cured the ailment.

CLAUSE 22-6

The patient suffers hysteria and tends to weep constantly as if she were haunted. She frequently stretches and yawns repeatedly. Decoction of Radix Glycyrrhizae, Fructus Tritici and Fructus Ziziphi Jujubae can be adopted to calm the patient.

Decoction of Radix Glycyrrhizae, Fructus Tritici and
Fructus Ziziphi Jujubae
(*Gan Mai Dazao Tang*):

Radix Glycyrrhizae	3 *liang*
Fructus Tritici	1 *sheng*
Fructus Ziziphi Jujubae	10 pcs.

Stew the drugs in six *sheng* of water until three *sheng* remain. Serve the lukewarm decoction in three doses. This decoction is also a tonic for the Spleen.

Explanation of the Prescription: This prescription is effective in treating syndromes of *Zangzao* (hysteria), which results from emotional depression and excessive worry. Symptoms and signs may include restlessness and irritability, insomnia and constipation. To strengthen the action of the prescription, the following can be added: Radix Angelicae Sinensis, Radix Paeoniae Alba, Poria, Semen Ziziphi Spinosae, Semen Biotae, Dens Draconis, Concha Ostreae, etc. (02-199)

CASES

Case 1 (66-246): Cases Recorded in Journal of *Chinese Medicine*, Vol. 2, 1960

The journal reported treatment of twenty-five cases of hysterical mania. Therapeutic results were as follows:

Total: 25 cases.
22 cases were cured;
2 cases had marked progress; and
1 case had certain progress.

Two cases among them had a recurrence.

Prescription:

Fructus Tritici	30 grams
Radix Glycyrrhizae	9 grams
Fructus Ziziphi Jujubae	7 pcs.

The decoction served two times a day. Ten to fifteen doses can be served successively in one period of treatment.

Case 2 (64-819): Case Recorded in *Collection of Case Studies of Veteran Doctors in Hunan Province*

Xiong, 22, had given birth to two children in two years. Excessive loss of blood and overexertion made her weak. Vertigo, dim vision, irritability palpitation, and severe insomnia resulted. The patient laughed and wept unreasonably. Pulse was slender and speedy. Tongue was red, covered with yellow and dry coating.

Decoction of Radix Glycyrrhizae, Fructus Tritici and Fructus Ziziphi Jujubae was prescribed:

Radix Glycyrrhizae	10 grams
Fructus Tritici	30 grams
Fructus Ziziphi Jujubae	20 grams
Os Draconis	10 grams
Bulbus Lilii	15 grams
Semen Ziziphi Spinosae	15 grams
Radix Paeoniae Alba	10 grams
Rhizoma Acori Graminei	6 grams

Radix Rehmanniae	10 grams
Caulis Polygoni Multiflori	12 grams

Second treatment: Five doses were given. The patient could sleep better and looked relaxed. Pulse and tongue condition remained the same. Another five doses were given.

Third treatment: The patient slept better, but appetite was not good. The other symptoms were subsiding. Prescription was given to regulate the Spleen and Stomach function and tranquilize the disturbed mental condition:

Radix Codonopsis Pilosulae	10 grams
Rhizoma Dioscoreae	10 grams
Semen Ziziphi Spinosae	12 grams
Radix Polygalae	6 grams
Radix Polygoni Multiflori	12 grams
Radix Glycyrrhizae	3 grams
Arillus Longan	5 pcs.
Endothelium Corneum Gigeriae Galli	3 grams

Fourth treatment: Three doses of decoction were served. Further treatment cured the trouble.

Case 3 (65-617): Male Hysteria, Case Recorded in *Collection of Dr. Yue Meizhong's Case Studies*

Dr. Yue once treated a man of thirty in Heze County Hospital, Shandong Province. The patient suffered from a mental disorder and wept and laughed unreasonably.

Decoction of Radix Glycyrrhizae, Fructus Tritici and Fructus Ziziphi Jujubae was prescribed:

Radix Glycyrrhizae	9 grams
Fructus Tritici	9 grams
Fructus Ziziphi Jujubae	6 pcs.

Seven doses of the decoction worked effectively. In the following three years, there was no recurrence.

CLAUSE 22-7

A woman patient salivates copiously, but the doctor prescribes a purgative for the patient, and Vital-energy Stagnation (1) in the epigastrium results. In treating the case, saliva should be dealt with first. Decoction of Lesser *Qinglong* can be adopted (see Clause 12-21). When salivation stops, Decoction of *Xiexin* (2) can be adopted to disperse the Vital-energy Stagnation (See Clause 16-17) (3).

NOTES

1. Vital-energy Stagnation (*Pi*): The ancient term for a syndrome commonly defined as fullness and stagnant sensation caused by stagnation of Vital Energy in the chest with no pain or swelling mass. (04-81)

2. Decoction of *Xiexin* (*Xiexin Tang*): According to *Qianjian*, this is Decoction of Radix Glycyrrhizae *Xiexin* (*Gancao Xiexin Tang*). For details, see Clause 158 of *Shanghan Lun*.

Decoction of Radix Glycyrrhizae *Xiexin*
(*Gancao Xiexin Tang*):

Radix Glycyrrhizae Praeparata	4 *liang*
Radix Scutellariae	3 *liang*
Rhizoma Zingiberis	3 *liang*
Rhizoma Pinelliae	0.5 *sheng*
Fructus Ziziphi Jujubae	12 pcs.
Rhizoma Coptidis	1 *liang*

3. This clause discusses the treatment of Vital-energy Stagnation caused by improper use of purgatives in a case with Cold Fluid-retention in the Upper Portion. Copious salivation is caused by Cold Fluid-retention in the Upper Portion, treatment for which is dispersion of the Fluid-retention by using warm and dispersive drugs. When a purgative is used instead, Interior Body Resistance is weakened, and Vital-energy Stagnation will follow. Although Vital-energy Stagnation continues, copious salivation does not cease. This shows that the Cold Fluid-retention is still resting at the Upper Portion. Decoction of Lesser *Qinglong* is adopted to disperse the Fluid-retention. Once the Fluid-retention is eliminated, salivation will come to an end. Decoction of *Xiexin* can then be used to treat Vital-energy Stagnation. (02-199)

Remark: According to *Interpretation of TCM Terminology*, p. 335, diseases resulting from Vital-energy Stagnation include acute and chronic gastritis and enteritis, and indigestion. Also see Clause 131 of *Shanghan Lun*.

CLAUSE 22-8

Deficiency, accumulation of pathogenetic Cold and stagnation of Vital Energy are the main causes of menolipsis, which may last as long as a year. Pathogenetic Cold intermingles with the Blood. The uterus is weakened, and the Channels and Collaterals blocked.

When the pathogenetic factors invade the Upper Portion, there will be copious salivation, which gradually evolves into pulmonary abscesses. Consequently, the patient loses weight.

While the pathogenetic factors invade the Middle Portion, pain caused by Cold appears in the region around the navel or in the costal regions with dragging pain moving in the direction of the Viscus (the Liver). Or the Cold may evolve into Heat and accumulate in the abdomen, causing pain around acupoint Guanyuan (RN 4). The pulse is speedy. This is not a case of skin sores or carbuncles. Scaly skin appears. The syndrome may also affect male patients.

When the pathogenetic factors invade the Lower Portion, amount of menstrual blood is less than normal. Other symptoms are irregular menses, menorrhalgia with dragging pains in the vagina, chills in the abdomen which may stretch to the waist and *Qijie* (1), and acute pain on Qichong (ST 30) (2), the knee and the shin. Syncopes and vertigo may suddenly occur, accompanied by melancholy, distress and indigestion. These symptoms are not caused by ghosts and spirits, but are rather symptoms and signs of gynopathy. They will make the patient weak and emaciated, and will be accompanied by Cold syndrome and deficient pulse (3).

The thirty-six varieties of gynopathy (4) may evolve into numerous syndromes. Diagnosis should be made to evaluate the Yin and the Yang, and whether the pulse is deficient, excessive, tense or tight. Relevant prescriptions and acupuncture should be prescribed to save the patient. Symptoms and signs may be the same in different cases, but different pulses will indicate different pathology. Diagnosis should be made carefully. Particular caution is advised.

NOTES

1. *Qijie*: According to *Dictionary of Traditional Chinese Medicine*, *Qijie* may refer to either of the following:

a) Channel where the Vital Energy flows;

NOTES

1. This clause discusses the treament of abdominal pain caused by various gynopathies. Pathology of such pain generally results from stagnation of the Vital Energy and the Blood. When complicated with Fluid-retention, symptoms and signs will include dysuria, slight abdominal distention and slight swelling in the head, face and extremities. Powder of Radix Angelicae Sinensis and Radix Paeoniae harmonizes the Vital Energy with the Blood and eliminate Fluid-retention. When it is taken, abdominal pain will subside. (02-203)

CLAUSE 22-18

Decoction of Lesser *Jianzhong* can be adopted to reduce the abdominal pain of female patients. (For prescription, see Clause 6-13.) (1)

NOTES

1. This clause discusses the treatment of abdominal pain in women caused by deficient and Cold factors. Symptoms and signs should include abdominal pain that eases when pressed, restlessness and palpitation, facial paleness, red tongue and hesitant-tight pulse. Decoction of Lesser *Jianzhong* is used to tonify the Vital Energy and produce more Blood. When the Stomach is tonified and functions normally, the Vital Energy and the Blood will flow smoothly, and abdominal pain will cease. (02-203)

Commentary: Clauses 22-16, 22-17 and 22-18 deal with abdominal pains in women. But the mechanism of the diseases are different.

Wine of Flos Carthami: removes blood stasis and regulates the Vital Energy and the Blood;

Powder of Radix Angelicae Sinensis and Radix Paeoniae: regulates the Blood and disperses Fluid-retention;

Decoction of Lesser *Jianzhong:* tonifies and harmonizes the Spleen and the Stomach.

The mechanism, symptoms and signs, and treatment of the different syndromes should be carefully differentiated.

CLAUSE 22-19

Question: The patient experiences restlessness and a fever that prevents her from lying quietly in bed. The patient must recline to breathe freely (the patient suffers from dyspnea). But she is eating normally. Please explain this.

Master: This is a case of dysuria due to pressure exerted by the fetus (*Zhuan pao*). The fetus is pressing the urinary bladder and the urethra, preventing them from voiding urine. A diuretic should be adopted. Pills of the Kidney Vital Energy can be used. (For prescription, see Appendix to Chapter V, "Pills of Eight-Ingredients.")

Powder of Fructus Cnidii is effective in relieving a cold feeling in the vagina.

Powder of Fructus Cnidii
(*Shechuangzi San*):

Fructus Cnidii

Pound Fructus Cnidii into powder. Blend it with rice powder. Wrap enough powder in a piece of silk to form a pouch the size of a date. Insert the silk pouch as a vaginal suppository. A warm feeling will be sensed.

Explanation of the Prescription: This treatment provides a cure for relieving a cold feeling in the vagina. Fructus Cnidii, warm in quality, dries up the Humidity, kills parasites and stops itching. (01-241)

CLAUSE 22-20

The pulse in the Cubit is slippery and speedy. Carbuncles are found in the pudenda. Decoction of Herba Agrimoniae can be used to cleanse the affected part.

Decoction of Herba Agrimoniae
(*Langya Tang*):

Herba Agrimoniae 3 *liang**

Stew the drug in four *sheng* of water until one half *sheng* remains. Make a ball of silk to resemble a silkworm cocoon. Soak this in the decoction and use it to wash the pudenda, four times a day.

*Or two bundles, according to another edition.

CLAUSE 22-21

When the cereal Vital Energy descends to produce flatus, it is emitted from the vagina with an audible sound. This is caused by an excessive state of the cereal Vital Energy. Decoction of Lard and Human Hair can be used to cure the syndrome. (For prescription, see Clause 15-17.) (1)

NOTES

1. This clause discusses the mechanism and treatment of vaginal flatus (*Yin chui*). Vaginal flatus results when fetid gas invades the pudenda. Constipation is the cause of such invasion. Decoction of Lard and Human Hair moistens the intestine and loosens the bowels. Turbid gas would follow its original route and be emitted from the anus. Vaginal flatus will cease. (02-204)

APPENDIX I
BIBLIOGRAPHY

1. Explanation of Synopsis of the Golden Chamber *(Jinkui Yaolue Yuyi)*, abbreviated as *Jinkui E*, Academy of Traditional Chinese Medicine, Beijing
金匮要略语译，中医研究院

2. Selected Readings of Synopsis of the Golden Chamber *(Jinkui Yaolue Xuandu)*, abbreviated as *Jinkui S*, Science and Technology Press, Shanghai, textbook for all medical colleges
金匮要略选读，全国高等医药院校试用教材

3. Treatise on Febrile Diseases Caused by Cold, abbreviated as *Shanghan Lun*, (English edition, New World Press, Beijing, 1985, translated by Luo Xiwen)
伤寒论英译本，罗希文译

4. Explanation of Treatise on Febrile Diseases Caused by Cold, abbreviated as *Shanghan E*, Academy of Traditional Chinese Medicine, Beijing
伤寒论语译,中医研究院

5. The Golden Mirror of Medicine (*Yizong Jinjian*), abbreviated as *Jinjian*, Wu Qian, et al.
医宗金鉴，吴谦等

6. Compendium of Materia Medica, Li Shizhen
本草纲目，李时珍

7. Records of Present-day and Ancient Proven Prescriptions, Zhen Quan
古今录验方，甄权

8. Concise Chinese-English Dictionary of Medicine, abbreviated as *DM*, Beijing Medical College
汉英常用中医词汇，北京医学院

103. Mr. Zhang Yuqing's Case Studies
张聿青先生医案

104. Dr. Ran Xuefeng's Case Studies
冉雪峰医案

105. The Great Wall Medical News
长城医讯

106. Journal of Zhejiang College of Chinese Medicine
浙江中医学院学报

107. New Chinese Medicine
新中医

108. Collection of Case Studies and Commentaries of Chinese Medical Doctors
中医医案医话集锦

109. Dr. Qian Boxuan's Case Studies of Gynecology
钱伯煊妇科医案

110. Commentaries on Ancient and Modern Case Reports, Yu Zhen
古今医案按，俞震

111. Selected Case Studies of Dr. He Ren
何任医案选

112. Journal of Beijing College of Chinese Medicine
北京中医学院学报

113. Journal of Bare-foot Doctors
赤脚医生杂志

APPENDIX II

DIFFERENT PULSES AND THE RESPECTIVE SYNDROMES THEY REPRESENT

(Excerpts from "The Pulse Studies of Binhu" by Li Shizhen)

1. Floating Pulse (*Fu Mai* 浮脉)

Floating pulse is the representation of a pathological condition at the Exterior caused by excessive Yang Vital Energy. Floating but also slow and tense signifies a pathological condition of a Wind and Cold nature, whereas floating with speedy pulse will indicate a pathological condition of a Wind and Heat nature. Floating and mighty always signifies Wind and Heat, but floating and strengthless will mean a syndrome with a Blood Deficiency.

2. Deep Pulse (*Chen Mai* 沉脉)

Stagnant Water and Fluid of the Yin Channel always brings a deep pulse. Deep but speedy indicates the existence of pathogenetic Heat at the Interior, while deep and slow may signify the existence of Cold at the Interior. As to a deep and slippery pulse, it always indicates stagnancy of sputum. A strengthless deep pulse shows the sinking of the deficient Yang Vital Energy. Deep but mighty can tell of the existence of stagnancy and Cold congelation at the Interior.

3. Slow Pulse (*Chi Mai* 迟脉)

Slow pulse always indicates diseases of the Viscera or an accumulation of sputum, Cold congelation, or a mass or stagnancy. Slow but mighty will always indicate pains caused by Interior Cold of an excessive nature. Slow but strengthless can indicate diseases of a Cold and deficient type.

4. Speedy Pulse (*Shuo Mai* 数脉)

Speedy pulse always indicates a syndrome of a Yang and Heat nature. Fire of Heart and Kidney should be eliminated. Speedy pulse of an excessive nature should be treated with cool and eliminating drugs, whereas speedy pulse of a deficient nature should be warmed and tonified. Speedy pulse in the late autumn would foretell a dangerous case.

5. Slippery Pulse (*Hua Mai* 滑脉)

Slippery pulse may indicate either excessive Yang or evanescence of the source of the Vital Energy. It also indicates: sputum, indigestion, nausea and vomiting, blood stasis at lower portion and pregnancy (for women).

6. Hesitant Pulse (*Se Mai* 涩脉)

Hesitant pulse always indicates an insufficiency of Blood or loss of sperm. When profuse perspiration has exhausted the Body Fluid and brought Stomach uncomfort, hesitant pulse is likely to appear. Hesitant pulse may also reflect pathogenetic Cold resting in the Blood, pregnancy, or abnormal menstruation.

7. Deficient Pulse (*Xu Mai* 虚脉)

Deficient pulse always reflects evanescence and loss of Body Resistance with symptoms of spontaneous perspiration, fright and irritation, or melancholia.

8. Excessive Pulse (*Shi Mai* 实脉)

Excessive pulse, of a Yang nature, reflects the congelation of Heat with symptoms of delirium, insanity, vomiting and anorexia, constipation, or pain caused by Vital-energy Stagnancy.

9. Long Pulse (*Chang Mai* 长脉)

A moderate long pulse is soft and even. When it is tight and tense, it will indicate diseases of the Greater Yang Channel. Long pulse may reflect Heat in the Blood, insanity caused by Wind sputum, and Interior excessive Heat (in the Stomach and Intestine).

10. Short Pulse (*Duan Mai* 短脉)

Short pulse is a reflection of evanescence and exhaustion of the Blood and Vital Energy. Short pulse with slippery and speedy pulse will indicate excessive Interior Heat-Humidity. Short-floating pulse will reflect insufficiency of the Blood. Chest and abdominal distention is reflected by deep-short pulse. Short pulse under the fore-finger generally indicates a headache caused by Deficiency of the Yang Vital Energy. Short pulse under the ring-finger will indicate abdominal pain when Yang Vital Energy is deficient at the lower portion.

11. Grand Pulse (*Hong Mai* 洪脉)

Grand pulse is a reflection of excessive Yang and Heat as well as Deficiency and insufficiency of Blood. When the Heart Fire is ascending, there will be a grand pulse. Grand pulse appearing with Stomach discomfort or nausea and vomiting will indicate a syndrome of an excessive nature, while grand pulse appearing with diarrhea will be an indication of a deficient syndrome with exhaustion of the Body Fluid and excessive Heat of a Yang nature.

12. Feeble Pulse (*Wei Mai* 微脉)

Feeble pulse reflects Deficiency both in the Vital Energy and Blood. Symptoms of chill, fever, and profuse perspiration (evanescence of Yang Vital Energy) will generally bear a feeble pulse. Feeble pulse also indicates various syndromes of an extreme deficient nature for men and abnormal menstruation for women.

13. Tense Pulse (*Jin Mai* 紧脉)

Tense pulse always indicates various pains caused by extreme pathogenetic Cold. It also reflects a cough caused by pathogenetic Cold in the Lungs, epilepsy caused by pathogenetic Cold in the Liver, or spitting of sputum caused by Cold in the Spleen.

14. Moderate Pulse (*Huan Mai* 缓脉)

Moderate pulse is a pulse that reflects the normal state of a healthy person. But moderate-floating pulse will indicate pathogenetic Wind at the Exterior with an insufficiency of the Nutrient Essence and an Excess of Body Resistance; moderate-deep pulse reflects Humidity on the Channels and Collaterals; moderate-slow-slender pulse indicates Deficiency and weakness of the Spleen and Stomach; moderate-floating and mighty pulse reflects Wind-Humidity at the upper portion with stiffness in the neck and back; moderate-deep and mighty pulse reflects Wind-Humidity at the lower portion with symptoms of paralysis.

15. Void Pulse (*Kou Mai* 芤脉)

After hemorrhage occurs, void pulse will appear, reflecting an insufficiency of Heart Blood with palpitation. Void pulse under the middle-finger is a proof that hemoptysis has taken place. If void pulse appears under the ring-finger, it will be a proof of loss of blood from gonorrhea, diarrhea, melena, profuse menstruation, or hemorrhea.

16. Tight Pulse (*Xian Mai* 弦脉)

Tight pulse is a pulse of the Liver and Gall Bladder. Tight-slippery pulse is a reflection of a syndrome of a Yang nature; tight-tense-slender pulse is a reflection of a syndrome of a Yin nature. Tight pulse may also indicate Water-fluid stagnancy, sputum congelation, intermittent fever and chill, and malaria.

17. Void-tight Pulse (*Ge Mai* 革脉)

Void-tight pulse reflects a Deficiency of Blood and sperm with the effects of

Exterior pathogenetic Cold. It is a pulse of a deficient and Cold nature.

18. Hidden-excessive Pulse (*Lao Mai* 牢脉)

Hidden-excessive pulse is a reflection of Interior Excess and long-term Cold syndrome with the presentation of symptoms and signs of abdominal pain of a Cold nature, imbalance of the Liver Vital Energy, or stagnancy of the Spleen and Stomach Vital Energy.

19. Soft Pulse *(Ru Mai or Ruan Mai* 濡脉)

Soft pulse generally indicates a loss of Blood and extreme Deficiency of Yin with the presentation of symptoms and signs of night sweat, restlessness and fever, hemorrhea, or diarrhea caused by Humidity in the Spleen.

20. Weak Pulse (*Ruo Mai* 弱脉)

Weak pulse always reflects a Deficiency of Yin and evanescence of Yang. Weak pulse may also appear with the following symptoms: fever and chill, paralysis, fright and irritation, spontaneous perspiration, and general malaise.

21. Loose Pulse (*San Mai* 散脉)

When loose pulse appears under the fore-finger of the left wrist, it may indicate melancholia caused by Deficiency of Heart Yang . When loose pulse appears under the fore-finger of right wrist, it indicates spontaneous perspiration caused by Deficiency of the Body Resistance. Loose pulse under the middle-finger of the left wrist may reflect Water-fluid stagnancy. Loose pulse under the middle-finger of the right wrist is an indication of edema on both legs. When the patient has been ill for a long time, loose pulse will foretell total collapse of the source of Vital Energy.

22. Slender Pulse (*Xi Mai* 细脉)

Deficiency of Blood and Vital Energy makes the pulse slender. Slender pulse reflects a Deficiency of Yang Vital Energy with Humidity intruding into the Kidney and spontaneous perspiration.

23. Hidden Pulse (*Fu Mai* 伏脉)

When a syndrome congeals at the Interior, normal circulation of the Blood and Vital Energy will be hampered. Hidden pulse will appear. Cholera and congelation of sputum will also bear a hidden pulse.

24. Moving Pulse (*Dong Mai* 动脉)

Moving pulse may appear to reflect the following symptoms and signs: pain caused by Cold prevalence, irritation and palpitation caused by abnormal movement of the Vital Energy, spontaneous perspiration caused by Yin prevalence, fever caused by Yang prevalence, diarrhea caused by an abnormal state of the Spleen and Stomach with intermingled Heat and Cold, spasms caused by pathogenetic Cold, and lost of sperm for men and hemorrhea for women.

25. Irregular-speedy Pulse (*Cu Mai* 促脉)

Irregular-speedy pulse reflects the congelation of pathogenetic Heat in the Three Portions of the Body Cavity. The congelation of Vital Energy, Blood (blood stasis), sputum, Water-fluid, and indigestion all may bear irregular-speedy pulse. Obstruction of the normal circulation of the Vital Energy and Blood is the cause of irregular-speedy pulse.

26. Slow-uneven Pulse (*Jie Mai* 结脉)

Slow-uneven pulse appears in cases with a congelation of the Vital Energy and Blood. The following cases may bear a slow-uneven pulse: Congelation of sputum, carbuncle, and swelling, etc. Compared with irregular-speedy pulse (of a Heat nature), slow-uneven pulse always foretells a case of a Yin nature.

27. Interval Pulse (*Dai Mai* 代脉)

Interval pulse appears in a case with evanescence of the Viscera Vital Energy and weakness of the Yang Vital Energy. It may appear in the following cases: abdominal pain and diarrhea caused by Deficiency at the lower portion, weakness of the Spleen and Stomach functions, and vomiting and diarrhea caused by Deficiency of the Interior Vital Energy.

28. Huge Pulse (*Da Mai* 大脉)*

Huge and mighty pulse will indicate an excessive case with a Heat syndrome. Huge and strengthless pulse will either reflect a deficient case or the dispersion of the Interior deficient Vital Energy.

29. Swift Pulse (*Ji Mai* 疾脉)**

Swift pulse is an indication of the extreme prevalence of Yang and exhaustion of Yin and the dispersion of the source of the Vital Energy. It is a pulse that generally foretells an acute case of febrile disease or a case with a severe Deficiency.

* According to *Concise Dictionary of Chinese Medicine*, p. 28.

***Ibid*, p. 742.

APPENDIX III

ORIGINAL PRESCRIPTIONS IN THE BOOK IN CHINESE

Clause 2-11

Decoction of Radix Trichosanthis and Ramulus Cinnamomi

栝蒌桂枝汤

栝蒌根二两　桂枝三两(去皮)　芍药三两　甘草二两(炙)　生姜三两(切)　大枣十二枚(掰)

Clause 2-12

Decoction of Radix Puerariae

葛根汤

葛根四两　麻黄三两(去节)　桂枝二两(去皮)　芍药二两　生姜三两(切)　大枣十二枚(掰)　甘草二两(炙)

Clause 2-13

Decoction of Greater *Chengqi*

大承气汤

大黄四两(酒洗)　厚朴半斤(炙去皮)　枳实五枚(炙)　芒硝三合

Clause 2-20

Decoction of Herba Ephedrae adding Rhizoma Atractylodis Macrocephalae

麻黄加术汤

麻黄三两(去节)　桂枝二两(去皮)　甘草一两(炙)　白术四两　杏仁七十个(去皮尖)

Clause 2-21

Decoction of Herba Ephedrae, Semen Armeniacae Amarum, Semen Coicis and Radix Glycyrrhizae

麻黄杏仁薏苡甘草汤

麻黄(去节)半两(汤泡)　甘草一两(炙)　薏苡仁半两　杏仁十个(去皮尖,炒)

Clause 2-22

Decoction of Radix Stephaniae Tetrandrae and Radix Astragali Hedysari

防己黄芪汤

防己一两　甘草半两(炒)　白术七钱半　黄芪一两一分(去芦)

Clause 2-23

Decoction of Ramulus Cinnamomi and Radix Aconiti Praeparata
桂枝附子汤
桂枝四两(去皮) 生姜三两(切) 附子三枚(炮去皮,破八片) 甘草二两(炙) 大枣十二枚(掰)

Decoction of Rhizoma Atractylodis Macrocephalae and Radix Aconiti Praeparata
白术附子汤
白术二两 附子一枚半(炮去皮) 甘草一两(炙) 生姜一两半(切) 大枣六枚(掰)

Clause 2-24

Decoction of Radix Glycyrrhizae and Radix Aconiti Praeparata
甘草附子汤
甘草二两(炙) 白术二两 附子二枚(炮去皮) 桂枝四两(去皮)

Clause 2-26

Decoction of *Baihu* adding Radix Ginseng
白虎加人参汤
知母六两 石膏一斤(碎) 甘草二两 粳米六合 人参三两

Clause 2-27

Decoction of Pedicellus Melo
一物瓜蒂汤
瓜蒂二十个

Clause 3-2

Decoction of Bulbus Lilii and Rhizoma Anemarrhenae
百合知母汤
百合七枚(掰) 知母三两(切)

Clause 3-3

Decoction of Talcum and Ochra Haematitum
滑石代赭汤
百合七枚(掰) 滑石三两(碎,绵裹) 代赭石如弹丸大一枚(碎,绵裹)

Clause 3-4

Decoction of Bulbus Lilii and Egg Yolk
百合鸡子汤

百合七枚(掰) 鸡子黄一枚

Clause 3-5

Decoction of Bulbus Lilii and Radix Rehmanniae

百合地黄汤

百合七枚(掰) 生地黄片一升

Clause 3-7

Powder of Radix Trichosanthis and Concha Ostreae

栝蒌牡蛎散

栝蒌根 牡蛎(熬)等分

Clause 3-8

Powder of Bulbus Lilii and Talcum

百合滑石散

百合一两(炙) 滑石三两

Clause 3-10

Decoction of Radix Glycyrrhizae *Xiexin*

甘草泻心汤

甘草四两 黄芩 人参 干姜各三两 黄连一两 大枣十二枚(掰) 半夏半升

Clause 3-11

Decoction of Radix Sophorae Flavescentis

苦参汤

苦参一升

Clause 3-12

Fumigating Therapy of Realgar

雄黄熏方

雄黄

Clause 3-13

Powder of Radix Angelicae Sinensis and Semen Phaseoli

赤小豆当归散

赤小豆三升(浸令芽出,曝干) 当归三两

Clause 3-15

Decoction of Rhizoma Cimicifugae and Carapax Trionycis

升麻鳖甲汤

升麻二两　当归一两　蜀椒(炒去汗)一两　甘草二两　鳖甲手指大一片(炙)　雄黄半两(研)

Clause 4-2

Pills of Carapax Trionycis

鳖甲煎丸

鳖甲十二分(炙)　乌扇三分(烧)　黄芩三分　柴胡六分　鼠妇三分(熬)　干姜三分　大黄三分　芍药五分　桂枝三分　葶苈一分(熬)　石韦三分(去毛)　厚朴三分　牡丹五分(去心)　瞿麦二分　紫葳三分　半夏一分　人参一分　䗪虫五分(熬)　阿胶三分(炙)　蜂窝四分(炙)　赤硝十二分　蜣螂六分(熬)　桃仁二分

Clause 4-4

Decoction of *Baihu* adding Ramulus Cinnamomi

白虎加桂枝汤

知母六两　甘草二两(炙)　石膏一斤　粳米二合　桂枝(去皮)三两

Clause 4-5

Powder of Ramulus et Folium Dichroae

蜀漆散

蜀漆(洗去腥)　云母(烧二日夜)　龙骨等分

Appended Prescriptions in Chapter IV

Decoction of Concha Ostreae

牡蛎汤

牡蛎四两(熬)　麻黄四两(去节)　甘草二两　蜀漆三两

Decoction of Radix Bupleuri subtracting Rhizoma Pinelliae adding Radix Trichosanthis

柴胡去半夏加栝蒌根汤

柴胡八两　人参　黄芩　甘草各三两　栝蒌根四两　生姜二两　大枣十二枚

Decoction of Radix Bupleuri, Ramulus Cinnamomi and Rhizoma Zingiberis

柴胡桂姜汤

柴胡半斤　桂枝三两(去皮)　干姜二两　栝蒌根四两　黄芩三两　牡蛎三两(熬)　甘草二两(炙)

Clause 5-2

Black Powder of *Houshi*

侯氏黑散

菊花四十分　白术十分　细辛三分　茯苓三分　牡蛎三分　桔梗八分　防风十分　人参三分

矾石三分 黄芩五分 当归三分 干姜三分 芎䓖三分 桂枝三分

Clause 5-3

Decoction of *Fengyin*

风引汤

大黄 干姜 龙骨各四两 桂枝三两 甘草 牡蛎各二两 滑石 赤不脂 白不脂 紫石英 石膏各六两 寒水石

Decoction of Radix Stephaniae Tetrandrae and Radix Rehmanniae

防己地黄汤

防己一分 桂枝三分 防风三分 甘草一分

Circular-rubbing Therapy for Head-wind

头风摩散

大附子一枚(炮) 盐等分

Clause 5-8

Decoction of Ramulus Cinnamomi, Radix Paeoniae and Rhizoma Anemarrhenae

桂枝芍药知母汤

桂枝四两 芍药三两 甘草二两 麻黄二两 生姜五两 白术五两 知母四两 防风四两 附子二枚(炮)

Clause 5-10

Decoction of Rhizoma Aconiti

乌头汤

麻黄 芍药 黄芪各三两 甘草三两(炙) 川乌五枚(㕮咀，以蜜二升，煎取一升，即出乌头)

Decoction of Alumen

矾石汤

矾石二两

Appended Prescriptions in Chapter V

Decoction of *Xuming*

续命汤

麻黄 桂枝 当归 人参 石膏 干姜 甘草各三两 杏仁四十枚 芎䓖一两五钱

Decoction of *Sanhuang*

三黄汤

麻黄五分　独活四分　细辛二分　黄芪二分　黄芩三分

Decoction of Rhizoma Atractylodis Macrocephalae and Radix Aconiti Praeparata

术附汤

白术二两　附子一枚半(炮去皮)　甘草一两(炙)

Pills of Eight-Ingredients

崔氏八味丸

干地黄八两　山茱萸　薯蓣各四两　泽泻　茯苓　牡丹皮各三两　桂枝　附子(炮) 各一两

Decoction of *Yuebei* adding Rhizoma Atractylodis Macrocephalae

越婢加术汤

麻黄六两　石膏半斤　生姜三两　甘草二两　白术四两　大枣十五枚

Clause 6-2

Decoction of Five Drugs with Radix Astragali Hedysari and Ramulus Cinnamomi

黄芪桂枝五物汤

黄芪三两　芍药三两　桂枝三两　生姜六两　大枣十二枚

Clause 6-8

Decoction of Ramulus Cinnamomi adding Os Draconis and Concha Ostreae

桂枝加龙骨牡蛎汤

桂枝　芍药　生姜各三两　甘草二两　大枣十二枚　龙骨　牡蛎各三两

Powder of Rhizoma Aconiti (*Tianxiong*)

天雄散

天雄三两(炮)　白术八两　桂枝六两　龙骨三两

Clause 6-13

Decoction of Lesser *Jianzhong*

小建中汤

桂枝三两(去皮)　甘草二两(炙)　大枣十二枚　芍药六两　生姜三两　胶饴一升

Clause 6-14

Decoction of Radix Astragali Hedysari *Jianzhong*

黄芪建中汤

于小建中汤内加黄芪一两半,余依上法。

Clause 6-16

Pills of Rhizoma Dioscoreae

薯蓣丸

薯蓣三十分 当归 桂枝 曲 干地黄 豆黄卷各十分 人参七分 芎䓖 芍药 白术 麦门冬 杏仁各六分 茯苓各五分 阿胶七分 干姜三分 白敛二 分 防风六分 甘草二十八分 柴胡 桔梗 大枣百枚为膏

Clause 6-17

Decoction of Semen Ziziphi Spinosae

酸枣仁汤

酸枣仁二升 甘草一两 知母二两 茯苓二两 芎䓖二两 深师有生姜二两

Clause 6-18

Pills of Radix et Rhizoma Rhei and Eupolyphaga seu Steleophaga

大黄䗪虫丸

大黄十分(蒸) 黄芩二两 甘草三两 桃仁一升 杏仁一升 干地黄十两 干漆一两 虻虫一升 水蛭百枚 蛴螬一升 䗪虫半升 芍药四两

Appended Prescriptions in Chapter VI

Decoction of Radix Glycyrrhizae Praeparata

炙甘草汤

甘草四两(炙) 桂枝 生姜各三两 麦门冬半升 麻仁半升 阿胶各二两 大枣三十枚 生地黄一升 人参

Otter Liver Powder

獭肝散

獭肝一具

Clause 7-5

Decoction of Radix Glycyrrhizae and Rhizoma Zingiberis

甘草干姜汤

甘草四两(炙) 干姜二两(炮)

Clause 7-6

Decoction of Rhizoma Belamcandae and Herba Ephedrae

射干麻黄汤

射干十三枚(一法三两) 麻黄四两 生姜四两 细辛 紫菀 五味子半升 大枣七枚

半夏(大者洗) 八枚(一法半升) 款冬花各三两

Clause 7-7

Pills of Fructus Gleditsiae Sinensis

皂荚丸

皂荚八两(刮去皮,用酥炙)

Clause 7-8

Decoction of Cortex Magnoliae Officinalis and Herba Ephedrae

厚朴麻黄汤

厚朴五两 麻黄四两 石膏如鸡子大 杏仁半升 半夏半升 细辛二两 小麦一升 五味子半升 干姜二两

Clause 7-9

Decoction of Herba Euphorbiae Helioscopiae

泽漆汤

半夏半升 紫参五两(一作紫菀) 人参 桂枝各三两 生姜五两 白前五两 甘草 黄芩 泽漆三斤(以东流水五斗,煮取一斗五升)

Clause 7-10

Decoction of Radix Ophiopogonis

麦门冬汤

麦门冬七升 半夏一升 人参二两 甘草三两 粳米三合 大枣十二枚

Clause 7-11

Decoction of Lung-purgation with Semen Lepidii seu Descurainiae and Fructus Ziziphi Jujubae

葶苈大枣泻肺汤

葶苈(熬令黄色,捣丸如弹子大) 大枣十二枚

Clause 7-12

Decoction of Radix Platycodi

桔梗汤

桔梗一两 甘草二两

Clause 7-13

Decoction of *Yuebei* adding Rhizoma Pinelliae

越婢加半夏汤

麻黄六两 石膏半斤 生姜三两 大枣十五枚 甘草二两 半夏半升

Clause 7-14

Decoction of Lesser *Qinglong* adding Gypsum Fibrosum
小青龙加石膏汤
麻黄 芍药 桂枝 细辛 甘草 干姜各三两 五味子 半夏各半升 石膏二两

Appended Prescriptions in Chapter VII

Decoction of Rhizoma Zingiberis Recens and Radix Glycyrrhizae
生姜甘草汤
生姜五两 人参三两, 甘草四两 大枣十五枚

Decoction of Ramulus Cinnamomi subtracting Radix Paeoniae adding Fructus Gleditsiae Sinensis
桂枝去芍药加皂荚汤
桂枝 生姜各三两 甘草二两 大枣十枚 皂荚一枚(去皮子,炙焦)

Baisan Powder with Radix Platycodi
桔梗白散
桔梗 贝母各三分 巴豆一分(去皮,熬,研如脂)

Decoction of Rhizoma Phragmitis
苇茎汤
苇茎二升 薏苡仁半升 桃仁五十枚 瓜瓣半升

Clause 8-3

Decoction of *Bentun*
奔豚汤
甘草 芎䓖 当归各二两 半夏四两 黄芩二两 生葛五两 芍药二两 生姜四两 甘李根白皮一升

Clause 8-4

Decoction of Ramulus Cinnamomi adding Ramulus Cinnamomi
桂枝加桂汤
桂枝五两 芍药三两 甘草二两(炙) 生姜三两 大枣十二枚

Clause 8-5

Decoction of Poria, Ramulus Cinnamomi, Radix Glycyrrhizae and Fructus Ziziphi Jujubae

茯苓桂枝甘草大枣汤

茯苓半斤 甘草二两(炙) 大枣十五枚 桂枝四两

Clause 9-3

Decoction of Fructus Trichosanthis, Bulbus Allii Aacrostemi and Wine

栝蒌薤白白酒汤

栝蒌实一枚(捣) 薤白半升 白酒七升

Clause 9-4

Decoction of Fructus Trichosanthis, Bulbus Allii Aacrostemi and Rhizoma Pinelliae

栝蒌薤白半夏汤

栝蒌实一枚(捣) 薤白三两 半夏半升 白酒一斗

Clause 9-5

Decoction of Fructus Aurantii Immaturus, Bulbus Allii Aacrostemi and Ramulus Cinnamomi

枳实薤白桂枝汤

枳实四枚 厚朴四两 薤白半升 桂枝一两 栝蒌实一枚(捣)

Decoction of Radix Ginseng

人参汤

人参 甘草 干姜 白术各三两

Clause 9-6

Decoction of Poria, Semen Armeniacae Amarum and Radix Glycyrrhizae

茯苓杏仁甘草汤

茯苓三两 杏仁五十个 甘草一两

Decoction of Pericarpium Citri Reticulatae, Fructus Aurantii Immaturus and Rhizoma Zingiberis Recens

橘枳姜汤

橘皮一斤 枳实三两 生姜半斤

Clause 9-7

Powder of Semen Coicis and Radix Aconiti Praeparata

薏苡附子散

薏苡仁十五两 大附子十枚(炮)

Clause 9-8

Decoction of Ramulus Cinnamomi, Rhizoma Zingiberis Recens and Fructus Aurantii Immaturus
桂枝生姜枳实汤
桂枝 生姜各三两 枳实五枚

Clause 9-9

Pills of Rhizoma Aconiti and Halloysitum Rubrum
乌头赤石脂丸
蜀椒一两(一法二分) 乌头一分(炮) 附子半两(炮)(一法一分) 干姜一两(一法一分)
赤石脂一两(一法二分)

Pills for Treating Nine Types of Pain
九痛丸
附子三两(炮) 生狼牙一两(炙香) 人参 干姜 吴茱萸各一两 巴豆一两(去皮心,熬,研如脂)

Clause 10-9

Decoction of Cortex Magnoliae Officinalis with Seven Drugs
厚朴七物汤
厚朴半斤 甘草 大黄各三两 大枣十枚 枳实五枚 桂枝二两 生姜五两

Clause 10-10

Decoction of Radix Aconiti Praeparata and Semen Oryzae Nonglutinosae
附子粳米汤
附子一枚(炮) 半夏 粳米各半升 甘草一两 大枣十枚

Clause 10-11

Decoction of Cortex Magnoliae Officinalis with Three Drugs
厚朴三物汤
厚朴八两 大黄四两 枳实五枚

Clause 10-12

Decoction of Greater Radix Bupleuri
大柴胡汤
柴胡半斤 黄芩三两 芍药三两 半夏半升(洗) 枳实四枚(炙) 大黄二两 大枣十二枚 生姜五两

Clause 10-14

Decoction of Greater *Jianzhong*

大建中汤

蜀椒二合(去汗) 干姜四两 人参二两

Clause 10-15

Decoction of Radix et Rhizoma Rhei and Radix Aconiti Praeparata

大黄附子汤

大黄三两 附子三枚(炮) 细辛二两

Clause 10-16

Chiwan Pills

赤丸

茯苓四两 乌头二两(炮) 半夏四两(洗)一方用桂 细辛一两

Clause 10-17

Decoction of Greater Rhizoma Aconiti

大乌头煎

乌头大者五枚(熬,去皮,不㕮咀)

Clause 10-18

Decoction of Radix Angelicae Sinensis, Rhizoma Zingiberis Recens and Mutton

当归生姜羊肉汤

当归三两 生姜五两 羊肉一斤

Clause 10-19

Decoction of Rhizoma Aconiti and Ramulus Cinnamomi

乌头桂枝汤

乌头实中者五枚,除去角 蜜二斤(千金原书作一斤) 桂枝汤五合

Appended Prescriptions in Chapter X

Decoction of Radix Bupleuri and Ramulus Cinnamomi

外台柴胡桂枝汤

柴胡四两 黄芩 人参 芍药 桂枝 生姜各一两半 甘草一两 半夏二合半 大枣六枚

Decoction of *Zouma*

走马汤

杏仁二枚 巴豆二枚(去皮心,熬)

Clause 10-24

Powder of Pedicellus Melo

瓜蒂散

瓜蒂一分(熬黄) 赤小豆一分(煮)

Clause 11-7

Decoction of Flos Inulae

旋覆花汤

旋覆花三两 葱十四茎 新绛少许

Clause 11-15

Pills of Fructus Cannabis

麻子仁丸

麻子仁二升 芍药半斤 枳实一斤 大黄一斤(去皮) 杏仁一升(去皮尖,熬,别作脂) 厚朴一尺(去皮)

Clause 11-16

Decoction of Radix Glycyrrhizae, Rhizoma Zingiberis, Poria and Rhizoma Atractylodis Macrocephalae

甘姜苓术汤

甘草 白术各二两 干姜 茯苓各四两

Clause 12-15

Decoction of Poria, Ramulus Cinnamomi, Rhizoma Atractylodis Macrocephalae and Radix Glycyrrhizae

苓桂术甘汤

茯苓四两 桂枝三两 白术三两 甘草二两

Clause 12-17

Decoction of Radix Euphorbiae Kansui and Rhizoma Pinelliae

甘遂半夏汤

甘遂大者三枚 半夏十二枚(以水一升,煮取半升,去滓) 芍药五枚 甘草如指大一枚(炙,一本作无)

Clause 12-20

Decoction of Ten Pieces of Fructus Ziziphi Jujubae

十枣汤

芫花(熬) 甘遂 大戟各等分 大枣十枚

Clause 12-21

Decoction of Greater *Qinglong*

大青龙汤

麻黄六两(去节) 桂枝二两(去皮) 甘草二两(炙) 杏仁四十个(去皮尖) 生姜三两 大枣十二枚 石膏如鸡子大(碎)

Decoction of Lesser *Qinglong*

小青龙汤

麻黄三两(去节) 芍药三两 五味子半升 干姜三两 细辛三两 桂枝三两(去皮) 半夏半升(汤洗) 甘草三两 (炙)

Clause 12-22

Decoction of Radix Stephaniae Tetrandrae

木防已汤

木防已三两 石膏十二枚(鸡子大)外台作鸡子大三枚 桂枝二两 人参四两

Decoction of Radix Stephaniae Tetrandrae subtracting Gypsum Fibrosum adding Poria and Natrii Sulfas

木防已去石膏加茯苓芒硝汤

木防已二两 桂枝二两 人参四两 芒硝三合 茯苓四两

Clause 12-23

Decoction of Rhizoma Alismatis

泽泻汤

泽泻五两 白术二两

Clause 12-24

Decoction of Cortex Magnoliae Officinalis and Radix et Rhizoma Rhei

厚朴大黄汤

厚朴一尺 大黄六两 枳实四枚

Clause 12-26

Decoction of Lesser Rhizoma Pinelliae

小半夏汤

半夏一升 生姜半斤

Clause 12-27

Pills of Radix Stephaniae Tetrandrae, Semen Zanthoxyli, Semen Lepidii seu